I0869120

RITUAL MEDICAL LORE OF SEPHARDIC WOMEN

ISAAC JACK LÉVY AND
ROSEMARY LÉVY ZUMWALT

Ritual Medical Lore of Sephardic Women

SWEETENING THE SPIRITS, HEALING THE SICK

UNIVERSITY OF ILLINOIS PRESS
URBANA AND CHICAGO

Publication of this book was supported by grants from the Sheldon Drobny Endowment for the University of Illinois Press and from the L. J. and Mary C. Skaggs Folklore Fund

© 2002 by the Board of Trustees of the University of Illinois
All rights reserved

♾ This book is printed on acid-free paper.

Library of Congress Cataloging-in-Publication Data
Lévy, Isaac Jack.
Ritual medical lore of Sephardic women : sweetening the spirits, healing the sick / Isaac Jack Lévy and Rosemary Lévy Zumwalt.
p. cm.
Includes bibliographical references and index.
ISBN 0-252-02697-7
1. Sephardim—Folklore. 2. Sephardim—Medicine. 3. Jewish women—Social life and customs—19th century. 4. Jewish women—Social life and customs—20th century. 5. Traditional medicine. 6. Medicine, Magic, mystic, and spagiric.
I. Zumwalt, Rosemary Lévy, 1944– . II. Title.
GR98.L48 2002
398'.353'089924—dc21 2001002079

To Catherine and Michael

Contents

Acknowledgments

We are enduringly grateful to all the Sephardim who took us into their homes, fed us, cared for us as family, and answered our numerous questions about medicines of the house with enthusiasm, alacrity, and, often, the added ingredient of patience. To thank them all would be impossible, but we hold each dearly in our hearts. Not to diminish the contributions of all, we would like to extend a special thanks to people who worked with us intensively. In Izmir, we are grateful to Uncle Yeoshua and Tante Rachel Musafir and their family for their generosity and extensive help. Leon and Jilda Benmayor of Salonika received us so kindly at their vacation home on the sea in 1985 and took us to a hillside restaurant where we ate in the open air; and in 1990, they took us to an elegant ice cream parlor in the heart of Salonika. In his capacity as president of the Jewish Community, Leon accompanied us to the Sephardic old age home in Salonika and facilitated our research there. In Skopje, Alexandar Matkovski, the esteemed author of *A History of the Jews of Macedonia,* met us at the faculty club of the Academy of Arts and Letters and shared with us his knowledge. In Istanbul, we were guests almost every Shabbat at the home of Suleyman and Beki Bardavid. Conducting a project of her own on life histories of Sephardic women, and having researched and written about proverbs, literature, and Sephardic customs, Beki was a crucial connection to the Istanbul Sephardic community. She would feed us sumptuous Turkish meals and help guide the dinner-table conversation of her guests to topics of our research. In Bat Yam, Israel, Ella Gross-Gefen, her family, and friends received us expansively and helped us with the translation of articles from Serbo-Croatian.

In Netanya, Albert and Luna Tuvi and their daughter, Margalite Tuvi, were gracious hosts and gave us rich information on village life in Turkey. Our Israeli colleagues and friends Avner Perez, Shmuel Refael, and Benni Nachmias were generous with their specialized knowledge and helpful in every way. Moshe Shaul, editor of *Aki Yerushalayim,* was ever ready to assist us and to share with us valuable information that he had collected on his Judeo-Spanish section of Kol Israel Radio. Robert Natal, director of the Yad Ben-Zvi Institute of Jerusalem, helped us immeasurably with his vast knowledge of the holdings of this remarkable library. We gratefully acknowledge the help of Shoshana Weich-Shahak of the National Sound Archives, Jerusalem, for her help with transcriptions of recordings pertaining to the customs surrounding birth. Estrella and Isaac Missistrano fed us sumptuously at their home, honored us at a reception of the Association of Turkish Jews in Bat Yam, and shared their deep knowledge about Sephardic customs. In Ashdod, Izahar and Julie Avzaradel invited us to their home to meet with a dozen Rodeslis for a delightful afternoon of recollections, served up, as always for the Sephardim, with a full banquet of delectable dishes. One of our major informants, Zimbul Maya Suzi of the Bet Avot Leon Recanati in Kryat Matalon, even though her voice was weak with age, talked with us patiently for hours.

Often we made crucial research connections through Sephardic organizations. In Belgrade, we worked with the Federation of Jewish Communities in Yugoslavia; and in Sarajevo, with Dr. Isaac Levi, president of the community. We are grateful to the officers of the Turkiye Hahambashi (Chief Rabbinate of Turkey) in Istanbul for giving us access to their archives. The staff members of the *Shalom Newspaper* of Istanbul also opened their archives to us and invited us to a Judeo-Spanish evening in which all discussion was conducted in Judeo-Spanish. It was here that we met Ester Alkanli, who so kindly invited us to her home and introduced us to Sara Nair, the Sephardic spirit medium. In Israel, through a serendipitous connection with the clerk in our hotel, who was originally from Turkey, we made contact with the Association of Turkish Jews, which led us to Sephardim in Bat Yam, Herzelia, Netanya, Tel Aviv, and Jerusalem.

Our friend and colleague Rabbi Howard Kosovske assisted us with translations and interpretations of esoteric Hebrew texts on magic and amulets. Rabbi Murray Ezring of Temple Israel and Rabbi Yossef Groner of the Lubavitch Synagogue, both of Charlotte, North Carolina, were always ready to help us. We are grateful to our friend and colleague Dr. Patricia Mason, who offered her wise interpretation of linguistic matters. Professors Zoran Kuzmanovich and Karl Plank, both of Davidson College, offered us their invaluable assistance. Rebecca Amato Levy, originally of

Rhodes, received us in her home in Los Angeles, offered us coffee and *biskochos* (sweet Turkish pretzels), and shared with us her vast wisdom on all things Sephardic. The Reverend Doctors Marc Angel, Alan Corré, and Mitchell Serels kindly helped us with materials and interpretive translations. We are particularly grateful to Sharon Byrd, Joe Gutekanst, and Suzy Yoder of the E. H. Little Library of Davidson College for ceaselessly helping us with interlibrary loan materials. We thank Carol Bolton Betts of the University of Illinois Press for her meticulous care in copy-editing our manuscript.

Our fieldwork in 1990 was made possible through the generous funding of the American Philosophical Society, the Atlanta Jewish Federation, the Lucius N. Littauer Foundation, the Program for Cultural Cooperation between Spain's Ministry of Culture and United States' Universities, the Southern Regional Education Board, the University of South Carolina, and Davidson College. Research leaves from our college and university in the fall of 1990 and the spring of 1991 were supported by the National Endowment for the Humanities with an Interpretive Research Grant, which was followed in 1992 by generous supplementary funding. We are immeasurably grateful to the funding agencies for making our work possible.

Final acknowledgment must be to Isaac's grandmother, Sarota Amato Musafir, and to his mother of blessed memory, Caden Lévy Israel, who died just as this manuscript was nearing completion. Our work is dedicated to our daughter, Catherine Ann Lévy Ott, and to our son, Michael Jack Lévy, who have the blood of the Sephardim in their veins. This book is to record for them, and for all the descendants of Sephardim, the spiritual pulse of life of their ancestors who lived so fully and vibrantly in the Ottoman Empire, as well as in the other lands.

Introduction

"Esto es melezina de muestras madres ke mos azian [This is the medicine of our mothers that they used to do for us]," one woman said, as she told how a pomegranate could be used to cure a stomachache. "Boil it a little," she explained, "and give it to the one whose stomach hurts."[1] An elderly Sephardic woman recounted this cure to us when we asked her about *melezinas de kaza* (medicines of the house).[2] It is appropriate that our work on domesticated religion should begin with the seemingly mundane use of the pomegranate. Just as the garnet-like, gleaming seeds encased in the thick-fleshed pomegranate are emblematic of its symbolic representation—the redness for the blood of life and the abundant seeds for fertility—so does this cure signal richly embedded knowledge drawn from a deep cultural reservoir.

While not intending to intimate an origin for the use of the pomegranate, still we would like to follow its roots in Jewish sacred history and trace them right back to the Holy of Holies, the Temple of Solomon in Jerusalem. In 1988, the Israel Museum acquired a small ivory pomegranate, dating to the late eighth century B.C.E., with a paleo-Hebrew inscription reading, "'Belonging to the Tem[ple of the Lor]d . . . , holy to the priests'" (Avigad 1989, 8). If, perchance, this delicate blossom of the pomegranate was not in fact "used by the priests in the service of the Temple of Jerusalem"—an interpretation disputed by some—still the *rimmon* (Hebrew, pomegranate) was one of the seven fruits that blessed the land of Israel: "For the Lord your God is bringing you into a good land, a land with streams of water, with springs and pools welling up in the valleys and on the hills; a land of wheat and barley, of vines, fig trees and pomegranates, a land of olive oil and of honey" (Deuteronomy 8: 7–8). The decorative symbol of the pomegranate also graced the hem of the high priest Aron's robe (Exodus 28:33–34) and the capitals of the pillars of the Temple (1 Kings 7:18, 42). In following the roots of the symbolic uses of the pomegranate, we are tied not only to Jewish sacred tradition, but also to other cultures, for the "juicy pomegranate fruit with its multitudinous seeds was a popular symbol of fertility from the earliest times" (Avigad 1989, 12).

Our work focuses on the Sephardim of the Ottoman Empire, specifically on those who resided in the Balkans, the Dodecanese Islands, and Turkey, as well as on their descendants who emigrated to other lands. The Sephardim of this area were linked together linguistically and historically. The language of the home was Judeo-Spanish, which dates to the time of the expulsion from the Iberian Peninsula in the fifteenth century and which has been richly embellished with vocabulary from the languages of the Ottoman Empire, including Turkish, Greek, Serbian, and Croatian, as well as Hebrew, Italian, and French. The events of history provide a further unifying bond: the Balkan countries, the Dodecanese Islands, and Turkey were part of the Ottoman Empire for over five hundred years. With geographical proximity and frequently with friendly borders, there has been a constant exchange and interaction among these Sephardim. They are a people with religion, folklore, language, and history in common. In sum, the Sephardim of this area form a subculture within the larger grouping of Sephardim. The renowned folklorist Dov Noy points to the importance of recognizing just such geographical units of study. Jewish folk religions, Noy writes, "differ from each other depending upon their ethnic and regional background" (1980, 273).

The research has been carried out—by Isaac Jack Lévy alone or with Rosemary Lévy Zumwalt—over the past forty years. Some of the earliest work, which began in 1957, was done by Isaac among the Rodesli community of Atlanta, Georgia, as well as in Sephardic communities elsewhere in the United States and abroad. Isaac's earlier research was part of a more expansive study of Sephardic language and culture. In a trip to Israel in 1985, Isaac and Rosemary together continued the study he had begun on Sephardic folk beliefs.[3] The most concentrated portion of the research came in 1990, when we undertook six months of travel to the Sephardic communities of Greece (Athens, Kavalla, Salonika, and Rhodes), the former Yugoslavia (Belgrade, Dubrovnik, Sarajevo, and Skopje), Turkey (Istanbul and Izmir), and Israel (Ashdod, Bat Yam, Herzelia, Jaffa [Yafo], Jerusalem, Kryat Matalon, Netanya, Rishon LeZion, and Tel Aviv).

The life and beliefs we describe in this book for the most part span the years from the beginning of the 1800s to World War II. We arrive at this time line by adding the age of our informants to the age of their parents and grandparents. The people with whom we worked were usually about eighty years old; they remembered most vividly the medicines of the house as practiced by their mothers and their grandmothers. We assume that the two ascending generations did not enjoy quite such a lengthy life span, and estimate sixty years for the parent and sixty years for the grandparent. Thus we arrive at a time depth of two hundred years. Assuredly, these medicines of the house reached much further back in time. As discussed in chapters 5 and 6, aspects of the humoral system of the Hippocratic School (800–50 B.C.E.) formed the symbolic basis for the evil-eye complex and for the belief system of *espanto* (fright). The prevalence of sugar as a cure for illness, as presented in chapter 7, linked the Sephardic folk medical system to the Arab pharmacopeia, which spanned "Persia to Spain" and whose specialists were "the major interpreters of humoral medicine to the Europeans" (Mintz 1985, 96). Specifically, we connect the Sephardic cure of *al sereno,* which involved putting sugar water in the night air, to a practice in Spain. In chapter 8, we draw parallels between the Sephardic *prekante* and the Spanish and Portuguese *ensalmo,* both used as ritual prayers for curing. Thus, while our focus is on the Sephardic ritual curing system, we make links, both historically and culturally, to related medical systems and beliefs. Nonetheless, we will eschew the attempt to suggest a date of origin for the customs and beliefs described in our work. Others before us have shown this a fatiguing and futile task.[4] World War II provides an end point for so much in Jewish life, and so it marks the demise of a way of life of the Sephardim in what had been, years earlier, the Ottoman Empire.

As a team, Isaac and Rosemary brought together the insider and outsider perspectives, sometimes referred to as the ideal combination for fieldwork.[5] Born on the Isle of Rhodes in 1928, Isaac is Sephardi. His native language is Judeo-Spanish; he grew up under the tutelage of two of the finest teachers of Sephardic life ways, his grandmother, Sarota Amato Musafir, born in Milas, Turkey, in 1888; and his mother, Caden Lévy Israel, born in Milas in 1905, who moved to Rhodes with her mother in 1920. His early years spent in Rhodes were firmly rooted in the customs, the ties of family and friends, the religious celebrations, in short, the total belief system, which so tragically unraveled with the destruction and upheaval of World War II. An outsider to Sephardic culture, Rosemary was born in Decatur, Georgia, in 1944, and grew up in Napa, California. However, among the Sephardim, one does not remain an outsider long. Thus, as Isaac's wife, she became an adopted Sephardi, or as Isaac's friend from Rhodes said on meeting her, "I will embrace you as *una ija mia"* (a daughter of mine).

The research we conducted was aimed at drawing together from all those with whom we spoke remembrances of their past. As we would say to the people, we were interested in learning about *"las melezinas de kaza* [medicines of the house]." While we worked in various locations, much of our research was conducted in *bet avot,* which is Hebrew for "house of parents," or old age homes, where we attempted to find people who could recall the ways in which their mothers and grandmothers had cured their ills, whether these were physical—a stomachache or toothache—or emotional and spiritual, which almost always was connected with *mal ojo* (the evil eye) or *espanto* (fright). To locate informants, we would start with personal contacts or with the administrators in the front office. Anxious to help, the latter would direct us to people they thought were likely to know about the old ways. Sometimes this was successful; other times, the people to whom we were directed wanted to know why they had been singled out. Did the administrators think that they were superstitious? Did they think that they had come from an uneducated background?

If we were at first unsuccessful in locating knowledgeable informants, we would simply keep asking. At times, it seemed that we were working ourselves through to the oldest of the old at the old age homes. We were constantly struck with what we intuitively knew, that there was a crucial need to complete the research when we did. The old people, those who knew what we had come to learn, often were very feeble or were dying. In the Salonika old age home, we had to curtail our interviews in order to participate in a prayer service for a deceased member of the home. At Bet Avot Leon Recanati—the Leon Recanati Old Age Home in Kryat Matalon, outside of Tel Aviv—our single most treasured informant, Zimbul Maya Suzi, had a voice so weak as to be barely audible. We were truly at the closing of an age. Those who remembered the past were becoming part of it.

Before we had left for the field, Rosemary had argued with Isaac about this point. Trained in folklore by Alan Dundes, she had learned that folklore was not disappearing, only changing. She was sure that Sephardic culture might be different from what Isaac remembered as a young child, but that it would be there as something new. In the course of the fieldwork, however, she became convinced that he was right. The distinctly Sephardic culture of his childhood was not just changing; it was disappearing. The children were not learning the language, and the culture was being supplanted by the majority culture in each of the countries we visited. It was the passing of an age that in 1990 existed only in the memories of the elderly. As the rabbi in Salonika told us, "You should have come here fifty years ago. In Salonika, there was everything. If you had come here fifty years ago you could have found a lot. There was a lot of material here then. Now, no." Even in the 1960s, Isaac recalls, there was rich material. Thus, in a real sense, our fieldwork was an endeavor to reconstruct the past. We were working with people's memories of what life had been like in their childhood.

To reach these memories of their childhood, we had to contend with more than just the passage of years. The lives of the people had been suddenly and tragically disrupted by the events of World War II. Some of the individuals we spoke with were survivors of the Holocaust; others, like Isaac's family, had been refugees, forced to leave their homes and communities in haste; others had gone into hiding, sequestered by Christian families for the duration of the war. So for the Sephardim, as for all Jews, the Holocaust runs like a bleak chasm through individual and collective memory. The disruption and dwindling of a way of life is for the Sephardim of the former Ottoman Empire a historical reality, not a romantic fantasy of a lost golden age.

In this work, our theoretical orientation is towards a gendered view of religion, a domesticated religion, with women at the center of this complex of beliefs. While many scholars have discussed this domesticated religion in the diminutive form of the "little tradition"—in contradistinction to the more grand "great tradition"—we prefer to emphasize the powerful position of domesticated religion at the center of the Sephardic community, the Jewish home. Others have also identified the strength of this domesticated religion. Laurel Kendall, in *Shamans, Housewives, and Other Restless Spirits: Women in Korean Ritual Life,* writes of the woman shaman whose *kut* (curing) rituals are performed in the homes. The shaman and her followers weave a colorful, vibrant religious display that is not a weak palliative to the official Confucian, male religious system. The *kut* ritual is female and it is focused: "The physical house is the primary metaphor for women's rituals. . . . It is from the perspective of *household,* not [patrilineal, patriarchal] *family,* that women deal with the ancestors of their own and their husband's house" (1985, 168).

Our intent, then, is not just to recognize and to document this domesticated religion of the Sephardim but also to celebrate it. By listening to the voices of the Sephardic women and men who have spoken enthusiastically with us about their recollections of the medicines of the house, by conveying the spirit of these people, we hope to capture the heartbeat of Sephardic life. While so much literature on the Sephardim has focused on the great writers, philosophers, and scientists of the Middle Ages of Spain and on their history in the Ottoman Empire, all too little has been written about those who have been the life blood of the Sephardic communities. In our work, we unabashedly privilege the Sephardic woman, whom we see as the center of this domesticated religion and as the keeper of the home. It is through her hands that the health of the community was maintained, a health that was not limited to the physical but encompassed the spiritual and required a sensitive attention to the maintenance of careful relations among themselves, with their non-Jewish neighbors, and with the denizens of the spirit world.

We have encountered from time to time the arrogant dismissal of the importance of women in the religious sphere. In Bat Yam, Israel, we spoke with a Sephardic rabbi who clearly conveyed not only that he was not interested in our research on Sephardic folk religion, but that he held in contempt anything he saw as "superstitious." In response to our questions about the role of women in curing and household religious rituals, he responded that we could find all the answers in "El livro de las mujeres, el livro de Rahel [The Book of Women, the book by Rachel]." To our inquiry as to which book he was referring, he laughed mockingly and said in Judeo-Spanish, "It is written in the book by Rachel [the Matriarch]. This book does not exist, it is all superstition!" Feeling the fools, we realized that he had dismissed not only our research interests but also the importance of anything to do with women's domestic religious rituals.

In our conversations with each other about our work, we have referred frequently to "El livro de Rahel," the book by Rachel, and to the attitudes conveyed in this rabbi's response to our questions. Happily, we acknowledge, there were other rabbis with whom we spoke whose attitudes were much more positive towards the religious rituals conducted by women at home. We are in agreement with Susan Sered, who remarks in *Priestess, Mother, Sacred Sister,* "In many societies women have active religious lives, yet ecclesiastic hierarchies rarely include women, and official or 'great tradition' religious concepts generally reflect men's and not women's priorities and life-experiences" (1994, 3). This exclusion of women in the religious ritual of the synagogue was clearly evidenced in the Bat Yam synagogue, as it is in other Sephardic and Ashkenazi Orthodox synagogues. After the rabbi had given us numerous copies of his books and told us to search for our answers in "the book by Rachel," he directed Rosemary to the women's section. In the far corner of the synagogue, behind a cloth screen, known as the *azara* (separation), were three rows of chairs. There sat the women, all save one with heads covered. There were no prayer books for the women. Why should there have been? They had no part to play in the service. They showed this exclusion by talking throughout the service. Before the prayers began, the men looked in the direction of the women and hushed them loudly, and one of the men banged on a chair. Then the women whispered quietly, but they still whispered. They did not even bother to watch the ceremony. In a few seconds, their whispers were at regular volume, scarved heads nodding together in enthusiastic conversation. Occasionally, one of the men would look with irritation towards the women. The only time in the entire service when the women quit talking was when they were involved in the service, when they had to stand for the *meldado,* the reading of the *kaddish* (the prayer for the dead). As soon as their part in the service was over, the women continued talking with as much enthusiasm as ever.

Here, in our book, we will document the religious life of women, the domesticated religion. While others before us have spoken of "domestic religion" (Myerhoff 1978; Sered 1992, 1994; and Eliade 1987), we prefer to speak of "domesticated religion," in order to convey the sense of the taming of religion. As Kerry Noonan notes, "domesticated" gives the sense of a religion "tamed or changed in order to serve a purpose," in contrast to the more situational sense ("in the home") of "domestic."[6] We will turn to *las buenas mujeres* (the good women), *muestras madres* (our mothers), who were the ones knowledgeable about the ways of divining illness and effecting cures. We will situate these women curers at the center of the domesticated religion, not at the periphery of the male power structure. This Sephardic domesticated religion provided a way of making sense of the perplexities of social life, and of shaping behavior to fit the narrow constraints of a tightly structured, face-to-face community. This "personalizing" of religion gave women access to—indeed, control over—specific rituals. Shaped to give expression to the concerns of women, these rituals were aimed at the heart of women's lives, the health and well-being of their family members and their neighbors.

In chapter 1, we discuss the categories of illness and develop the concepts of the folk society, folk religion, the great and little traditions, as these apply to the Sephardim of the Ottoman Empire. Most important, we present our concept of domesticated religion and introduce las buenas mujeres of the Sephardic communities. Chapter 2 gives a history of the Sephardim in Spain and in the Ottoman Empire. Chapter 3 details the manner in which we gathered our material, specifically the fieldwork that we conducted in 1990 in the Sephardic communities of Greece, the former Yugoslavia, Turkey, and Israel. Chapter 4 focuses on the power of the spoken word as articulated thought. In chapter 5, we discuss the beliefs and customs surrounding *mal ojo* (evil eye). Chapter 6 presents the narratives about *espanto* (fright) and *echizo* (witchcraft) as a means of delineating social boundaries. In chapter 7, we discuss the simpler cures for illness; and in chapter 8, we explain the more complex ritual prayer of *prekante.* Chapter 9 details the most serious cure, *saradura,* the ritual of enclosure.

1 *Keeping the Spirits Happy, Keeping the Family Healthy*

For the Sephardim, as for so many other peoples, the relationship with the spirit world was fraught with danger. One's health, good fortune, fertility, happiness, love life, the length of one's days, all could be diminished by actions of the spirits. One needed, therefore, to take special precautions to protect oneself and one's family against contact with the spirits. The first such precaution was simply not mentioning them by name, for to name them was to give them power. Rather, they were referred to by euphemisms. In Hebrew, they were the *sheddim* (spirits), a term used also by the Sephardim. As defined by Nehama in his Judeo-Spanish dictionary, the *shed* was a "demon, revenant, the shadow of the dead which the popular imagination believes is seen moving about in solitary quarters in the shadows or in the light of the moon, during the night" (1977, 533). Zimbul Maya Suzi, originally from a small village near Istanbul, explained to us that the shed (spirit) was "*una mejor de mozotros* [one (female) better than us] who injured children, made them sick, and did not breast-feed them."[1] In Judeo-Spanish, they belonged to *la buena djente* (the good people), *los buenos de mozotros* (the good among us), and *los mejores de mozotros* (the best among us), complimentary references that might have the effect of assuaging the spirits. They were also called *los ke no se nombran* (those who should not be named) and *los ke vienin i van* (those who come and go). There were occasions, however, when the reference would be less than complimentary: the spirits would be referred to as *los negros* (the bad ones), *los ke danyan* (those who do harm), or *los de abasho* (those from below), the latter a directional term with an implicit negative connotation of *basho,* or low in moral character.

The anthropologist George Foster notes that euphemisms function in all cultures as a way to avoid direct mention of sensitive or taboo topics (1966, 57).[2] Moshe Shaul, editor of *Aki Yerushalayim* and former director of the Judeo-Spanish section of Kol Israel Radio, said in response to the question "Why do they call it mejores de mozotros?": "In order not to insult them. This, I think, is a belief of the Jews. To do the reverse. That is to say, someone who is blind, is called *vistozo* (one who can see). *Bet ahayim* (house of the living) instead of *bet akevorot* (house of the graves). Los mejores de mozotros, we think they are not the best. They are the worst, but for more security they are called the best."

There was reason to appease the spirits by euphemistic reference: they were frightening and they were deadly. As Lea Amram, originally from Kuskunjuk, Turkey, related, the people of her community believed in the evil spirits. "The older ladies would tell stories that would scare us. The old people, yes, about los mejores de mozotros. They would walk here, they would walk there, like prints of duck feet. The old ladies would talk a lot about it!" She added, "When I remember this, whew!" and she made a face of fear. Zimbul Maya Suzi also recalled los buenos de mozotros (the good among us) as having the feet of a chicken. And one man remembered an incident that happened to his wife's father: "'He used to go [to] the villages to sell shoes. They would give him a guest room. As he went to sleep he felt pressure on his body. The spirits were congregating and taking their place. He then took . . . the book of prayers and said the *Shema* and the weight disappeared. He saw on his quilt footprints like a rooster'" (Stern 1980, 146).

Sol Azuz and Korin Madem told of one child who had been stricken with *espanto* (fright) and who was taken (died). Isaac asked the two women if the child had died because the cure had not been accepted by the spirits. The answer, repeated as if in litany response is, "*La tomaron*" (they [the evil spirits] took her):

> Isaac: They performed something for fright for the child, and she died? That's because the buenos de mozotros [good among us, evil spirits] didn't accept—
> Sol: Didn't accept it, they took her [she died]—
> Isaac: —and they took her.
> Sol: They took her.
> Isaac: Therefore, the curse was still there.
> Sol: Yes, they took her away.
> Korin: The *ruha* [Hebrew, spirit], the ruha was there.

Sol: They took her—
Korin: They took her, they took her. The ruha, the ruha.
Sol: They took her, they took her.
Korin: They took her, they took her.
Sol: The ruha was there.
Isaac: The ruha yes.
Sol: They took her away.
Isaac: They took her.
Sol: They took her for themselves.

For the Sephardim, illness was seldom simply the result of physical causes; usually there was a spiritual basis. Thus, in order to determine the nature of the illness, one had to determine the source of contact with the spirit world, whether it be through *mal ojo* (also rendered as *ojo malo*, both meaning evil eye), espanto, or *echizo* (witchcraft). The first two sources of contact—mal ojo and espanto—were brought about mainly through unintentional thought, speech, or action, as well as through accident or happenstance; the third category, echizo, was the intentional use of magical incantations and objects for malevolent purposes. In all three categories, whether the source of contact with the spirit world was unintentional or intentional, the illness or misfortune came about through the actions of the spirits.

Mal ojo, also associated with *la avla mala* (evil speech), was brought forth through the expression of envy or greed in thought or word. This could be, and usually was, entirely unintentional. For instance, one's passing compliment could bring illness to a baby. It was the spirits who heard the praise and who brought illness to the little one. Why would they so willfully cause pain to an innocent? Because they, themselves, were envious of beautiful, healthy children. They were given power to act out their envy through the agency of human beings. Thus, while the person, in thought or word, might intend no harm, the spirits did. As Simha Hen of Trachia, Greece, explained, "The *ojo malo* [evil eye] should be taken as one understands it. It is the work of the evil eye, it is not the eye that causes it, it is what comes of it." Espanto might result from an accident, a shock, or a bad dream. It was also believed that when one was in contact with the dead, one was ever so close to the spirits. The sheddim could be set in action by one person seeing another killed, or by a person lingering in a cemetery or even passing through it without taking the proper precautions. Since sleep was considered one-sixtieth part of death,[3] one would come in close contact with the souls of the dead through dreaming, and, thus, a nightmare could give the spirits power. Through accidental pollution, an individual could rouse the spirits by insulting them.

One might become ill oneself, or cause another to fall ill, through the unintentional, careless disposal of polluting fluids, often bodily fluids, such as menstrual blood or urine, or even dirty dishwater. With echizo, the source of contact with the spirit world was the direct, conscious use of powerful incantations and manipulation of objects to bring about a desired end. In this instance, the volition was intentional, and the subject of illness or misfortune was specified. The spirits were aroused with echizo by design, to cause harm.

The results of these three sources of contact with the spirits were the same: illness and misfortune. Those afflicted were sick; they lost their appetite, they could not sleep, they tripped or fell frequently, vomited continuously, cried constantly. The degree of affliction, however, might vary in all three of the categories from a mild problem to a serious disorder. The treatment would vary accordingly from a simple cure to a complex remedy. The simple and slightly more complex cures were, for the most part, interchangeable, whether the cause of illness was mal ojo, espanto, or even echizo. A person who was seriously ill was said to be *asolumbrado* or *asolumbrada,* which meant that he or she was overtaken by a shadow, or possessed by evil spirits.

For all cures, regardless of the simplicity or the complexity, the treatment itself provided for a lessening of tension. Nothing else might be needed to make the stricken one feel better, simply attention, rest, special care. The folk medical system allowed one to blame bizarre or unacceptable behavior on the mal ojo, espanto, or echizo, and ultimately on the spirits. By deflecting blame onto the spirits, one could act out at least some hostility and, at the same time, deny the responsibility for the behavior—both of which were crucial considerations for life in a community where each individual was personally known to all.

In a conversation about the customs for announcing a birth, our mother, Caden Lévy Israel, led us directly and succinctly to a core feature of life in a Sephardic community—indeed, to the central aspect of life in any community based on face-to-face interaction:

> Rosemary: Mother, do you do anything to a house when the baby is born? Like [placing] a bow. You don't put anything outside?
> Caden: We don't put anything outside.
> Isaac: How do they know a baby has been born? Do they know from the street when a baby is born?
> Caden: In Rhodes, the whole world knew already.

The anthropologist Robert Redfield speaks of precisely this aspect of connectedness in what he refers to as "the folk society," or "the little society": "The communication upon which understanding is built . . . takes place among neighbors, within the little society itself" (1947, 296). For the Sephardic communities of which we speak, just as for the folk society discussed at length by Redfield (1934, 1941, 1947, 1956), there was a predominantly personal character of relationships, or, expressed another way, "a strong sense of belonging together" (1947, 297).

The personal was also the familial, since the social organization of the community was based on kinship; it was "an organization of families" (Redfield 1947, 303). An individual was nested in the ties of kinship as is evidenced in the following excerpt from an interview Isaac conducted in 1965 with Bohora Biton and with his step-father, Baruch Israel. Mrs. Biton, who was born in Rhodes, was attempting to identify a woman who knew how to do *livianos* (divination by reading the shapes of molten lead that had solidified in cold water):

> Bohora Biton: Do you know who may know it? . . . Miriam di Yako Buchuk.
> Isaac Jack Lévy: Is she still alive?
> Bohora: What?
> Baruch Israel: Miriam di Yako Buchuk. The daughter of Eliau Alkana?
> Bohora: The daughter of David Lehem—[correcting herself] the sister of David Lehem. She is your relative.
> Baruch: Miriam di Yako Buchuk!
> Bohora: Yes. She is your relative.
> Baruch: The daughter of *Mana* [Mrs.] Sara Notrica?
> Bohora: No. The daughter of *La Tia* [Aunt/Mrs.] Bulisa. She was the daughter of the *kumadri* [midwife], Tia Bulisa, of Natan Hason. You are relatives.
> Baruch: Of the daughter, the sister of the *kumadri*.
> Bohora: This one is the grandchild of the *kumadri*. She is the wife of Yako Buchuk.
> Baruch: I know, I know who it is.
> Bohora: Son of *El Tio* [Uncle/Mr.] Buhor Levy.
> Baruch: Buhor Levy, yes. . . . The brother of Yehuda Levy. The brother of Yehuda Levy.
> Bohora: Father.
> Baruch: The brother of Yehuda Levy.

While the two could not concur on the relationship—it was the father; no, it was the brother—Bohora Biton was able to identify the individual through a complex tracing of the web of kinship, a kind of litany of kinship relationships with Baruch Israel as the independent-minded echo.

This aspect of the personalized life was part of the "contained" nature of Sephardic communities in the Ottoman Empire. Though these communities did not suffer the extreme and enforced ghettoization of their coreligionists, the Ashkenazim of Eastern Europe, still there was a recognizable Jewish community within established boundaries. While some Sephardim might elect to live outside the Jewish quarters, most chose to reside in close proximity with friends and relatives of their faith. Thus, even in the larger urban centers, Jewish life was set apart, by the physical markers of the community and the spiritual markers of membership in the group. In the smaller towns, this was also the case. The Sephardic communities were contained, not dispersed. The constraints and restraints characteristic of small groups worked, then, even in the larger population centers.

Since relationships were situated in personal, kin-based, religiously and culturally centered networks, an outward semblance of harmony was crucial to the functioning of the group. The intensity of this interconnectedness was reflected in the Judeo-Spanish formulaic saying about awakening in the morning: "Primero si vei la kara dil Dio, despues si lava la kara, i al fin si vei la kara del vezino [First, one sees the face of God, then one washes one's face, and finally, one sees the face of the neighbor]." Disruptions of this apparent harmony and cohesiveness would pose threats to the social fabric of the community. There was an explicit attempt, when problems could not be avoided, to keep them within the Jewish community, and thus to protect the reputation of the Jews against criticism from the outside. Eager, even adamant in this regard, the rabbis and officers of the *kahal* (community, synagogue) often enacted laws to ensure that, whenever possible, legal arbitration and judgments remained within the Jewish jurisdiction.

Greed, envy, resentment, jealousy, all would be perceived as social and moral evils that would undermine the good of the whole. One could not openly admire or praise the possessions or achievements of another without a protective disclaimer, since this might call attention to another's good fortune, to the imbalance of limited good, as this concept was developed by George Foster (1965) and linked so artfully to the evil eye by Alan Dundes in "Wet and Dry, the Evil Eye" (1981). In his essay on "The 'Uncanny,'" Freud remarks on this aspect of the evil eye: "Whoever possesses something at once valuable and fragile is afraid of the envy of others [and] . . . projects on to them the envy" that she or he would feel in their place. Freud continues, "A feeling like this betrays itself in a look even though it is not put into words" (1959, 393).

While ideally the balance in material and spiritual goods had to be maintained, ultimately, this could not be. The reality of living in a close-knit community where individuals interacted intensively on a day-today basis meant that misunderstandings and resentments simply had to occur. When social disruption arose within the family, or within the community, the cause was attributed not only to the misbehavior of individuals, but also to the malevolence of the spirits who had been alerted through some careless word or action by the people involved. *Mal ojo* (evil eye) and *avla mala* (evil speech) were often perceived as the cause of the social disruption, and the spirits were the ones to blame for unpleasantness.

As the source of malaise, illness, physical handicaps, mental disturbances, poisoned relationships, and death, the spirits had to be controlled. This attempt to control them, to maintain a working balance between the world of the spirits and the world of the living, was effected through a complex belief system, a Jewish folk religion, or a Jewish "domesticated" religion that provided a way of making sense of perplexities—of illnesses and rashes, of love-struck children and irascible neighbors—as well as a way of shaping behavior to fit the narrow constraints of a tightly structured, face-to-face community.

While the people in their daily lives felt a need to domesticate their religion—to make it fit the exigencies of navigating the narrow and twisting alleyways of both physical and emotional space—there was still the standard, in Judaism as in other religions, of the pure, the doctrinaire, the correct religious tradition. Credited as the first scholar to use the term "folk religion,"[4] Joshua Trachtenberg, in the opening to his 1939 *Jewish Magic and Superstition: A Study of Folk Religion,* remarked on the tension and interplay between the religion of the folk and that of the "Synagogue":

> But alongside this formal development there was a constant elaboration of what we may call "folk religion"—ideas and practices that never met with the whole-hearted approval of the religious leaders, but which enjoyed such wide popularity that they could not be altogether excluded from the field of religion. Of this sort were the beliefs concerning demons and angels, and the many superstitious usages based on these beliefs, which by more or less devious routes actually became a part of Judaism, and on the periphery of the religious life, the practices of magic, which never broke completely with the tenets of the faith, yet stretched them almost to the breaking-point. If we call these "folk religion" it is because they expressed the common attitude of the people, as against the official attitude of the Synagogue, to the universe. (1939, vii–viii)

While first in using the term, Trachtenberg was not alone in his work on folk religion. The transcendent and the pragmatic, the official and the folk, these are terms that emphasize the dichotomy between doctrinal religion and the religion of the common people. The division between the two is more than what might be perceived as a separation of the lettered from the unlettered. Rather, it slices into the ways in which the community of believers is organized—through kinship, economics, and education—and how this community is linked to other communities. The division has a temporal dimension, as well. For "official Judaism"—often referred to as "rabbinical Judaism," or simply as Judaism—the temporal dimension is linked quite consciously and with great pride to a historical lineage through the development of accepted doctrine and dogma. This sacred history becomes, as it were, a religious "pedigree." For domesticated or folk religion, the temporal dimension has little import for the adherents, but it is there, nonetheless: it is the historical connections with other cultures and blendings from other belief systems, which result in a religious "mélange." This mélange was revealed in the response of ninety-four-year-old Regina Arogeti of Atlanta, Georgia, originally from Rhodes, to our query about where she had learned all the customs about which she was so knowledgeable: "Esto es traer agua di venti mulinus [This is to bring water from twenty windmills]."

In this mélange of domesticated religion, there was a sharing of beliefs about the spirit world, and of illnesses and cures. The Sephardim blended religious elements taken from Spain and Portugal with those of the Ottoman Turks and of the Orthodox Christians. All of these folk medical beliefs—whether Jewish, Muslim, or Christian—were overlaid on the ancient Greek humoral system. For example, the Sephardim carried with them from the Iberian Peninsula various cures for illnesses brought on by contact with the spirits, from their cure for espanto, which involved, among other things, placing sugar or another substance *al sereno,* in the night air, to the complex *prekantes,* or curing formulas, which had existed among Catholics in Spain and Portugal. The evil-eye belief system, so strong among the Sephardim, was threaded throughout the entire Indo-European world. The people with whom we spoke would often acknowledge this "shared" nature of their beliefs. To Isaac's question "Once in a while, did you go to the Turkish people for them to write *kemiyas* [amulets]?" Sol Azuz, originally of Istanbul, responded, "Turkish, even Turkish people used to write. And the Turkish people pay a lot of attention to this. *Muy, muy, muy mucho* [Very, very, very much]! They give more credit to it than we do. . . . Turkish believe a lot in it." At times this acknowledgment of shared beliefs also reflected political alliances and factions. For example, Sol Azuz and Korin Madem, who was also originally from Istanbul, both agreed that the Sephardim did not seek assistance for cures from the Greeks:

Isaac: You didn't go to Greek people? To Christians?
Sol: No. Not to Greeks, not to Greeks.
Korin: Not to Greeks. . . . To Arabs, yes, to Arabs, yes.

Sol Azuz told about going to Turkish women for a cure against the evil eye. The woman would take a long chain of maroon beads, put it over the head of the stricken one, and draw it down to the legs: "Three times. With the words that they used to pronounce. In Turkish they used to say words. . . . And the beads, they used to count them, and they used to blow on us. They used to count the beads. . . . They would stop, they would blow on the complete body." She imitated blowing over the entire body. "And they kept doing it until the beads were complete." Then Sol and Korin recounted the efficacy of the cure:

Sol: And they would count them, and they would blow on us. The Turkish women.
Isaac: After they count seven . . .
Sol: The Turkish women.
Korin: Sick we used to go . . .
Sol: We would return well.
Korin: We returned well. We returned well [spoken from the background].
Sol: We returned well, we returned well. Immediately, on the spot, the body felt light. We used to go heavy, and the women used to make everything light.
Isaac: The Jews also used to utter words? Blessings?
Sol: Yes, yes. They used to talk a pure Turkish, not the words that we used to use. They used to speak another type of language.
Korin: Koran, Koran.
Isaac: Of the Koran.
Sol: Yes, of the Koran they used to speak, that we couldn't understand.

In *Peasant Society and Culture,* Robert Redfield elects to use the terms "great tradition" and "little tradition" to refer to what in other writings had been designated as high and low culture, classic and folk culture, learned and popular tradition, and hierarchic and lay culture. For him, the great tradition is connected with the "reflective few" and is "cultivated in schools or temples" (1956, 41–42). The little tradition is the domain of "the largely unreflective many," and it "works itself out and keeps itself going in the lives of the unlettered in their village communities" (42). In short, as Barbara Myerhoff so aptly summarized, the "'Great Tradition' refers to the abstract, literate, often impersonal and formal set of usages . . . associated with civilizations. The 'Little Tradition' is the local, oral, often more concrete set of ideas and practices, which is authoritative because it is ancient and indigenous; it is what might be called the folk culture, associated with community rather than civilized social forms" (1978, 287 n. 4).

Redfield characterized the two religious traditions as interdependent, with each affecting the other: "Great and little tradition can be thought of as two currents of thought and action, distinguishable, yet ever flowing into and out of each other" (1956, 42–43). While viewing both as "dimensions of one another," ultimately Redfield conceptualized a hierarchical relationship between the two: the little tradition was subsumed under the great tradition. He stressed that there was consensus on this point: "Those people who carry on the lower layers and those who maintain the high alike recognize the same order of 'highness' and 'lowness'" (50). Don Yoder, in "Official Religion Versus Folk Religion," similarly writes of folk religion, "as those traditional levels of folk belief, those folk attitudes to life, death and the universe which, at least in certain regional societies, exist partially alongside, partially underneath the official levels of religion" (1965–66, 38).

In *Unity and Variety in Muslim Civilization,* Gustave von Grunebaum notes that the interrelationship between the two currents is not unproblematic: "The little tradition is the catchment of the popular undercurrent; its effectiveness is still felt by the intelligentsia, but 'officially' it will be denied or deprecated. Where the hypotheses of the great tradition are considered beliefs, the hypotheses of the little tradition will be considered superstitions. In fact, the social position of a person may depend on which of the two traditions he determines to live by" (1955, 28). To appraise the relationship between these two realms, one selects a vantage point. Those adhering to the folk religious system usually perceived no contradiction between their beliefs and practices and those embodied in the doctrinal religion. If there was to be conflict, it would likely come from the attitude of those in the doctrinal religion who might either reject outright folk practices that they viewed as heretical, or look askance at what they judged as harmless, though misinformed, beliefs. In his work, von Grunebaum notes precisely these two approaches. Islamic teachers may disparage the popular traditions as "the religion of the ignorant," or they may tolerate the local practices by, in some instances, adopting them as part of the great tradition (28–29).

In Judaism, the custom of changing one's name to improve one's health did, indeed, pass from folk religious practice to acceptance by rabbinical Judaism. As Hayyim Schauss records in *The Lifetime of a Jew throughout the Ages of Jewish History,* Franco-German Jews in post-Talmudic times began this practice, and eventually it was accepted as "a universal Jewish custom." "Even a special ritual was evolved for effecting the change of the name. A ritual quorum of ten assembled in the synagogue. . . . The Holy Ark, containing the Scrolls of the Torah, was opened. One man, who sometimes held in his hand a Scroll of the Torah, recited a special prayer in which he emphatically notified the heavenly authorities of the change in the name of the person who was ill and requested them to no longer identify the person bearing the old name with the person bearing the new name" (1950, 76).[5] There was, of course, biblical precedent for this practice, for God changed Abram's name to Abraham (Genesis 17:5), and Sarai to Sarah (Genesis 17:15). Among the four things that "cancel the decrees of Heaven," the Talmud lists "change of name" (RH 16b).

Among the Sephardim, this practice is known as *pidyon.* Zimbul Maya Suzi told us of the time when her husband was very ill. A cousin asked her, "'Why don't you open a book in the synagogue?' In the synagogue, they open the door of the ark and ask for *refua shelema* [good health]. They read whatever it is to be read, they open the book and they look. They opened the book and they found the name 'Eliezer,'" [by which he was to be called]. She concluded, "In the morning, he asked for his shoes, and he was well." The executive director of a Sephardic synagogue in Atlanta, Georgia, wrote to Isaac in 1988, on behalf of the rabbi, explaining this practice as follows: "When a child is critically ill, his or her name is changed (some give an additional name to the child of someone else who lived a very long life). This custom has esoteric meanings but none of which we consider to be magic or superstitious." The blessing for this is listed in *Book of Prayer, According to the Custom of the Spanish and Portuguese Jews,* under the section, "Change of Name for One Who Is Dangerously Ill":

> When it is desired to change the name of the one who is ill, after the mention of the name in the preceding prayer, the following declaration is made:
>
> With the permission and approval of the supreme King of kings, God of the universe, blessed be He; and with the approval of the heavenly and earthly tribunals, we definitely change and supersede the name of this sick person which was heretofore. . . . From this day on his name shall no more be. . . . but. . . . By that name of. . . . shall he be known and called, and by that name may he live [ellipses in the original]. (Sola Pool 1936, 455)

The new name was to be used in addition to the previous name for all religious purposes, such as being called to the Torah, for marriage, divorce, and even inscription on one's tombstone.

From the perspective of those adhering to folk religious practices, the element of tension with the official religion does not necessarily exist. As Don Yoder noted in his discussion of the Protestant Pennsylvania Dutch practices of *Braucherei* (powwowing, occult folk healing) and *Hexerei* (witchcraft), "On the people's level of understanding these things were accepted. They were, in fact, looked upon by Pennsylvania farmers as part of their religion" (1965–66, 39). Thus, while according to Yoder, "folk religion exists in a complex society in relation to and in tension with the organized religion of that society" (1974, 11), the folk, themselves, are but little disturbed, if even aware, of this tension. In his work on Jewish folk religion, Dov Noy is in accord with Yoder. The people, Noy says, see their beliefs and practices as their religion; they do not separate what might be categorized by outsiders as "folk" from "religion." As Noy wrote, "The element of tension which exists between folk and official levels of religion in the complex societies, dealt with by Don Yoder, is absent in Jewish folk religion, as the observers and performers see their views and practices as part of the official religion; for the most part, they are not even aware of the fact that their units are local or limited to their ethnic group" (1980, 285).

From the perspective of official Judaism, this equanimity and easy acceptance was not always the case. In "Transcendental and Folk Aspects of Judaism," David Siskin remarked on this ambivalent attitude of the rabbis: "The attitude of rabbinic authority toward folk beliefs and practices which violated sacrosanct norms was ambivalent. At different times and places they disclosed a variety of responses. Some denounced the beliefs and usages of the popular religion, others did not approve but refused to condemn, while still others showed a surprising toleration. And there were those who, while recognized as mentors of the transcendental faith, themselves participated in the rites and practices of the folk" (1987, 289). From our fieldwork, we have an example of Siskin's latter point, a rabbi who participated in the practices of the folk. Rivka Sarfati, originally of Salonika, told the following story about a rabbi in Izmir: "A friend of mine who was always fighting with her husband, went to see a rav [rabbi]. He gave her some powder and told her to put it under the doormat so that her husband would step on it when he entered the house." Mrs. Sarfati explained, "The idea is that as the powder is getting closer to the feet, so should the husband get closer to the wife."

Controversy over magic and idolatry can be traced to the sacred source of Judaism, the Torah. As Siskin noted, early Judaism, revealed in the Bible, was "both an elite religion and one rooted in popular belief and practice." The conflict between the two was like a clash between the worlds of the wholly sacred and the thoroughly profane. Labeled as idolatry, popular beliefs and practices were associated with magic, divination, necromancy, and idol cults (1987, 285). Still, while the Bible condemned the magicians and soothsayers of the neighboring peoples, the staff of Moses turning into a snake was religion. Thus, that which was designated as religion was sacred; and that which was designated as popular was blasphemy.

In some instances, the rabbis, as Trachtenberg noted, attempted to eradicate the folk religious practices. Abraham Danon chronicled the efforts of a series of rabbis who worked to combat the practice of "fantastic healings," which they viewed as against mosaic law. Rabbi Judas Lirma of Belgrade in the seventeenth century and Rabbi Isaac Navaro of Izmir in the eighteenth century objected to "the superstitious practice called 'Indulcho' [and] they promised in persuasive terms divine healing to those who abstained from such practice" (Danon 1897, 261). In 1852, the rabbinical body of Aleppo under the leadership of Rabbi Abraham ben Isaac Antibi (1765–1858), the Syrian Talmudist, expressed "with a rare vehemence the horror that [the practice of Indulcho] inspired" (262).

In other instances, the rabbis felt, as we learned in the course of our research, that if the practices did not hurt anyone, if there was no evil intent involved, then there was no real harm. Isaac was told precisely this by a Sephardic rabbi in New York in 1964: "What does not hurt us, does not hurt our religion, *si es por bueno* [only if it deals with good]." A Sephardic rabbi in Jaffa, Israel, told Isaac in 1990 of his wife's amulet against the evil eye: "She was warned not to speak of it, and she did not tell me about it," but he saw it on her. While he did not believe in the use of amulets, he didn't forbid their use either. As he said, "Each one to his custom." In the same vein, Hayim Palache (1788–1868?), a prominent rabbi from Izmir, wrote concerning magical remedies in opposition to a Hebron rabbi: "Even the *indulko* [magical cure] which the women here in our town, Izmir, are doing by throwing water and sweet [sugar] and other kinds [of ingredients] . . . and while doing it they mention 'God, Lord of Israel,' and the name of our Holy Fathers, in order to compensate [appease] the *Sheddim* [demons] and to bribe them in order for them not to cause harm or injury, there is no prohibition against it. . . . And we saw also that all the rabbis in time before us, and before, before that they did not oppose it. . . . According to the Halakhah, there is no prohibition of this *indulko* that the women in our town are doing. And it is well established on all statements of the rabbanim" (1874, 7).[6] Violette Alkalay, originally from Bulgaria, summed this up quite succinctly in response to Isaac's question, "The rabbis of Sofia, were they against the use of livianos?" "No," she responded, "they didn't interfere with this." Isaac persisted, asking, "Why not?" She replied, "Why should they interfere? Each one would do what they believed."

Barbara Myerhoff, in *Number Our Days,* linked Redfield's concepts of the great and the little tradition to the people whom she studied at a Jewish retirement center in Venice, California. The Great Tradition was "the formal [literate] expression of Jewish learning"; it was the use of Hebrew language for prayer and sacred study; it was the link to the shared history of the Jews. Myerhoff wrote: "This aspect of Judaism gave the old people at the Center—and probably most Jews anywhere—the experience of being One People, despite their geographical dispersion and cultural heterogeneity. Each Sabbath since the Diaspora Jews all over the world study the same portion of the Torah together and celebrate the same holidays in the same language, acknowledging their common membership with other Jews, and this forges an identity among them, *Klal Yisroel,* One People" (1978, 96). Important as it was to their identity as one people, this great tradition fed into and from the little tradition, which had the force of "early, strong emotional experiences." The people of the center whom Myerhoff studied, coming as they did from Eastern Europe, spoke of this as *Yiddishkeit* (flavor of Yiddish, flavor of Judaism). This was the people's "most influential and powerful identification as Jews." Drawing from the words of one of her most important informants, Myerhoff explained: "As Shmuel had put it, 'Yiddishkeit is our culture,' the slowly grown, beloved result of long, intimate relationships, 'not a thing of nations,' not grand or exalted but associated with family, nurturance, and survival. Yiddishkeit was inflected most powerfully in the *mamaloshen* [mother tongue, Yiddish]. . . . With this layer, all Center people had the most positive and sustained experience. It was the warp and woof of what held them together, the stuff of their common childhood in Eastern Europe; in it they were equals and equally comfortable" (96).

In like manner, the Sephardim distinguished between *lashon hakodesh* (Hebrew, the holy language) and *la lengua de la leche* (the language of the milk, mother tongue). Hebrew, as the language of the synagogue and of formal learning, was in the sphere of the men. Judeo-Spanish, known simply as *espanyol,* was the language of the home, and the first language spoken between the parents and the child. A Sephardi would identify another as a member of the group by the possessive, *uno di los muestros* or *una di las muestras,* meaning he or she is one of us, a Sephardi. Language and identity with the group merged in the explanation about the origin of Judeo-Spanish. If asked, "Di andi avlavash espanyol? [Where did you learn Judeo-Spanish?]," a Sephardi would reply, "Di muestros padres [From our ancestors]." When Isaac asked this question of an elderly woman with little formal education, she linked this to religion, as if among the ancient Hebrews, Judeo-Spanish was the language of discourse: "Di muestros padres. Di Avraam, Itzhak i Yako [From our Fathers. From Abraham, Isaac and Jacob]." Along with inclusion in the group went a certain assumption that this individual shared a Sephardic parentage and a religious and cultural identity with all the Sephardim. Additionally, as Myerhoff so eloquently details for the Ashkenazim, so for the Sephardim, the jewel in this crown of ethnic identity was the emotional component: it was the heartbeat of the Sephardic culture, the sounds and the smells of *la judería* (the Jewish quarters), the rhythm of life, the inflections of speech, the mannerisms that gave speech its nuanced meaning.

Rachel, another of Myerhoff's informants, referred to this emotional layer of religion—this Yiddishkeit, or little tradition—as "domestic religion." Expanding on what others had said in a group discussion of women's position in Judaism, Rachel said, "'What the girls had is different from the boys. Now what ideas Moshe and Nate got, they come to through the schooling. We girls had another kind of a religion. . . . We girls had what you could call domestic religion, that means it comes into you through the rituals'" (Myerhoff 1978, 234). Rachel explained that in the *shtetl* of her youth, her brothers left in the morning to pray, while the girls gathered around their grandmother to say their morning prayers in Hebrew. Since they had not formally studied Hebrew, they did not understand the words, but they understood the beauty. Then the grandmother switched to Yiddish to divide up the chores among the girls. Hating the task of wiping dishes because the cloth was so rough, Rachel would do a poor job of it. One day, her grandmother gently corrected her by telling her that she had a holy name and that she always had to be perfect to live up to it: "And always before me, when I was wiping the dishes was the name of the holy mother Rachel, and I thought, 'She's right. I am that woman.' That, that is what I call domestic religion. It makes the adrenaline flow. It changes your entire view on things. . . . These things were injected into you in childhood and chained together with that beautiful grandmother, so ever since infancy you can't know life without it. The boys in the cheder could learn the words and forget them, but in this domestic religion, you could never get rid of it. . . . When it goes in this way . . . , Jewish comes up in you from the roots and it stays with you all your life" (235).

Just as Rachel would recall the words and the beauty of her grandmother, so for Basha, the warmth of the Shabbat candles would bring back the memories of her mother: "When I was a little girl, I would stand this way, beside my mother when she would light the candles for Shabbat. We were alone in the house, everything warm and clean and quiet with all the good smells of the cooking food coming in around us. We were still warm from the mikva. . . . To this day, when the heat of the candles is on my face, I circle the flame and cover my eyes, and then I feel again my mother's hands on my smooth cheeks" (Myerhoff 1978, 256). This domestic religion was centered on the emotional link of mother and daughter and was fused through the weekly ritual of ushering in the Sabbath. As Myerhoff remarked, its strength came from drawing together "nurturance and ethnic specificities, and it was this blend that gave hearth-based religion such endurance and depth" (256).

In *Women as Ritual Experts: The Religious Lives of Elderly Jewish Women in Jerusalem,* Susan Sered develops the concept of the domestication of religion as a means for women "to personalize the rituals, institutions, symbols, and theology" as a means "to safeguard the health, happiness, and security" of their loved ones (1992, 10). This "personalizing" of religion gives women access, indeed, control over, specific rituals. Shaped to give expression to the concerns of women, these rituals are aimed at the heart of women's lives, the health and well-being of their family members and their neighbors. As Sered remarks, "In numerous rituals—spontaneous, formal, private, and communal—they guard over the living, dead, and unborn people with whom they have close relationships" (10).

Relationships, Sered argues in *Priestess, Mother, Sacred Sister,* are "often the core element of women's daily experiences." Thus, for women, rituals and belief systems are "designed to strengthen bonds among people" (1994, 121). Sered further develops the focus in domesticated religion on the interpersonal: "An intense concern with the well-being of their extended families characterizes the religious lives of many women. Women who have a great deal invested in interpersonal relationships, and are denied access to venues of formal power, tend to be associated with religious modes that stress relationship" (6).

Domesticated religion, then, gives primacy to the relationships that are at the center of women's lives. Excluded as they are from the more formal level of religious hierarchy, the women "modify and reinterpret Jewish rituals, symbols, institutions, and beliefs in directions that give meaning to their role as mothers and protect the children for whom they, as mothers, are responsible" (Sered 1994, 65). Still, while domesticating and personalizing their religion, the women do not believe themselves to be acting *outside* their religion. They perform their cures in the name of one God, and in the names of the archangels, and the patriarchs and matriarchs of Israel. Of the elderly Jewish women in Jerusalem with whom she worked, Sered remarks: "The women's religion is not independent of normative Judaism; the little tradition does not exist in a vacuum; and the women's beliefs do not radically differ from those of their fathers, husbands, and brothers. Rather, the . . . women, seeing themselves as good and pious Jews, subtly alter, elaborate, reinterpret, reshape, and domesticate selected aspects of Jewish belief and law into a form that is meaningful to and consistent with their perceptions, roles, identities, needs, and experiences" (1992, 50).

A gendered view of religion is necessary, then, for recognizing the sacred spheres of male and female power and control. For the Sephardim, the men undeniably were at the center of the synagogue: they led the services from the *teva* (Hebrew, altar, pulpit) in the sacred language of Hebrew, which the women were never officially taught. The men claimed this sphere; it was theirs, doctrinally according to Jewish law, and in actuality, according to practice. When included at all in the services, the women were marginalized, quite literally at the periphery, in the women's section. In most Sephardic synagogues, this was in the *azara*, a plain, unornamented balcony overlooking the central area of worship that was ornately decorated with crystal and brass candelabra, and shining ritual paraphernalia.

To stop with the ritual space of the synagogue, however, would provide a truncated and misshapen view of Sephardic religious life, for the women's religious sphere was at the heart of the Jewish families, in the homes. Here the language of the prayers was Judeo-Spanish, and those presiding over the rituals were *muestras madres* (our mothers), *las buenas mujeres* (the good women). Mary Algrante, whose father was a biblical scholar in Izmir, provided a succinct summation of these two spheres: "My father knew *ayin arah* [evil eye] in Hebrew, while I know *kozas de mujeres* [things of women]." Regina Arogeti remarked of the women who knew the medicines of the house, "They did not know how to read or write, but these words [of the ritual verses] they knew quite well, and they did help." While most could not read Hebrew—though there were some who recited the *Shema* in Hebrew from memory—most women said a prayer in Judeo-Spanish before going to bed, seeking protection from evil spirits throughout the night:

> Kuatro kantonadas ay en esta kaza,
> Kuatro malahimes, kuatro anjelines,
> Ke mos guadren de fuego, i de flama,
> I de palavra mala, i de muerte subetania. Amen.

There are four corners in this house,
Four angels (in Hebrew), four angels (in Judeo-Spanish),
May they protect us from fire, and from flame,
And from evil speech, and from sudden death. Amen.[7]

In "What's a Life Story Got to Do with It?" Karen Brodkin Sacks posits the term "centerwomen" for "women who initiate and sustain informal workplace social networks, and who are often keystones of family and kinship networks as well." While Sacks's research focused on women in the workplace, her concept is useful for a discussion of las buenas mujeres precisely because she delineates the core and unofficial position that such women occupy. Sacks continues, "They tend to initiate activities that maintain group cohesiveness. People expect them to know the events, opinions, and needs of those in the network, and to use that information for their shared well-being." Other people keep the centerwomen well informed about what is happening on the personal and family level. "As a result," Sacks emphasizes, "centerwomen are likely to know everyone's business, not least because people seek them out to discuss it" (1989, 91).

Sephardic women curers were, in Sacks's term, centerwomen. Not only were they in possession of the knowledge of the cures, but they were also closely linked to those they were treating. As Caden Lévy Israel of Milas, Turkey, and Rhodes remarked, "They were part of the community, well-known women. These women knew about everything." They had intimate knowledge about people's problems, about their worries and their pains, and they were trusted by the people. Their central position in the community and their knowledge about medical and emotional problems facilitated treatment. They often knew the sources of tension and could address these by traditional medicine in an accepted way.

Muestras madres (our mothers), the keepers of Sephardic health and home, answered to other names as well, some of which stressed feelings of kinship, such as *las madres di mi madre* (the mothers of my mother), *las bavas* (the grandmothers), *las tias* (the aunts), or *las ermanas* (the sisters), the latter two used as honorary titles for an older person. A woman from Edirne, Turkey, explained that these were "Mothers who knew. [Like] Aunt Rosa, she performed for espanto. We used to go to Aunt Rosa, and she used to show us what to do." Isaac's grandmother, Sarota Amato Musafir, originally from Milas, Turkey, and Rhodes, used to remark, "Of course, what our mothers did was successful! They knew what they did." Julie Alajef, from Rusçuk, Bulgaria, said, "My mother used to tell me those things in Bulgaria. 'You know that Esterika, Rahelika came and put the eye.' When things like that would happen, my grandmother would point them out." A man from Sarajevo recalled, "There were some old women who [prepared the medicines at home]. They used to come [to the houses]. An Aunt Luna came. 'We are going to call her,' people said." He emphasized that these women were neighbors. When needed, those who were known for their cures were summoned to the home, "Come, Aunt Luna, Aunt Hanna, Aunt Hannucha . . . Come Hannucha, come." Samuel Elazar referred to "Tija [Aunt] Hana di la ruda (who cured with rue), [and] Tija Rahelona Papo-Sason (an expert in cupping)" (1966, 156). A woman from Brusa, Turkey, explained that the knowledge of certain cures was generally shared; but when an individual was not aware of a cure, the source was always there: "Whoever didn't know how to do it, the mother could teach her. And if the mother didn't know it, she would say, 'Aunt, please come and *pase la mano* [pass the hand, *prekantar*]. The child is yawning a lot [a sign of the evil eye]. Please come and pass the hand.' And she came and passed the hand. . . . The mothers knew already how to do it. When they didn't know, they called the neighbor."[8] As this remark suggests, closeness of residence could come into play, as with *la vezindad* (the neighborhood).

Kinship and neighborhood proximity were not the only links to the keepers of Sephardic tradition. Age could also be a factor. *Las viejas* (old ladies) described elderly women. A man from Izmir, Turkey, explained, "In Turkish [these medicines are called] *koja kari ilaji*. . . . Women who are old and about to die are called *koja kari*. These are their medicines." Not age but the passage of time was conveyed in *las mujeres del pasado* (the women of the past). *Doktora sin chanta* (doctor without a bag) gave a humorous but respectful appraisal of the woman's skill. As one woman explained, "My grandmother . . . was doktora sin chanta. She was an old woman. She performed certain things that truly worked right away. She used to know about medicines."[9]

There were certain women who would be sought out for their specialized cures and knowledge. Those from Izmir and Rhodes were sources for the powerful *mumia* (mummy) made from dried bones of corpses or, preferably, the dried foreskin of the circumcision. As we were told, "There are special women who sell it." In Istanbul, there was a woman who was known for her ability to tell the reason for an illness through the traditional method of *prekantar*, which involved a ritual prayer. She added her own novel touch, a red fez with little stones in it. As Lea Amram explained, "She passed it over the head. She would put about five stones, and then she would pass it over whatever part of the body that hurt. And there was a benediction." From his childhood in Rhodes, Izachar Avzaradel remembered gathering baby mice for a woman who was known for curing earaches by using an oil in which they had been soaked:

> There was a lady, she was called la Ermana Rahel di Chikurmiji [Sister/Mrs. Rachel of Chikurmiji]. . . . This woman, for every newborn little mouse that was brought to her, she would give us a marzipan or a *travado* [sweet pastry]. We used to go to the warehouses of the Alhadefs, which were full of mice. Then we would just lift the boxes. We used to find mice just born, transparent. We brought a handful. She had a large jar where she made *trushi* [pickles] full of oil and full of mice. There was not a person in Rhodes in the Jewish quarter who had an earache who she would not put three or four drops of this and it would pass as if it were nothing. Better medicine than that didn't exist.

Certain women were skilled in all aspects of curing. As Caden Lévy Israel, told us, "These women knew about everything. They used to do it for the evil eye, they did it for *nazar* [casting the evil eye], for espanto, for many other things. And they were always respected, and they in turn did such things." In addition to being respected by all, often the women were regarded as saintly. They were called *mujeres santas* (saintly women), *mujeres bendichas* (blessed women), and *almas dil Dio* (souls from God, saintly people). They were *buenas di alma i korason* (good of soul and heart). Luna Tuvi spoke of two such women in Chanakali, Turkey: "We had two old ladies who were *sadikas* [holy], they were like *malahas* [saints], these two. . . . They were considered quite saintly." Lili Avraami told us about la Tia Rifka Natan of Pazarjik, Bulgaria, who was an expert in home remedies: "She was *una de las primeras maestras* [one of the best practitioners]. She was known as *la doktora* [the doctor]." As true for saintly people, Rifka Natan knew when she was to die, and she selected as her successor Lili's mother, Fortune Sibi. Rifka Natan said, "I am going to die, and I want someone to learn these things, in order for them not to be lost." Lili added, "She wanted my mother to learn it because she was sincere, honest, and believed in things like this, otherwise Aunt Rifka would not have given it to her. This is not a thing that you give to just anyone."

The women with this specialized knowledge would gladly visit the sick and the stricken as a mitzva, an act of kindness. They would not accept monetary payment for their cures, though they would accept presents. One woman remarked on her years of helping people, "I didn't charge them. I did it because they were Jews." After she treated them, people would bring her flowers and other little things. While not really wanting to accept the gifts, she felt compelled to do so, otherwise she would insult the people. Lili Avraami said of her mother, "Everything she did, she did without pay. Everything she did was for a mitzva." On the day of her death, Lili's mother had treated a man for pain in his leg. That evening, with no warning and no discomfort—the mark of a sainted person—she died. The next day, the man came to the house to give the mother a *bonbonyera* (silver candy dish) as a present. The children were insulted by this man bringing a gift to their dead mother, because one was not supposed to bring such things during *las sieti* (seven-day period of mourning). "We didn't understand why the man was there. He explained to us that he had come to thank her for what she had done the previous day." Her mother's mentor, Rifka Natan, was so renowned for her cures that even Christians from the surrounding villages came to see her. Since it was known that she would not accept any payment, they would bring her eggs, chickens, butter, and fresh produce from the farm.

Knowledge of the cures, of the events in the community, and of the problems of individuals, and their good, kind actions, earned these curers a position of respect in the community. The women were honored by those they treated. In response to our question, "And these women were highly respected?" Julie Alajef said, "I'll give you an example. There are children that my mother cured. And the women would say, 'Tia Buka, when Avramiko will have his bar mitzva, . . . you are going to be the first that we are going to sit at the table.' And the heart of the baklava, they would give it to her." These women exercised power as well, at least during the duration of the cures, for they could tell people what to do; and if the stricken ones wanted to be cured, they had better follow the advice of the experts.

The designation *las buenas mujeres* gave a positive evaluation of those who were willing to help, often when doctors had found no remedy. Rosa Avzaradel, originally from Rhodes, recalled a mysterious ailment that had afflicted her mother when she was a young girl: "There was no doctor that didn't see her. There was no solution. They would say that she had nothing. That she was O.K. But there were buenas mujeres. They used to do good deeds. Of free will, no? They were good women. Well, they told my mother, 'We are going to do something for [you].'"

The cures themselves were associated with the women, for these were *melezina de mujeres* (medicines of women), *koza de las nonas* (thing of the grandmothers), and, in French, *secrets des bonnes femmes* (secrets of good women). The practices were fixed in place as *melezinas de kaza* (medicines of the house) or *kozas de kaza* (things of the house). This link between the woman and the home was clearly made in one woman's explanation: "Es muy viejas personas ke azen en kaza kozas [It is very old ladies who do things at home]." The following exchange between Isaac and Avram Matia of Salonika delineated the connection between customary practices, women, and the home:

Isaac: Did you have any amulets against the evil eye?

Avram: Ah, yes, I remember it. They put it on. When I would put on new clothing, my mother would put one on me. They used to put here paper with things of women. I don't know what was inside.

Isaac: Who used to write these things? The rabbis?

Avram: Na! The women did it. It was the business of the women. No, it was not *hahamim* [rabbis, learned men]. They didn't occupy themselves with such things. The only thing they did to us was when we were going to put on new clothes, they would pin a little paper right here. What was inside I don't know.

Isaac: *Una nuska* [an amulet]?

Avram: Yes, *di kaza, di mujeres* [of the house, of women], not from hahamim. For evil eye.

People relied on the medicines of the house—the herbal cures, charms, incantations, divinations, and amulets—and they believed in their efficacy. As one woman said, "All these are cures of the women of our city. Everyone believed in it."[10] For the people, this was no idle or amusing pastime. Their lives depended on the results. There was little other option, for doctors either were not readily available or were unable to effect a cure for specific ailments, often for those caused by the spirits. Of her time in Rhodes, Regina Arogeti recalled, "There were no doctors, nothing!" Rosa Avzaradel concurred, "There were no doctors in Rhodes. Years ago, before one hundred years or more ago, there were no doctors. We did not have any doctors. A doctor Turiel came to Rhodes in 1908." Lisa Dasa recalled,

> Once upon a time, in our Jerusalem, we did not use too many doctors. But, we had a certain number of old women living around the courtyard. When the child was sick, we called Aunt Samalto, Aunt Rosa, Aunt Alegria. We used to go to their house, "The child is crying, what should I do?" She would check him up, "Aman, Aman, Aman [Woe, woe, woe]. He is [in some state], he has the evil eye." The child was nicely fat, handsome, with blue eyes. "It seems that so-and-so came to your house?" "She did." "She gave him the evil eye, darling. There is nothing to worry about." "What should I do for him?" "Take a little water and salt, in the name of the baby [and] in your name. Put some water on him. Wash his face three times from the bottom to the top, from the bottom to the top, three times, and then the legs, and then the feet, then the hands, then the body, and then by yourself take this water, go where three streets meet, pour it and say, 'As you [the stricken] are not looking at this water, so the eye that the neighbor has cast on you will not affect you.'" . . . She came home. The child was crying, I did [what the old lady told me], I covered him well and put him to sleep. What should I say? We believed in this.

Of their recourse to doctors, she concluded, "Aunt Sinyuri acted as a doctor for us. There was no need to go to the doctor. When did we go to a doctor? When we were quite sick. . . . When the doctor came, the child was already gone. This is the way that we spent our life in Jerusalem."

Medicines of the house, then, were just that. They were medicines that were readily available—herbs, ointments, poultices—as well as incantations, blessings, and prayers that one's mother could use to bring relief. Simha Hen remarked on the need to use anything at hand: "They would grab from the straw; they would grab from the cobweb." A woman recalled the necessity for such cures: "There weren't too many doctors. Everything was cured by the mothers. The child had a pain, they used to put warm oil on the abdomen. We used to boil chamomile . . . for tea. We gave it to drink. This kind of thing we did at home. There weren't too many doctors. People went to the doctor, for fever they went to the doctor. But a little pain that they had, or because the child was crying, right away they rubbed oil."[11]

To care for her family, the mother of the house would have to know when to apply a cure and what to select. Sometimes this would involve divining the cause of the illness with livianos. Other times, a simple herbal tea would be given. As a woman from Bulgaria recalled, "When we were sick, my mother used to perform livianos of lead. Also she used to boil mint, a little rue, a little lemon. All mixed. She would boil it like a tea, strain it, and give it to us to drink for stomachache. There we didn't go too much to the doctor, as we do here. Things of the house, they did things to us at home. All the medicines that were prepared were for different pains. Everything helped."

Sometimes even when a woman had access to a doctor, she preferred to use her own home remedies. A woman from Salonika said, "When we were children, and something happened, 'Ya mos espantimos! [We took fright!].' We didn't easily go to the doctor. We had a doctor, and the children used to treat him like a monkey. . . . Why did they think he was a monkey? Because from the street . . . before he even entered the house, he was already writing the prescription. Without even checking you!" Another woman said, "I told my daughter-in-law, the little one, I told her, don't take to the doctor. Everything is not resolved by doctors." In fact, she distrusted the cures of doctors and shielded her own children from them: "I had two children. I didn't allow that [treatment by the doctors]. And I was successful, because I learned from my mother, because I learned from my grandmother." Both children had developed hernias, she said, from crying too much; she used a treatment she had learned from her grandmother, belts for hernias. Of her son, she said, "I would take him to the doctor. He would just give any kind of an answer. I said, 'I am not taking him to a doctor anymore. I will take care of him at home.' I did what I learned from my grandmother."[12]

There were also instances of mutual acknowledgment of the skills of the other. The women would know when they could not treat an illness and would direct the afflicted to a doctor. A woman said that after a treatment, "If it didn't improve, they would immediately say, 'Go and call such a doctor. I cannot handle it.' There were certain things that she couldn't help." Doctors would also make recourse to the skills of certain women. Kalina Alvas recalled, "Well, our doctors believed in them in Bulgaria. They used to tell us, 'Try, try some of the things of the home.'" Julie Alajef spoke of her mother, Rachel Cohen: "She liked to help the poor a lot. And she put together medicines with which she cured people. And this compress, she learned from her mother. Even the doctors who knew her, when it happened that a woman was sick, they would call her. And my mother would say, 'Well, one can see that you had a cold.' She would *echar ventozas* [put small glasses for suction] on the back. There were some cases where women had pneumonia. First, the doctor would come and would check her. And [he] would tell the patient, 'Let's call Aunt Bulko, I will mark the spot where she could put the *ventozas,* where she could remove the blood.' And this way, she would cure her from the sickness."

In some instances, doctors were unable to help because of the nature of the illness. If an individual was sick through offense caused to the spirits, then medical treatment might only exacerbate the symptoms while doing nothing to affect the root cause of the disorder. One woman recalled the sufferings of her brother when he was a young boy living in a small village in Turkey. "We started to fool around with doctors. We called a doctor. He gave him a shot, he made him worse. Another doctor came, one said that he had typhus, the other one said that he had such-and-such sickness. More injections, more cures, time passed, eight days passed, the son instead of improving, he went crazy. He got crazy. He took off his underwear, he undressed himself completely, and he started to go into the streets. Now, what had actually happened? The cures that the doctor gave him had a negative result, because he was not [physically] sick." As the son became more disturbed, the father identified the cause of the problem. Accompanied by his son, he had traveled to a village on business. During the night, the son had sleepily gotten up to relieve himself. He told his wife, "Nissim wanted to urinate and I yelled at him, 'Here you are going to urinate, you are going to urinate on them [the spirits].' Since then he does not feel well." Two old women, who understood the nature of the malady—that the spirits had been offended when the boy had started to urinate on them—undertook a complicated cure. This involved blessing the boy and giving him a drink of water and sugar, visiting a Muslim holy man in the village who read from the Koran, returning by horse cart with an item of his clothing to the spot where the young boy took fright, washing this spot with water and sugar, washing the shirt, and returning to put the shirt on him. As soon as the boy put the shirt on, he said, "'Mama, all those who wanted to do harm were killed, they were all killed. They cannot do any more harm, they are not doing me any more harm. They were all killed.' Once he wore the undershirt, he felt better." Thus, according to this informant's account, not only were the doctors unable to cure the young boy, their ministrations intensified his bizarre behavior; the spirits had him in their grip and would not release him until the proper procedures had been followed.

Sephardic domesticated religion concerned women tending illnesses predominately of other women, of children, and of babies. In the hundreds of interviews we conducted, rarely did the discussion focus on the illness of a man. It was almost always that of a woman or a child. This was conveyed not just in the content of the narratives, but also linguistically, in the use of the feminine, such as "kayo una hazina," meaning "a woman fell sick." As Bohora Biton expressed it, often the women fell ill from "a sickness of the body," such as mal ojo or espanto. When a man was ill, often it had to do with echizo, mainly love magic performed by women, frequently with the intention of changing the object of affection; thus, ultimately, echizo linked back to women.

With this focus on spiritual health and gendered illness, gifted women curers with *manos livianas* (light hands) cured the ills of women and children, ills that could not be remedied—and indeed could be worsened—by the scientific approach of the doctors. Perhaps this was conveyed most acutely to us in our fieldwork when Isaac went alone without Rosemary to interview a woman who was known as a *maestra* (teacher, expert) of medicines of the house. Throughout the interview, Bienvenida Gabay kept insisting, "You're not going to understand it, you're not going to understand it. You're a man." When Isaac had trouble following her explanation, she exclaimed, "See, you can't understand! You're a man!" Through a large portion of the interview, she thought that Isaac wanted to collect this material so that he could perform it, thus her insistence that he would not be able to do these things because he was a man. She told him that some of the "heavy *endulchos* [complex cures]" could harm a person if not done correctly. As she explained the procedures to him, she emphasized, "These are difficult, they are difficult. You are not going to be able to do them."

While the focus of domesticated religion was largely on the threats to women's health, specifically to her fertility, the concern was almost always articulated in terms of the male infant. To a pregnant woman, one would say, "Eskapamiento bueno! Parida de ijo! [Good delivery! May you give birth to a boy!]," or, "Ijo de buena ventura ke te se aga [May you have a son with a good future]." The custom of offering food to visitors and the belief about its acceptance or rejection reflected the positive valuation on the male. For example, one informant told us that if a guest came to visit and did not take something to eat or to drink, this was a bad sign; it meant that the hostess would give birth to a baby girl. According to Regina Arogeti, if a pregnant woman offered something and no one took it, a girl would be born; if she offered something and it was taken, a boy would be born. Mrs. Arogeti reported, "The expectant mother used to say, 'Toma ke me naska ijo' [Take it so that a son will be born to me]." She added, "Boys were more precious." In this light, it seems that the woman's fertility was important in order for her to produce a son.

The cognitive model for a child may have been the son, but the affective, nurturing source was the daughter. As one woman would say in expressing her regret at having two sons and no daughter, "No ay mejor amigas komo la madre kon la ija [There are no better friends than the mother with the daughter]." Following this proverb, the emotional bond would be stronger between the mother and her daughter than with her son, on whom she might need to depend for financial security. The parents could count on the daughter for their old age: "Ijo es ijo, ma la ija es para la vijes [The son is a son, but the daughter is for old age]."

The differing attitudes towards the baby boy and the baby girl were summarized in the rituals following the birth. Lea Amram from Turkey commented, "When a woman gave birth, she would not come out of the room for eight days. That's for those who had people to take care of them. . . . For those who could, they took good care of [the mother], and after eight days, they would have the *brit milah* [ritual circumcision]." Another woman described the same ritual of enclosure for eight days after the birth of a baby boy, and then added, "All this is for a boy. It is not needed for a girl."[13] Madame Lea continued, "And for the girls, they would have the *viola* [party, watching of the child]. For the *viola,* they invited people, the haham would come, they picked up the child. They would dress her like a *novia* [bride], and they would put her in the hands of the haham, who would bless her. 'Lo bueno de Sara, de Rifka, de Lea' [The goodness of Sara, of Rebeca, of Lea]. He would bless her and name her."

The focus in the home and in the neighborhood involved a delicate balance of spiritual, familial, and social interactions, yet there were factors outside of the control of las buenas mujeres. The interface between the Jewish and non-Jewish communities, particularly during times of economic and political upheaval, often resulted in a total disruption of the Sephardic way of life. No amount of domesticated religion could counter the forces of the Spanish Inquisition, for instance, or of the economic disintegration of the Ottoman Empire during its later years, or of the deadly destruction of the Third Reich.

2 *The Sephardim of the Ottoman Empire*

Writing in the sixteenth century, Rabbi Eliyahu Capsali (1483–1555) told of the expulsion of the Jews from Spain, and of their reception into the Ottoman Empire: "So the Sultan Bayezid [1481–1512], king of Turkey, heard of all the evil that the Spanish king had brought upon the Jews and heard that they were seeking a refuge and resting place. He took pity on them, and wrote letters and sent emissaries to proclaim throughout his kingdom that none of his city rulers may be wicked enough to refuse entry to the Jews or expel them. Instead, they were to be given a gracious welcome. . . . Thousands and tens of thousands of the expelled Jews came to Turkey and filled the land. Then they built innumerable righteous communities in Turkey and gave generously to redeem captives" (Barnai 1990, 19).[1]

The Sephardim left a land in which they had flourished during the Moorish rule and alternately prospered and suffered under Catholic dominion. Their ties to the Iberian Peninsula had been long and deep. Indeed, Enrique Saporta y Beja, a Sephardi and a scholar, recorded one origin story that linked the ancient presence of Jews with the very designation for Iberia: "According to ancient tradition, the presence of the Jews in Hiberia (which some people wished to see derived from the Hebrew word '*hebria*': Jewish) dates from time immemorial. The Jews were already living in the Iberian Peninsula in the time of Solomon" (1979, 11). Other explanations for the term "Sepharad" also offer tantalizing tales of origin. In the Book of Obadiah, verse 20, the prophet spoke of those Hebrews who were captive in Sepharad, believed by many biblical, Hebrew, and linguistic scholars to be Ispania, Spain. While some have proposed Sfard—now Sardis—the capital of Lydia, as the origin of the term "Sepharad," other scholars have suggested that *Sefard* derived from the legendary Garden of Hesperides, a part of Hispanic Mauritania, where a third contingent of the Hebrew slaves in Egypt, who did not follow Moses to the Promised Land, had settled. Whatever the derivation of the term, it is believed that Jews came to the peninsula with Phoenician traders and settled in Cadiz, the biblical Tarshish, in 1500 B.C.E. They were later to be found in Malaga in the twelfth century B.C.E.; in Toledo, where exiles from the Tribes of Benjamin and Judah settled after the destruction of the First Temple (c. 586 B.C.E.); and in Seville around the same period (Lévy 1989b, 17).

Many of the exiles from the Iberian Peninsula found their way to the Ottoman Empire, where there were diverse and well-established Jewish communities, including the Romaniot, Karaite, Ashkenazi, and Arabic-speaking Jews. While all of these groups shared in the same faith, each had distinct cultural and religious backgrounds, and each had followed a complex path to the Balkans. The Jewish presence in the Balkans, Asia Minor, and the Dodecanese Islands can be traced back to the first millennium B.C.E.[2] While it is believed that many Jews were brought to the Ionian Islands as slaves by the Phoenicians, it is more plausible that they came as merchants alongside the Phoenicians. Jews came to Sfard (Sardis, Turkey) in the fifth century B.C.E. The Ptolemaic and Seleucid rulers (c. 312–165 B.C.E.) urged the Jews to continue their emigration throughout the Mediterranean. Victor Tcherikover notes that "2000 families were transferred from Babylonia to Asia Minor approximately in the years 210–205 B.C.E. These families settled in Lydia and Phrygia, as military *Katoikoi* (colonists)" (1961, 288). Jews fanned out along the Thracian and Aegean coast and settled in Salonika prior to 140 B.C.E. Jewish communities extended also to the islands of Delos, Samos, Cos, and Rhodes. By the second century C.E., an important Jewish community already had been established in Cyprus.

This early Jewish group, known as Romanim, and later called Romaniots or Gregos, settled not only in large centers but also in villages. Noting the literary and commercial activities in Bulgaria during the golden age of 800–900, Tamir remarks that "large numbers of Greek Jews emigrated to Bulgaria and settled in Nikopol, Vidin, Silistra, and Sofia" where they found religious freedom and prosperity (1979, 21). Romaniots in other areas were not quite so fortunate. Survival for them was not easy, even in the best of times. Their well-being depended on their relationship with the local peoples, and on the whims of the ruling classes and the church. In order to secure religious unity and to strengthen the political solidarity of the empire against Islamic attacks, the Byzantine emperors—Heraclius in 632, Leo III in 721, and Basil I in 874—decreed that all Jews were to be baptized, by force if necessary. Many Jews, out of fear, were induced to accept baptism; "still, they were suspected of potential acts of blasphemy and were therefore subjected to periodic persecution, as was later the case in Spain" (Shaw 1991, 21). In the main, the efforts of the Byzantine emperors failed, since the legal code, the *Basilica,* recognized the rights of the Jews to regulate their religious and communal affairs. Nonetheless, the efforts of the Christian rulers did not abate. When Emperor Romanus I Lecapenus (919–44) renounced his sinful ways and took up life as a monk, he "banished from the empire all the Jews and Armenians who would not embrace Orthodox Christianity" (Tamir 1979, 21). Under his rule hundreds of Jews were murdered and their synagogues desecrated. The Crusaders with their fanatic anti-Semitism repeatedly burned the Jewish quarters in Salonika and attacked the Jewish population of Constantinople and of other major cities. The religious fervor of the Sixth Crusade (1248–54) and the labeling of the Jews as heretics also "caused a major dislocation in European Jewish life, terror, and a continual search for asylum" (Haskell 1994, 75).

While the Romaniots suffered the vagaries of persecution by the Orthodox Christians, the Ashkenazim of northern Europe fled to the Balkans to escape the persecution ravaging their communities. During the spread of the bubonic plague in northern Europe (1334–51), Jews were accused of poisoning public wells and of spreading pestilence. Vicki Tamir writes, "In 1376, exploiting the prevailing superstitious popular belief (peculiar to all of medieval Europe) that Jews were sorcerers, heretics, and miscreants, Louis I [king of Hungary and Poland] expelled the Jews from Buda and loaded them on barges on the Danube" (1979, 45–46). Many found refuge in Kavalla and Siderokastron. Among these was Rabbi Shalom Ashkenazi, who took shelter in Vidin and founded the first rabbinical school in Bulgaria (Haskell 1994, 75). As chronicled by Avigdor Levy, the persecutions continued into the fifteenth century: "In 1421 Jews were burned in Vienna and expelled from Austria, then from Cologne (1426), Augsburg (1439), Bavaria (1452), Franconia (1453), and other German lands" (1992, 152). Tamir continues the record of persecutions: "A blood libel in Baden and a renewed air- and water-poisoning allegation in the 1470s in Regensburg led to forced confessions, torture, and eventual expulsion. Excluded from city after city, a number of Bavarian Jews turned to southern Europe. Jewish sources report that in 1470–1471 Bavarian

Ashkenazim came from Regensburg to Sofia, Vidin, Pleven, and Nikopol, and established an Ashkenazi synagogue in Sofia, which would absorb subsequent Hungarian immigrants" (1979, 54). Emigration to Bulgaria, Greece, and Asia Minor also took place from the Italian provinces and from Sicily.

Religious fervor was not the sole driving force for the persecution of the Jews in Christian lands. There were also political and economic concerns. Byzantine rulers and their subjects accused the Jews of assisting the Muslim conquest in the fifteenth century. The Christian merchants and professionals objected to the position of Jews as bankers, artisans, lawyers, and physicians.

With the Ottoman conquest of Asia Minor and the Balkans in the fourteenth and fifteenth centuries, the life of the Jews improved greatly. Recognizing the importance of the Jews and their contribution to the empire, the sultans "actively propagandized throughout Europe to attract Jewish emigrants to their newly expanding state" (Shaw 1991, 31). Sultan Orhan (1324–59) issued a *firman* (royal order) protecting the Romaniot Jews, who had actively helped him capture Bursa, the city from which they had been uprooted by the former Greek rulers. No longer under harsh laws, Jews voluntarily returned to Bursa and settled in a special *Yahudi mahallesi* (Jewish quarter). To reward them, Orhan brought Jewish craftsmen and money changers from Edirne and Damascus. As the conquest proceeded westward in the Middle East and in southeastern Europe, the Jews felt free to return to their former cities and villages in Byzantium and Anatolia.

Members of the Jewish communities were also active in attracting their coreligionists who were fleeing the persecutions in the European principalities and kingdoms. In 1454, Cohen and Kalmann, two Jews from Istanbul, urged Isaac Zarfati, originally from Germany, to write a circular letter to the Jews of Bavaria, Moravia, the Rhineland, northern France, and Hungary urging them to escape the anti-Semitic tyranny in these countries and to join them in the Ottoman Empire, where the sultanate granted them peace and tranquility. Zarfati, aware of the situation of his coreligionists, called "upon them to escape from the German House of Bondage and to migrate into Turkey . . . , a land wherein nothing is lacking . . . [and] every man may dwell at peace under his own vine and his own fig-tree" (Graetz 1941, 273).

In spite of all the freedoms accorded the Jews, as non-Muslims they were not considered on an equal basis with the Muslims. They were allowed to live freely throughout the land as *zimmis* (non-Muslim protected people), following the limitations and privileges set down by early Islam in the Pact of Umar, dating to the ninth century. With the mode of dress guided by the sultan's decrees, there were restrictions on the color, type of materials, cut, and size of garments. While only Muslims were allowed to wear green turbans, the typical headgear of the Jews was yellow. Jewish women were forbidden "to wear green garments, to use fabric embroidered with metal thread, or to wear gowns made of expensive furs" (Juhasz 1990, 122).[3] Jewish authorities, themselves, forbade the public display of excessive finery, such as expensive jewels and furs, in order to minimize restrictive governmental edicts and to avoid arousing the jealousy of non-Jews. Unlike the Christians, who were also subject to the decrees for non-Muslims, the Jews did not have any objections to these regulations since they "helped them distinguish themselves from non-Jews" (122). They also had to pay through their *millet* (religious administrative unit) a *cizye,* an annual poll tax assessed according to the income of each head of household. There were other taxes levied: the *avariz* (for army expenses), the *harac* (on agricultural produce), the *rav akçesi* (for the appointment of the chief rabbi), and the *resm-i kismet* (for inheritance) (Shaw 1991, 75).

After winning Constantinople on May 29, 1453, from the Christian defenders, Sultan Mehmed II moved the capital of the empire from Bursa to the newly conquered city. A visionary, he allowed each different group, regardless of origin and faith, to maintain its own social life, religion, and economic pursuits. The Jews, as well as the other minorities, were permitted to practice every occupation and profession and to be governed by their own community leaders, with very little interference from the ruling authorities. Although Islamic laws prohibited infidels (non-Muslims) from constructing new houses of worship, the sultan permitted the Jews to build synagogues on the foundations of existing houses (Shaw 1991, 29). Rabbi Eliyahu Capsali recorded that in Constantinople, under the rule of Sultan Mehmed, the Jewish population multiplied and flourished so that its synagogues increased from the two or three during the Byzantine kingdom to more than forty congregations (Shaw 1991, 30–31).

To repopulate and reinvigorate the conquered urban areas, and to develop and expand local commerce to other regions of the Ottoman Empire and abroad, the sultans transferred large portions of the Jewish population to important centers.[4] Of great significance to the subsequent development of the Sephardim, Mehmed II moved thousands from Edirne, Bursa, and other localities to Constantinople, which he had renamed Istanbul on his conquest of the city.[5] In the early decades of the sixteenth century, Selim I continued the policy of *sürgün* (uprooting) by deporting "segments of the conquered population to Istanbul. . . . In order to strengthen the economy of the Ottoman capital, most of the expatriates were chosen from among experienced Jewish craftsmen and merchants of Cairo and Alexandria" (Shaw 1991, 34). In 1523, Suleyman the Magnificent (1520–66) also moved 150 wealthy Jewish families from Salonika, Izmir, Istanbul, and Jerusalem, to Rhodes, because he recognized the island as a major geographical and commercial center. "In order to entice the Jews to emigrate, the Sultan accorded them a *firman* (edict) assuring them protective privileges not enjoyed previously by any minority. . . . Some of the enticements were the right to exploit the sulphur mines, a one-hundred year tax exemption, safe conduct through Moslem quarters when accompanying the dead, the guarantee that kosher meat would be available at competitive prices, free housing, and the privilege of exercising the profession of their choice. They were also allowed to practice freely their religion, to be governed by their own duly elected leaders, and to organize special schools and tribunals" (Lévy 1989b, 26). In the process, the sultans destroyed entire communities—often the very ones that they had previously ordered settled—and created new ones. For example, after the conquest of Cyprus in 1571, an order from Istanbul, dated October 1576, was dispatched through Suleiman Cha'ush, a member of the Palace Corps of Pursuivants, demanding the transfer of colonists from Rhodes to Cyprus. These waves of displacement were not restricted to Asia Minor and the Balkans. Bernard Lewis refers to an order of 1576 addressed to the *sanjek* of Safed, Palestine, instructing him "to send '1000 rich and prosperous Jews . . . with their property and effects and with their families' to Cyprus" (1984, 123). This was followed one year later with an order for five hundred families "'from the rich and wealthy among the Jews of Safed' to be transferred to Cyprus" (123–24).

It was to this prosperous and culturally complex empire that the Spanish Jews came. Their arrival at the end of the fifteenth and the beginning of the sixteenth century coincided precisely with the sultans' efforts to invigorate the empire, indeed, to create commercial cities through deliberate and enforced movement of populations. Decidedly, the sultans did not invite the Spanish Jews out of compassion but rather for pragmatic reasons. As Jacob Barnai remarks, "The Sephardi Jews constituted a positive element, economically and technologically, and [as the Romaniot and Ashkenazic communities had in the past] were likely to prove loyal subjects—unlike the large Christian minority, who were backed by Christian Europe" (1990, 19). Thus Sultan Bayezit's alleged remarks about the exile of the Jews from Spain makes perfect sense: "Spain's loss is my gain." Immanuel Aboab (1555–1628), a forced convert to Christianity who returned to Judaism, quoted the sultan as saying that the Catholic monarchs "were considered wise, [and] wrongly so," when in reality they impoverished Spain by expelling the Spanish Jews, and in the process enriched his empire (*Encyclopaedia Judaica* 1971, 4:349). Some add to these remarks the even more inviting touch, that Bayezit sent ships to the harbors to bring the exiles to his empire.

Medieval Spain, from the tenth to fifteenth centuries, was the cradle of Jewish literary, philosophical, biblical, and Talmudic luminaries, such as Hasdai ibn Shaprut, Samuel ibn Nagrela, Shelomo ibn Gabirol, Moshe ibn Ezra, Yehuda Halevi, and Moses son of Maimon (Maimonides). These were illustrious renaissance figures whose works had, and continue to have, a profound influence on the intellectual lives of Jews and Gentiles. There was no profession, no scientific discipline, no commercial endeavor where the Jews of the upper class did not participate and often dominate. Among them were ambassadors, financiers, astronomers, medical doctors, and cartographers. Many were wealthy and employed a retinue of servants. They owned buildings and vineyards, as well as olive groves and herds of cattle and sheep. They were admired and respected for their intellect, erudition, and commercial astuteness. The rulers, both Christian and Muslim, impressed with their ability, afforded them positions of trust, including administrative and financial posts in the government and the military. With the relative safety of the *juderías* (Jewish quarters) and the protection of the national and municipal governing bodies, the considerable influence of the Iberian Jews spread abroad—to France, England, the Netherlands, Germany, Italy, North Africa, Greece, Turkey, Egypt, and the Near East (Lévy 1989b, 24).

Along with the intellectual luminaries and the wealthy merchants, there were those who earned an adequate fare and those who were totally impoverished. The majority worked as small shopkeepers, artisans, and laborers. Among these were blacksmiths, coppersmiths, dyers, engravers, harnessmakers, locksmiths, ritual slaughterers, scribes, shoemakers, silk dealers, tanners, and peddlers. In spite of these economic pursuits, not all Jews were able to support themselves. Many, such as the old cloth dealers and the porters, eked out a meager income. For those unfortunate enough not even to have meager employ, each Jewish community had charitable organizations to assist the poor, the widows, and the orphans. Indeed, such organizations were not restricted solely to the Iberian Peninsula but were also to be found wherever the Sephardim found refuge.

According to Américo Castro, during the Judeo-Christian symbiosis of the Middle Ages, the reputation of the more prestigious Jews was such that a great number of prominent Christian families not only socialized with them but also were linked to them by marriage (Castro 1948, 537–38).[6] Due to the virtues attributed to them—Hebraic ancestry, wealth, gentleness, and knowledge—the Jews themselves felt proud of their own lineage and of their contributions to their communities and to Spain. This feeling of *hidalguía* (nobility, haughtiness) was perpetuated in their exile after departure from Spain and Portugal.[7]

The Jews of medieval Spain did not live in isolation but rather coexisted with the Muslims and Christians (Gerber 1992, xi). As Américo Castro says of medieval Jewish life, "One cannot fragment this history in watertight compartments . . . because each of the three cultural groups was . . . integrated in the events planned by the other two" (1948, 471). This *convivencia,* or intermingling, was based on tolerance and often on the need of the Christians for the support of the Jews. It was not limited to intellectual and commercial circles as portrayed by students of medieval Spain, nor was it restricted to the male sphere, but encompassed the whole family, and extended to people of varying economic classes.[8] Jews, Christians, and Muslims visited one another in their homes and met in the plazas and in the marketplace. Christians even attended synagogues, where they listened to the sermons of famous rabbis, such as Rabbi Samuel ibn Cuellar. As Renée Melammed writes, "On the social level, there were places where women, Jews as well as non-Jews, would come to execute chores such as obtaining drinking and cooking water at the spring, laundering at specified spots, using the oven, utilizing the water mill for processing grain, or spinning and weaving in courtyards. An additional meeting place was the bathhouse which was attended by Jewish, Moslem, and Christian women together. . . . Attending the bathhouse was definitely a social event; for the Spanish lady, regardless of her religion, was often accompanied by her daughters, servants, and neighbors" (1991, 119–20).

Jewish life shared much with that of the Muslims and the Christians—even in terms of sexual laxity. As Assis remarks, the latter was particularly a problem "among members of the upper social stratum . . . as it was among their non-Jewish counterparts" (Assis 1988, 51). This permissive behavior was forbidden by the crown, the Catholic Church, and, of course, by the rabbis. Assis continues, "What is clear is that despite the legality of polygamous marriage [and] concubinage, extra-marital liaisons and homosexual relations were widespread. . . . [The Jews] led an extremely permissive life, notwithstanding criticism from pietists and ascetics" (27). Moreover, Jewish men kept Muslim, and to a lesser degree Christian, mistresses, while some Jewish women became the mistresses of Christian men. The children born from these relationships posed a problem for the recognition of religious lineages, since only the offspring of Jewish mothers were considered Jewish. While less concerned about the newborns of Jewish women, the rabbis were quite preoccupied with the children of Jewish fathers and Christian and Muslim mothers (41). Ironically, in order to discourage sexual relations between Jewish men and Gentile women, the rabbis adopted a tolerant attitude towards prostitution and concubinage with Jewish women. They maintained, however, that the first wife was to be protected financially by her husband according to their marriage contract, the *ketuba,* and that the husband had to keep his obligations, including intimacy, with all his wives (Alfasi 1781, 31).[9]

The officers of the church as well as a great number of the Christian populace found the interaction between the Jews and Christians disturbing and repeatedly tried to impress upon the rulers that the presence of the Jews in Spain was abominable. From time to time, the church and the local courts would pass laws confining the Jews to ghettos in order to secure the separation between the infidel Jews and the faithful Christians, and to ensure that the Christian faith would not be weakened or broken (Fernández 1964, 583). They also ordered the removal of the Jews from all positions of influence, and they exacted from them exorbitant taxes. These persecutions were not unique to the sixteenth century; they had occurred throughout the Iberian Peninsula since Christianization. The persecutions became more intense in the Middle Ages (1280 in Aragon and Tarragona; 1288 in Gerona; 1322, again, in Tarragona; 1348 in Barcelona; and 1391 in Seville, Toledo, Valencia, and other cities) (Lévy 1989b, 24–25). When it was to their economic advantage, the monarchs, the dignitaries of the church, the nobles, and the local government officials rescinded the original edicts and offered protection to the Jews against the popular anti-Semitism (Castro 1948, 211).[10]

In the last decades of the fifteenth century, the ecclesiastic ranks with a new zeal urged the Catholic monarchs to join their fight against the infidels. While thousands of Jews converted to Catholicism "for reasons of sincere commitment,"[11] many more did so as a result of overwhelming pressure. For them, baptism was their only assurance of safety. Still, the fathers of the church knew well that any contact between the New Christians (*conversos*) and their former coreligionists would tempt their return to Judaism (Ríos 1984, 282). In spite of all the efforts by the church, contact between the converts and Jews persisted. From the archives of the Inquisition, Encarnación Marín Padilla traces the continuing interaction between Jews and conversos during the fifteenth century, specifically for religious holy days such as Shabbat and Yom Kippur; for family celebrations, such as marriage, birth, circumcision, the naming of a newborn girl; and for family crises, such as sickness and death.[12]

At the instigation of the officers of the Inquisition, and with the support of the pope and the Christian populace, Isabella and Ferdinand finally ordered the expulsion of the Jews in 1492. Some scholars posit that they acted reluctantly and were pressured to pronounce the Edict of Expulsion either by the powerful religious forces who clamored for the protection of the Holy Mother Church, or by the politicians who sought to bring about the unity of Spain. We suggest that it was both the religious and political forces that brought the monarchs, though reluctantly, to this declaration. As Luís Suarez Fernández writes, "Ferdinand and Isabella were not on principle hostile against the Jews. To attribute to them a diplomacy of antisemitism in the modern sense of the word would be an error" (1964, 13). The Jews, after all, had served the monarchs in numerous and vital capacities. From the archival documents of the Registro General del Sello, which were the official documents of the crown, it appears that the king and the queen were loath to sever their relationship with the Jews, many of whom had been their closest advisors in the court. Time and again, they attempted to protect the *aljamas* (self-governing Jewish communities, Jewish quarters) and individual Jews from the furies of the officers of the church, the representatives of the municipalities, and members of the nobility.[13] Isabella herself gave voice to this in 1477, when she pronounced, "All the Jews in my kingdom are mine and are under my refuge and protection, and it is up to me to defend and shelter them, and maintain their rights" (Fernández 1964, 13).[14]

The efforts of the monarchs and of some nobles and clergymen to protect the Jews were for naught. In the last decades of the fifteenth century, the arm of the inquisitional Supreme Council reached out to all parts of Spain. Neither the payment of the poll tax or other expenditures for the maintenance of the wars and of the Holy Fraternity, nor the promise to pay a ransom of millions of *maravedís* for the Jews' safety, nor the intervention of prominent Christian and Jewish individuals could secure the repeal of the royal order. All their efforts were in vain; their sole choices were conversion, exile, or death. They knew that some of their ancestors had suffered callous cruelty and intense brutality, that they had been banished from their cities and provinces. Indeed in 1280, Jews from Spain, fleeing the persecution and atrocities committed in the Iberian Peninsula, had sailed from Tarragona. Some had taken refuge in Rhodes, then under the rule of the Saracens, and were, thus, the first Sephardim to join the ancient Jewish population of the island (Lévy 1989b, 20). Again, in 1391, Hispanic Jews had escaped the recurring massacres by taking refuge in Palestine, Egypt, the Balkans, and Constantinople.

At the end of the fifteenth century, the persecution returned in full force. The juderías were repeatedly ransacked and burned; thousands of Jews were tortured and put to death. As mentioned above, thousands were forced to embrace Catholicism in order to save their lives. Still, conversion had not saved even those who desired to remain faithful to their new religion. *Marranos*, or pigs, as the converts were called, were always under suspicion of Judaizing.[15] Thousands of marranos—those who had relapsed and those who had genuinely embraced Catholicism—were seized and thrown into the dungeons, where they were ruthlessly tortured. Vast multitudes watched as the priests marched "the heretics" in a solemn procession to the *quemaderos* (pyres), where it is estimated that from the foundation of the Inquisition to 1808, "the total number of heretics burned . . . in Spain totalled 31,912" (C. Roth 1964, 123). Even those who had fled or who had died (17,659) did not escape, for they were symbolically burned in effigy. The property of those burned was acquired by the Holy Office. Tens of thousands suffered in the torture chambers; and 291,450 repented and were accepted back into the fold of Christianity after they had been publicly punished and humiliated.[16]

Under these circumstances, as Luís Suárez Fernández remarks, "The order of expulsion did not produce among [the majority of] the Jews any inclination toward baptism but rather a religious exaltation; the rabbis declared that as God had taken Moses out of Egypt, He would help them also" (1964, 49). Rabbi Abraham Bivach of Huesca, the author of *Derek-'emunah* (The road to faith), urged his people, forced convert or Jew, not to abandon the Jewish faith and its practices: "Only through loyalty to our faith were we able to survive the exile; . . . had we not placed our hope in this truth and in this perfection, how could we have been capable of enduring so many difficulties and so much suffering" (Méchoulan 1992, 43). Thus, for the most part the Jewish people—the rich and the poor with the financial backing of their prosperous brethren—chose exile from the land they had loved as a second Jerusalem in order to continue worshiping the God of Abraham.

Scholars hardly agree on the number of Jews who abandoned their homes in that fateful year of 1492 and in subsequent years.[17] The estimates range from 100,000 to 800,000. Norman Roth, quoting an anonymous chronicler, states that "'more than one hundred thousand, besides the children they took,' left the realm" (1995, 286). On the other hand, Salo Whittmayer Baron reports, "The celebrated sixteenth-century Spanish historian Juan Mariana, . . . wrote: 'We do not know the number of

Jews who left Castile and Aragon. But most authors claim that they were up to 170,000 families. One will not err in saying that they amounted to 800,000 souls'" (1967, 23).[18]

Between 100,000 and 120,000 Jews found refuge in Portugal after their expulsion from Spain in 1492. They were granted an eight-month stay in the country upon payment of a tax of eight gold cruzados to King John II, whose son, King Manoel, issued the edict of 1497 forcing these refugees to embrace the Catholic religion or abandon Portugal. Their children between the ages of four and fourteen were taken from the parents and forced to convert. Several thousand Jews also took refuge in the northern province of Navarre where their quasi-independent aljamas initially prospered. However, at the instigation of forces in Spain, King Johan and Queen Catalina of Navarre also ordered the expulsion of the Jews in 1498. It is believed that with them left the last Jews of the Iberian Peninsula (Beinart 1997, 93).

The exiles fled Spain by land and by sea: some overland to Portugal and southern France, and others by sea to northwestern Europe, North Africa, Italy, and the Ottoman Empire. The priest Andrés Bernáldez recorded his own observations of the departure of the Jews: "They went out from the lands of their birth, boys and adults, old men and children, on foot, and riding on donkeys and other beasts and in wagons. . . . They went by the roads and fields with much labor and ill-fortune, some collapsing, others getting up, some dying, others giving birth, others falling ill, so that there was no Christian who was not sorry for them. . . . The rabbis were encouraging them and making the women and boys sing and beat drums and tambourines, to enliven the people. And so they went out of Castile" (Sachar 1994, 73). Arriving at the Spanish harbors, the exiles found numerous Spanish, Muslim, Genoese, Venetian, and Greek vessels to carry them, for a price, to their various ports. Some of the exiles found their way to Seville where nearby in the small harbor of Palos de la Frontéra, Christopher Columbus was preparing for his own voyage. Columbus watched the vessels taking on the refugees and wrote in his log about the "'fleet of misery and woe'" (Sachar 1994, 73).

Some exiles reached the Ottoman lands directly; others settled first in Naples, Genoa, and Venice, and then continued on to the empire years later. For many decades, the preferred route of the Spanish and Portuguese Jewish expatriates was eastward, toward the Ottoman lands, to the existing Jewish communities of Istanbul and to Belgrade, Smyrna, Monastir, Nicopolis, Philippopolis, Ragusa (Dubrovnik), Rhodes, Sarajevo, Sofia, Spalato (Split), Uskub (Skopje), Valona, Vidin, Salonika, and Asia Minor. While many reached their destination safely, for others, the tragedy continued. Many unscrupulous captains reaped the benefit of the expulsion by exacting exorbitant fares. They often demanded additional payment once the Jews were aboard, confiscated their possessions, sold them as slaves, abused the women and young girls, or drowned the exiles in the Mediterranean. In some instances, those who reached port either were not permitted to land or were allowed to settle at the pier only until they found sanctuary elsewhere. As a result of the long voyage and the overcrowded ships, many of the passengers contracted diseases and were greeted at their intended destination by an alarmed populace who, believing the new arrivals were the cause of epidemics, demanded their expulsion.

While initially the established Jewish organizations came to the immediate assistance of the Spanish Jews, there subsequently developed a great deal of tension between the groups over issues of politics, economics, and claims to cultural uniqueness. The Romaniots, especially those of the major centers, desired to retain their own identity and not to be absorbed by the Sephardim. They felt threatened by the Iberian immigrants, who were granted more privileges than they had received in spite of their long and proven loyalty and contributions to the Ottomans (Ankori 1977, 21). The Sephardim, on the other hand, maintained a sense of cultural exclusiveness. In his 1454 letter to Ashkenazi brethren in northern Europe, Zarfati remarked on the Sephardi exiles, who, once in Turkey, displayed "their grave demeanour, extreme piety, and peculiar apparel at once distinguishing them from the Jews of Greece and the Orient" (Graetz 1941, 295). In a similar vein, Abraham Danon noted that "the Sephardim, far from mixing with their indigenous brethren or immigrants from other provinces, kept away from them." Danon continued, "They imagined being of a more noble origin and they believed [themselves] to be superior to the other co-religionists. They manifested disdain especially toward the Ashkenazim, who did not appreciate, as did the Sephardim, good manners, elegance in behavior, and a pure language and correctness" (1899–1900, 210).

In all likelihood, the Sephardim would have concurred with these assessments of their exclusivity. After all, in their view, they were the descendants of the tribe of Judah. In Spain, they had been physicians and counselors to the Christian and Muslim courts, and their communities had been the glory of Zion. Additionally, from their own perspective, they had suffered more than other Jews from the fervor and flames of the Inquisition, from the forced conversions, abduction of their children, ritual murders, and, finally, expulsion from their homes.

Regardless of their passion for what had been a remarkable past, and however secure they were in their new homes, the Sephardim must have felt abandoned and dejected. Just as Yehuda Halevi and Maimonides in medieval Spain had yearned for the return to the Promised Land, their descendants, now in the Ottoman Empire, yearned for their juderías and for their peninsular way of life. As Howard Sachar writes in "The Long Good-bye," for generations after their expulsion, the Sephardim would lament "the departed glory of an idealized race of Jewish hidalgos [noblemen], they would manage also to embellish and romanticize their former homeland." But their yearning was for, as Sachar said, "the bejeweled and enameled Spain of folklore, not for the rapacious zealots who had left them . . . plundered, and broken in mind and heart" (1994, 73). Stripped of the essence of their lives, the Sephardim clung to what they could of their past—to their language, customs, and religious practices. As Esther Benbassa and Aron Rodrigue write, "By perpetuating their customs and traditions in their new host country, they would be able to recreate the 'paradise lost' and their suffering would assume some meaning. If they had made sacrifices in order to remain Jews, they also had the sacred duty to hand on this Hispanicity which was inseparable from their Jewishness" (1995, 13).

To perpetuate their sense of separate identity, the Jews from the Iberian Peninsula formed their own synagogues, established according to their places of origin—Andalusia, Aragon, Catalonia, Castilia (*Gerush* Castilia or *Gerush* Sepharad), Cordova, Gana (Jaen), Evora-Portugal, Lisbon, Saragossa, Seville, Spain, Toledo.[19] As new immigrants joined them, the congregations further divided themselves according to their date of arrival—Old Catalan and New Catalan, Old Sicilian and New Sicilian—or their former homes—Calabria, Corfu, Messina, Ohri, Provence, Pulia.[20] Some synagogues were named after important families, such as the Hamon, established by the members of this family from Granada.[21]

Each immigrant group was organized into a *kahal,* a self-governing congregation in charge of the administration of the community, including the synagogue, the court, schools, hospital, cemetery, slaughterhouse, and charitable organizations.[22] To maintain their sense of identity, the kahals conducted their religious rituals and legal rulings based on the procedures of their communities of origin, such as those of Aragon, Catalonia, and Castile, but with modifications necessitated by their new environment. The rabbis and the officers of the kahal had the duty as ruling members to govern every aspect of the daily life of the community with leniency, objectivity, and fairness. Hardly any personal or communal activity was outside their purview.[23] Only a few members of the kahal, such as the rabbis and the beadle, also known in Hebrew as a *samas,* were paid. One of the most important officials, the samas attended to all aspects of the synagogue. He served as the messenger for the rabbi and the *Bet Din* (religious court), the enforcer of the laws, and the collector of the taxes. Functioning also as a town crier, he passed through the streets on the eve of Shabbat and of holidays, calling to the men to close their stores and come to services, and to the women to light the lamps.[24]

The members of the Bet Din, comprising the rabbi and the officers of the community, had the right to punish offenders by inflicting corporal punishment, levying fines, and confiscating part of their wealth. It was also within their power to sentence transgressors to prison, an area located near or within the grounds of the synagogue. Today such a jail still stands in a ruined house of worship in Balat, Turkey. In serious cases, the judicial body could impose the *herem* (ban of excommunication), the most powerful and terrible weapon, to maintain discipline, to check insubordination, to enforce their regulations, and to impose their authority.[25] The Bet Din also was responsible for settling disputes between one community and another.

The Sephardim, who were spread, as Mayer says, "from the Aegean Sea in the South, to the Danube in the North, and from the Adriatic in the West, to the Black Sea and Marmora in the East" (1913, 14), kept in touch with one another through family relationships and shared economic interests. Despite the distance, the regional divide, and the different kahals, the Sephardim often found it convenient to represent themselves as a group before local ruling classes and to work together as one single community, particularly for matters pertaining to *Halakhah*, the rabbinic rulings on Jewish legal traditions and rules of conduct. In order to prevent rivalry among themselves, to protect the small Jewish merchants, and to avert any controversy with the non-Jewish mercantile society, they established common rules to regulate local and international commerce. Safe from persecutions and hostilities, the Jewish merchants engaged in free trade and transacted business not only with their former communities, but also beyond their southern borders and north of the Danube.

In the earlier decades of the sixteenth century, the Sephardim, Ashkenazim, and Romaniots remained separate groups, though living in the same neighborhoods. Each united within its own group, with its particular leadership and governing apparatus. The various kahals dealt with matters of *halakhic* rulings (religious law), *minhagim* (customs), and communal decrees as these affected their own communities. There were differing interpretations on the matters of dietary laws, ritual slaughter, adultery, polygyny, extramarital affairs with non-Jewish and slave women, and the treatment of the offspring of such unions. Another major disagreement was over the Jewishness of the *anusim* (marranos, forced converts), who, once distant from the Iberian Peninsula and the shackles of the Inquisition, longed to return to Judaism. While the Romaniots and particularly the Ashkenazim were against accepting them as Jews, the Sephardim were elated and embraced their Iberian brothers and sisters into their fold.[26]

In Istanbul, Salonika, and the cities of the Balkans, the sheer numbers of the Sephardim engulfed the Ashkenazim and the Italian Jews by the sixteenth century.[27] Yet the community of Romaniots in Istanbul held fast to its identity. In the Greek-speaking centers of Janina and Chalcis, the Romaniots remained the dominant group, with Greek as their language, up to the twentieth century. Here it was the Sephardim who integrated themselves with the Romaniots. Elsewhere, by the seventeenth century, most of the Romaniots had been absorbed by the Sephardim (A. Levy 1992, 62).[28]

Eventually, the groups were drawn together by social, economic, and legal factors. These included the following: the closeness of living quarters and daily activities; the intermarriage among the children; the need to adopt standard legal practices, such as inheritance and divorce; and the codification of Jewish laws by Joseph Caro (1488–1575). Some of the other considerations for the merging of the groups were the need to organize collective guilds to regulate international, regional, and local business; the collection of the taxes demanded by the state from the total Jewish community;[29] the importance of a common national entity; and the necessity for a common representation in external affairs, whether within the Ottoman Empire or with other nations. Judeo-Spanish became the dominant language of the Jewish community, and the Sephardic rituals, the common religious practice.

Among the refugees arriving from the peninsula were not only celebrated diplomats, jurists, scientists, doctors, but also philosophers, Talmudic scholars, poets, and writers.[30] With them, Sephardic scholarship flourished in the sixteenth and seventeenth centuries, especially in the important centers of the Ottoman Empire. Prominent families, such as the Alatun, Hamon, and Nahmias, and individuals, such as Don Joseph Nasi and Doña Gracia, became patrons of scholars and supported the publication of important books.[31] During this period, schools were founded and libraries and presses established. The sixteenth and seventeenth centuries were mainly known for the printing of religious works, both in Hebrew and, in the case of translations from the Hebrew, in *aljamiado* (Spanish with Hebrew characters). Most of the publications written in Judeo-Spanish did not appear until the eighteenth century.[32]

The Sephardic immigrants did not live isolated from their coreligionists in other lands, including their converted relatives in Spain, Portugal, and the Netherlands. In their new land, they were not restricted by laws nor limited to any specific profession, except those few controlled by the state and by their own guilds or communities. Their knowledge of numerous languages—of Hebrew, French, Spanish, Italian, Greek, Turkish, and Arabic—as well as their expertise in international commerce, their connection with fellow Jews in other countries, their family ties, and common economic interests and cultural attachments made it possible for them to contribute to the international and domestic trade of the region. Many played prominent roles as bankers and industrialists. As merchants, they practically monopolized several sectors of commerce; the international trade was essentially in their hands. As Shaw remarks, the Jews in the Ottoman Empire sent "their ships through the Aegean and Adriatic to Venice and through the Red Sea and Persian Gulf to the Indian Ocean, to India and China and beyond. They created major markets for Ottoman goods and raw materials both in Europe and the East. . . . Jews set up branch banks and hostels which were managed by other Jews" (1991, 95). The harbors of Salonika, Izmir, Rhodes, and Dubrovnik sent Jewish ships throughout the world and rivaled the leading ports of Ancona, Genoa, Marseilles, and Venice. This was the golden age of Ottoman Jewry, not only in commerce, but also in diplomacy and scholarship.

The Christians, unable to compete in areas monopolized by the Jews, such as in diplomacy, manufacturing, and printing, resented their prosperity in the local and international markets. They begrudged the newcomers' considerable influence on the courts of the sultans as counselors, interpreters, physicians, and tax collectors. Moreover, they knew that they could not rival the acclaimed erudition of a great number of those who had first arrived from Spain in 1492 and from Portugal in the early decades of the sixteenth century, but especially of the marranos who followed in the later part of the same century.

In the seventeenth century, the supremacy of the Ottoman Empire began to crumble. As the political and commercial power of the western nations increased, that of the Ottoman Empire waned. The empire was overpowered from without and disintegrating from within. There was extensive abuse of power from governmental mismanagement and despotism, including the corruption of the judges and local governors, and the pillaging and massacres by the Janissary Corps, which continued until Mahmoud II crushed it on June 15, 1826.[33] These disintegrative forces had been set in motion in 1535, when Suleyman the Magnificent, following the permissive governance of Mehmed II toward minorities, initiated the agreements of capitulation. These were treaties between the Ottoman

Empire and the Christian states of Europe that allowed "foreigners to be ruled by their own laws within the Empire" (R. Lewis 1971, 16). Many Jewish merchants, even those with no foreign nationality, also found protection under these treaties. These same rules also were in existence in the nineteenth century and the early decades of the twentieth century when French and British citizens came under the protection of their own governments.

Eventually, the capitulation agreements contributed to a fraying of the Ottoman rule, for identity, allegiance, and compliance were so fractured. An example of just such "capitulated" identity can be seen in the encounter recorded in 1888, between a Turk, Ebüzziya, and a Franco-Jewish merchant in Istanbul. Ebüzziya called on the Jewish bookseller to conduct some personal business; his visit followed the news of the defeat of the French in the Franco-Prussian War. "The following conversation took place between us: 'I [Ebüzziya]: What is the matter with you. Is something afflicting you? The bookseller: Don't you know of the misfortune which my country has suffered? Can there be any greater affliction? I (smiling): But you are not a Frenchman. What is it to you? The bookseller: How? If I am not a Frenchman, then what am I? I: But aren't you Jewish? The bookseller: Excuse me sir! In France everything is French" (B. Lewis 1984, 224 n. 45).[34]

While many Ottoman Jews enjoyed the protection of the capitulation agreements, the majority, with no link to European governments, lost their competitive economic prominence to the Catholics, Armenians, and Greek Orthodox, who came under the protection of the western Christian states (Shaw 1991, 110). Except for the large centers such as Salonika, Istanbul, and Izmir where the situation was not so extreme, the economic condition of the smaller Jewish communities deteriorated, and their members were in the main poverty-stricken. In time, however, even those in the large centers suffered. Bernard Levy observes, "The occupations most frequently listed in the *Alliance* school records for the parents of children are hawkers, ragmen, tinkers, bootblacks, match vendors, and water carriers" (1952, 179). Aron Rodrigue notes, "The economic state of the Jewish masses in Turkey was dire indeed. David Cazès reported in 1873 that out of 3500 Jewish families in Izmir [Smyrna], 1000 were entirely destitute and survived through begging. Misery had become 'chronic' in Edirne, where there were thousands of men without any regular means of subsistence: beggars, smugglers, porters, peddlers of fruit and vegetables" (1990, 101).

Traveling in Turkey at the time of this economic hardship, Lucy Garnett wrote of the conditions in Salonika, where the Jewish population was crowded into a slum. Garnett noted, "In other cities and towns of the Empire, however, where the Jews exist in less disproportionate numbers, their quarters present a less squalid and unsightly appearance" (1891, 5). Impoverished as they were, the Sephardim existed chiefly on a diet of bread, salt fish, and leeks. In spite of this, Garnett observed, they remained healthy because of their fondness for being out-of-doors. In their courtyards or at their doorsteps, the women and girls "do the washing, making and mending; their mothers rock their cradles, and comb the little ones' heads; and the children play, quarrel and indulge in their amiable national propensity of stone-throwing" (6).

With reverses in the economy of the Jewish communities, the obligations of the synagogues to the indigent became insurmountable. The officials were forced to raise taxes and demand more from the affluent, which exacerbated the existing tensions between the rich and the poor. In spite of all the efforts of the governing body, the coffers were exhausted. As Shaw concludes, "schools, orphanages, and hospitals closed or operated on such reduced budgets that the poor were unable to secure any appreciable benefit from them (1991, 125).

There was by no means a complete cessation of Jewish economic activity. Those Ottoman Jews who came under the capitulation agreements continued to prosper and lived a lavish life. For example, Abraham and Isaac Camondo of Istanbul, who represented several prominent Jewish bankers in Europe, established their own Bank Camondo, with branches in London, Paris, and Vienna (Rodrigue 1992, 184). Sephardim founded lucrative department stores in the nineteenth century. The Bohor Alhadeff's branch was to become the Maison Alhadeff Fils with divisions in Izmir, Mersina, Athens, Rhodes, and Milan. The Rhodian families of the Notricas, the Menasches, the Amatos, and the Surmanies had similar successes; some of their enterprises had branches in Anatolia.

With the crumbling of the Ottoman Empire and the rise of nationalism, accusations and attacks against the Jewish population also became more common. The *Tanzimat* imperial decrees of 1839 and 1876, conferring equal rights to all the citizens regardless of religion or nationality, did not appease the Christian minorities. Largely because of the recurring economic rivalry, they complained that the Jews should not have been granted the same reforms. The attacks from the Christian population continued to increase in the first decades of the twentieth century even in the Turkish towns where the Jews were still under the protection of the Ottoman Empire. The new leaders in areas no longer under the Ottoman rule were indifferent in the face of rising anti-Semitism. As a consequence, a large number of Jews from Salonika and other cities were forced to emigrate to major centers of Turkey.

For the Sephardim of the Ottoman Empire, the twentieth century dawned with only faint promise and with three foes—anti-Semitism, economic hardship, and isolation from the West. Education became the key to the counterattack. As Aron Rodrigue remarks, "Western education [and the acquisition of French and other European languages] came to constitute for the Jews a major tool for the re-establishment of economic links with the West that had been lost in the previous two centuries" (1992, 184).[35] Founded in Paris in 1860, the Alliance Israélite Universelle taught courses in French language, sciences, humanities, and in Hebrew language and Jewish religion. The program was extended to trade courses for the benefit of those who were not able to pursue an academic curriculum.[36] However, education alone was not enough; people needed work. The young, especially the impoverished, looked for better economic opportunities in Western Europe, the Americas, and Central and South Africa. With the news of their success, more young people and heads of family joined them.

With the sad irony of history, the Sephardim had found their way to the Ottoman Empire to escape the fires of the Inquisition but four centuries later again met the flames of destruction.[37] This time it was the forces of the Third Reich that desecrated their synagogues, disemboweled their communities, and deported them to the death camps. Only the Sephardim of Turkey escaped the wrenching disruption of the war, since their country alone of those that had been home to the Sephardim in the Ottoman Empire had not been drawn into the conflict. Not only were thousands of Sephardim transported to Hitler's death camps—some to die there, others to suffer the agonies shared by all those interned—but their way of life was killed also. In brief, there was no going back. Even for those who did return to Belgrade, to Janina, to Kavalla, to Rhodes, to Salonika, to Sarajevo, to Xanthi, there was nothing to return to. Their homes were gone, either destroyed or occupied by people who had been their neighbors. Their property had been taken as spoils of war. The familiar faces were nowhere to be seen. How could one expect to step back into the rhythm of a familiar life when nothing left was familiar? All this is not to say that people did not reconstruct their lives after the war. They did, and they did it with courage. They moved back into their gutted communities and forced a life to emerge, though there were communities that were never revived, that remained as shells, empty husks with few signs that showed a Jewish people had once lived there. After the war, many

Sephardim continued the emigration that had begun earlier in the century, to the Americas, to the southern nations of Africa, and especially to Israel, to begin a new life in a new land.

As if in echo of the endless cries of the refugee, a Sephardi told Isaac in 1968, "From the day we were the Chosen ones, our destiny was to be hated, to be expelled from place to place. Naked, we ran, but not without our traditions, our beliefs, and the labor of our hands. This is our legacy."[38]

3 *Memories of Time Past*

Our fieldwork among the Sephardim took us to the heart of the culture, into the people's homes, where sustenance and friendship were offered in generous measure. For the Sephardim, food and hospitality are the necessary components for friendly conversation. Our interviews and research were not clinical investigations—as they should never be—but lively interactions, laughing exchanges of ideas, mixed with food and drink. In Kenneth Goldstein's words, this was the "natural context" for collecting folklore (1964, 80–81). Isaac remembers this setting for storytelling from his childhood in Rhodes: "I recall that on wintry rainy evenings, men and women gathered in a neighbor's house, shared a meal, and told one story after another until they had to retire for the night" (Lévy 1989b, 69).

Often our fieldwork was a chain of visits to people's homes. This meant that to be polite, our hosts had to offer us food, and to be polite, we had to eat it. The food was a delight to the eye and the stomach. The quantity of the food and the frequency of the service, however, was a challenge. For example, on May 19, 1990, we visited Lea Amram at Bet Avot Kryat Segal in Ramat Efal, Israel. As Isaac observed, she was a typical Sephardic grandmother in talk, in mannerisms, even in coiffure, with her hair pulled back in a wispy bun and a scarf tied round her head. When we arrived, she wore her apron; Isaac told her she reminded him exactly of his grandmother, who always had her apron on. As with all Sephardim, Mrs. Amram greeted us with sweets. She offered us grapefruit peels preserved in a heavy, sweet syrup and pressed candy on us when we left. Her hospitality was an enactment of the blessing, "May you come in *dulsuria* [sweetness], may you go in *dulsuria.*" Not that it was enough to come and go in sweetness; in between she served sponge cake, soft drinks, and wanted to serve us watermelon. Twenty-four hours later, as we learned from her daughter, Mrs. Amram was still upset because she had not served us coffee. And this was simply for an afternoon visit.

The next day, we were dinner guests in Bat Yam at the home of Ella Gross-Gefen, originally from Skopje, Macedonia, whom we had met through the Judeo-Spanish group in Tel Aviv. She had arranged for us to talk with her mother and her aunt. We were plied with food throughout our time in the house. Before dinner, we were served snacks. During dinner, we were urged to fill our plates from a table of numerous wonderful dishes. After dinner, we were offered dessert and then a variety of nuts. Ella was upset when we left because she had prepared a fruit salad for us that she had not yet been able to serve. In parting, she said to Isaac, who worked intensely and ate only some of the proffered food, "You scare me." He asked why, and she explained, "Because you work so hard and you don't eat."

From Ella's house, we went in search of Yakov and Fortuna Mizrahi, the latter the daughter of Lea Amram whom we had visited the day before. We found them with friends seated at an outdoor café in Bat Yam. We stopped to say hello and ended up collecting a rich body of information. This was the perfect collection situation, save for the noise of the passing traffic. Everyone was relaxed, and for Turkish Jews it was the perfect social setting, around a table at a café in the evening.

The following day, we were in Netanya, visiting with Luna and Albert Tuvi, and their daughter, Margalite, who, herself a doctoral student of Sephardic culture, had arranged the interview. They received us on their balcony and served us nuts and cool drinks. Then we moved to the living room where we began the interview. Margalite had been especially keen on our talking with her mother because of her remarkable memories from her childhood in a small village in Turkey. We were transfixed by Mrs. Tuvi's account, and all of us were joined in a web of conversational exchange. However, talk can never be separated from food. Luna Tuvi spread a crisp linen cloth on the coffee table and covered it with dishes prepared in the Turkish-Jewish culinary tradition, each more delectable and beautiful than the other. To our eye, she must have baked and cooked for days in preparation for our visit. We ate and talked for hours, and we finished neither the food nor the recollections, but we were left with delicious remembrances.

Thus, these three days of fieldwork in our months-long endeavor took us from an afternoon visit in an old age home to a dinner in a home in

Bat Yam, to an evening reunion in an open-air café, and then to an afternoon gathering in an apartment in Netanya. The common thread was food, hospitality, talk, and friendship.

The fieldwork situation would vary, then, from the friendly, social gathering around the dinner table of our hosts to the interview in the lounge or room in an old people's home. We gathered information from individuals, from two people or more, and from larger groups of people, numbering from twenty-five to over one hundred. In each situation, the dynamics varied, of course, simply because different people were involved, with different ideas and attitudes towards our topic. However, there were also certain aspects of interviewing that were associated with the number of people included in the interview. Often, it was better strategy to begin an interview with only one person present. The individual was free to recall aspects of the past without the critical assessment of a friend sitting by her side, who might or might not have heard the story before. Certainly it was flattering for one person to have the attention of two professors focused on her own thoughts and memories. Many of the women wanted to be reassured that the information they gave us was worthy of our attention. Often, they would conclude the interview with a question that was really a search for approval: "I have given you more than anyone else, haven't I?"

Frequently in old age homes, we conducted interviews at the same time with two friends. Depending on the relationship between the two, and their attitudes towards the topic of conversation, this could be a productive, rich experience or a limiting, frustrating one. In some interviews such as this, one friend would serve as a catalyst for the memories of the other. Ideas and recollections would bounce from one to the other. At the outset, the women sometimes would claim quite convincingly that they knew of no customary beliefs: they could not remember, or they were not raised to follow such beliefs. However, when they sat with a friend and began reminiscing about the past with us, the memories returned. And with the recollections came an electric excitement. It was a special moment when the talk of two friends with the periodic questioning from us revived memories long dormant.

In other interviews that we conducted with two friends present, the result was not so scintillating. In the old age home in Salonika, we interviewed two men. Solomon Sephiha, who spoke first, was very learned in Jewish law. The second man was self-conscious about speaking in the presence of his friend. He was careful not to disagree with anything Mr. Sephiha had said. When Isaac asked him about his opinions on amulets—did they work or not?—he replied, "The same thing, the same thing as

Solomon." In an old age home in Israel, we were talking with one woman who was a strong believer in the evil eye and in the cures she had learned from her mother and her grandmother. As she was enthusiastically recounting stories about her life in Bulgaria and her illnesses, which she attributed to the evil eye, her friend joined us. Scornful of such beliefs, her friend had her own cure for the evil eye. She simply dismissed it, thus essentially bringing to an end what had been up to that point an engaging interview. In this situation, and in others like it, we simply made arrangements to return later and to talk alone with the individual who had wanted to relate memories to us. Such clashes of views, however, were never a waste, for we were able to see how one who believed in the medicines of the house and the inhabitants of the spirit world would defend her beliefs, or abandon them for the moment, and then later recount them confidentially to us.

In New Belgrade, we met with a combination of the above components of the interview, both positive and negative. We began the interview with two older women, both of whom enjoyed talking about their memories of their childhood and the medicines of the house. They spoke of ways of divining illness (*livianos*), of treatment for colds (*ventozas*), and of herbal cures. To Isaac's question, "Did you use any herbs, like *mayorana* [marjoram] or *ruda* [rue]?" one of the women replied, "Ah! Ruda yes. When the eye hurt, this I remember from my grandmother, they washed the ruda, they mashed it well, they put it with a little sugar in a thin rag, and it was placed on the eye. And it was good. It is good even today." The other woman immediately added, "It is also used for *ayin arah* [evil eye]." Both of the women continued discussing the beneficial aspects of the herb, rue.

The daughter of one of the women had joined the interview as it was in progress. She sat silently, listening, and refusing Isaac's invitations to participate with, "I am young for this." When the discussion turned to garlic as a protection against the evil eye, the daughter recalled with a smile that her father had put it on her son when he was a baby. However, when we asked about fortune-telling practices, about divining from coffee grounds, the daughter responded, "This is not only restricted to the Jews. It is done by everyone." She was alternately scornful of these practices and apologetic about the Sephardim's following them. Her attitude had an immediate effect on the response of the two older women. Instead of offering responses with alacrity and humor, they, too, became defensive. When asked if the Sephardim had used cards to tell the future, one of the older women responded in a way as if to dismiss the question, "Of course!" The other agreed, "Yes. And such a thing, is it not found among yourselves?" Her daughter promptly added in an apologetic tone, as if to dismiss the practice, "We are part of the world, as all Jews are." In this instance, it was the daughter, as the third participant in the interview, who acted as a damper on the enthusiasm of the two older women. When she began participating, the two older women spoke less and punctuated their responses with self-conscious laughter. With the arrival of the daughter, they had a spectator who did not approve of their sharing what might be regarded as superstitious practices with others. So the elder two edited their remarks and apologized for what they did say with their laughter, and the daughter acted as a guardian of her people's reputation. If, indeed, the Sephardim had engaged in such frivolous pursuits as reading coffee grounds and cards, so did other people. It was not unique to them, and therefore they were not alone in their "superstitious" practices.

We encountered this defensive attitude from others as well, once from an upper-class Sephardic woman in Salonika, and another time from a scholarly Sephardic gentleman in Istanbul who expressed shame that his ancestors could be so ignorant and follow beliefs that were so against Jewish Law. Our response in these instances was to assure the individuals that we viewed these practices as part of the lives of the people; and that as part of the wisdom of "*muestras madres* [our mothers]," these should be recorded before they were totally forgotten. Often we would point to the extensive record of elite literary and philosophical achievements of the Sephardim during the time in the Iberian Peninsula, specifically to Yehuda Halevi, Shelomo ibn Gabirol, and Maimonides. This, we said, was certainly part of the proud heritage of the Sephardim, but only a part. And from our perspective, it was the practices in the homes, carried on largely by the women, that had sustained the Sephardim over the centuries. Sometimes, our explanations as to why we thought our research important eased the anxieties of the interviewees; at other times, individuals remained unconvinced.

Large group interviews posed particular challenges. Usually, we tried to avoid such gatherings simply because it was difficult to record the information when, as invariably happened, everyone began talking at once. However, there were instances where we could make no other arrangements, and where, on occasion, we were able to obtain information that probably would not have come to us in another setting. Sometimes the group simply gathered spontaneously. In Istanbul, we visited the old age home where we had hoped to talk individually with women. Isaac singled out a nice empty sun room where we could work with the first woman. Gradually people came in to sit down to hear what was going on. Soon more and more people had entered. Try as we might, at a certain point, it was no longer possible for us to quiet them all. Our usual technique in such a circumstance was for Isaac to ask the group to be quiet and to assure them that each would have her turn to talk; and for Rosemary to keep people occupied by talking with them quietly away from the tape recorder. In this instance, however, the enthusiasm of the group for the subject matter simply laid waste our plan. Instead of one person answering Isaac's question, the whole group would shout answers at once, none of which could be understood. At one point, in exasperation, Isaac asked, "Could you please give me slowly in Turkish the name of the plant. Please give it to me slowly. One person, please!" In this instance, he was able to get the answer. However, soon it became apparent that if they could not all talk at once, then they would carry on conversations about medicines of the house with the person sitting next to them in their own small groups. Clusters of individuals began talking with great animation about medicines. In spite of our efforts, we could neither follow the thread of these multiple conversations, nor cajole them into silence. Certainly we were assured of the obvious: the topic of medicines of the house was of intense interest to these women.

Other group settings were more organized in format. In Istanbul, and in Herzelia, Israel, we were asked to address Judeo-Spanish organizations. After we finished telling about our research, people spontaneously began recounting events from their own lives. Here the difficulty was also in keeping everyone else quiet while one person spoke into the tape recorder. Even if we succeeded in conveying the need for silence, often the sounds of everyone reinforcing our requests with "Shhhhh!" made recording problematic. In Istanbul, this was not quite so difficult because there were about fifty people. In Herzelia, it was much more challenging since the gathering included over a hundred people. As requested, individuals would come up before the group, give name, age, biographical information, and tell their stories. The amount and quality of the information we were given astounded us. Neither of us would ever have anticipated being able to conduct interviews with an audience of over a hundred people. Still we would not recommend this technique on a regular basis. The frustrations were plenty. We could not ask the individuals to stop, pronounce a term more carefully, spell it for us; nor could we probe for details. We had to take the information as it was given and attempt to follow up questions later in person. In addition, people were understandably reticent to speak about certain things in front of a large group. Whereas some topics came up easily and with great rapidity, we have only an inkling of the materials that were not covered. At the Nochada Judeo-Espanyola in Istanbul, one woman said, as she was walking out the door,

"Au revoir. We already have given you much. I have many things, but I have things that I do not like to tell. Had it been otherwise, I would have told you many things."

The pattern of topics discussed was in itself interesting, since one person's story was the impetus for another's account. On occasion, an individual would come to sudden cognizance of the meaning of a past experience. In a humorous incident of this nature at the Judeo-Spanish evening in Istanbul, a young man who had listened intently to a discussion about beliefs in the curative properties of urine, especially the urine of a young child, was finally able to make sense of an experience he had had over twenty years earlier. Laughing and blushing slightly, he recounted to the group how as a young boy of three or four, he was playing at the beach. A woman had come rushing up to him with an empty jar and had told him to urinate in it. He did, but he never knew why she had wanted him to until that night—that as a young child, he had urine with curative powers.

The large gatherings were also excellent sources for informants. We never left such a group without names and telephone numbers of those who were willing to work with us. In effect, the evening had provided them with an introduction to us and to our research. When we contacted them in their homes, they had had time to reflect on their experiences; they were primed for the interview. Thus what had begun as talks about our research opened into group interviews and led to further individual contacts.

In beginning the interviews, we would ask if the people recalled any *melezinas di kaza* (medicines of the house). This term was understood by all the Sephardim we interviewed. It was, as anthropologists would refer to it, an "emic," or native term for precisely what we were researching: folk medicine, folk beliefs, and folk religion. Usually, we would begin by discussing herbal cures. This was advantageous for two reasons: first, herbal cures were often easy to recall, and second, people did not feel self-conscious or uncomfortable talking about how herbs might be used for medicines, as they might have felt had we begun immediately with a question about more esoteric, or magical aspects. Next, we would attempt to find how herbs might be used as protection against evil spirits. Was rue used as a protection against the evil eye? Were there other things, such as garlic, that might be used to protect a newborn against the evil eye? Throughout the interviews, we encouraged the people to tell their own stories, their recollections of how their mothers and grandmothers used these cures, and of how they might have used them with their children. It was the personalized element that made the memories come alive. It was not, for example, the abstract concept of the evil eye that was important to us, but rather, how the people themselves experienced the effect of the evil eye. There is a sea of emotional difference between the calm recollection of a concept and the passionate remembrance of its grip on one's own life.

While Isaac and Rosemary both participated in the interviews, Isaac was responsible for conducting the interview, always in Judeo-Spanish, for jogging the informant's memory by talking about customs with which he had been familiar as a small child in the Sephardic community in Rhodes, and for helping to guide the discussion back to our interests when the conversation ranged too far afield. Rosemary often served as an excuse for Isaac's persistence in pursuing a line of questioning when he would explain, "Rosemary is very interested in knowing about this practice." In addition, this division of labor allowed Rosemary to watch for details that Isaac might miss, involved as he was either in tending the tape recorder or in taking notes. Rosemary was able to listen intently to the responses, and to see how these were keyed to accompanying gestures and facial expressions. Often such nonverbal communication, not captured on tape or in notes, was as revealing of a person's feelings and emotions as the words themselves.

Since interviews were such a crucial component of our research, we developed a fine art of encouraging an informant, of triggering the flow of memories, guiding the discussion, prodding, and tactfully broaching taboo topics. Often, the informant simply needed to be praised for what she had given and for how fine her memory was, since forgetting was always an issue for the old people with whom we spoke. At the Istanbul Old Age Home, we interviewed an eighty-five-year-old woman who punctuated her responses with remarks indicating she could recall no more: "All this we know, but if I can remember more things I don't know." Isaac encouraged her, "You are doing very well." And she replied, "Well, of course, I am so old." In formulaic response to the mention of one's age, Isaac wished her good luck, "*Muchos i buenos* [many (years) and good (years)]. Do you remember anything for evil eye?" Throughout the interview, there was this exchange, her apologizing for her age and her lack of memory, and Isaac praising and encouraging her. "Should I remember more?" she asked. "Yes," Isaac responded. "If I can. I am already old," she said. "You may be old, but you remember better than I do," Isaac added.

At times, people's memory had to be primed with a little information, and then the recollections flowed. Isaac would ask a question, and then if he received no answer but sensed that the people knew something, he would answer his own question. The recollections often would follow. Precisely this situation occurred in Bet Avot Leon Recanati, in Kryat Matalon, Israel, where we were interviewing two women, Dina Danon and Duka Nar, originally from Izmir and Salonika, respectively. Mrs. Nar recalled, "When someone falls, they sprinkle a little sugar where the person fell. And they take three pinches. They put some on the ground, and take some to taste." Isaac asked if any words were spoken. Mrs. Danon said, "I don't remember"; and Mrs. Nar simultaneously added, "Nothing." "Didn't they say," Isaac replied, "'*Kon el nombre del Dio* [In the name of God],' or something?" Mrs. Danon immediately added, "*Soltura, soltura* [release from all evil]." And Mrs. Nar affirmed, "Yes, they said things."

Of course, this triggering of the memory is not unique to the interview situation. Lily Arditti wrote to the editor of the *Sephardic Home News:* "My favorite part [of the newsletter] is your 'Ladino Reverie.' Events which seemed to be forgotten, childhood memories, which are really safely stored in our minds, are easily triggered by a word, a tune, a scent, or a 'Reverie.' The poem, recited when something was sewn on [a garment you were wearing,] triggered a cascade of recollections" (Arditti 1988, 2). This "cascade of recollections" was precisely what we sought.

On the premise that there is no need to provide an answer if the person already knows it, Isaac would sometimes feign ignorance. When a woman at Bet Avot Bulgaria in Rishon LeZion, Israel, spoke of what was to us the well-known practice of *echar livianos* (divination by reading the shape of molten lead), Isaac asked, "Ah, what is this?" and received a much more amplified response than he would have had he indicated prior knowledge.

At times, the people themselves would dismiss a practice with a simple shake of the head, because they regarded it as unimportant. Here it was crucial to reassure them that the practice was important. An eighty-four-year-old woman, daughter of a very learned man, Mary Algrante of Izmir did not want to acknowledge the practice of divination. When Isaac asked if there had been women in Izmir who had foretold the future with cards, she shook her head no. Isaac emphasized, "But it is important," and she immediately responded, "*Filjan* [divination with coffee grounds]." "How was it?" Isaac asked. And Mrs. Algrante described the procedure: "Well, with filjan, when we drank the coffee, we shook it, we would think of something, we turned the cup over and it would settle. And they looked and said '*La bonne aventure* [good fortune],' as it is said in French." Then she answered Isaac's original question, "There were also cards."

Sometimes people had an idea either of what we would like to hear or of what we should know. Usually this was a subject that they judged as important or which reflected well on their knowledge. The challenge was to guide them back to our topics of study, but to do this without giving offense. To Isaac's question "What else do you remember? About medicines of the house," a ninety-year-old woman, living in Seattle, Washington, but originally from Rhodes, responded, "Well, I don't know about medicines, but I used to read a lot. I read on the Inquisition. I also know when the Alliance Israélite was founded. Rothschild came to Rhodes. Do you want me to tell you about that?" Isaac, using an excuse that would be understood by a ninety-year-old woman, said, "Well, later, but now, I have a bad memory, I forget a lot. When someone died in Rhodes, what did they do when they came home from the cemetery?"

At an old age home in Israel, we encountered a new twist on this sidetracking of our interview questions. Here a woman interpreted our research in light of her own interests. She assumed that we were focusing on mysticism, and her own special concern was about the connection between the physiognomy of the face and one's destiny. As she brought out stacks of books on the topic, all written in Bulgarian, which we do not read, she kept looking intensely and deeply into Rosemary's eyes as if she read something about the soul's intent through the eyes. Since Rosemary's eyes probably did show that she was indeed interested in this new wrinkle on the spiritual, Isaac had a difficult time bringing the discussion back around to our corner of the spirit world.

At times, tact was needed to broach a topic. For instance, we were interested in *echizos*, witchcraft practices, but one can hardly ask directly, "Did your people practice witchcraft?" Isaac would indicate that he had heard that other Sephardim practiced echizos, those living, for instance, in a neighboring country. This usually brought laughing acknowledgment that, yes, they, too, in their own country had practiced echizos. Isaac would pose the question in another way, as he did with a woman, originally from Izmir, who had emigrated to Israel when she was eighteen: "One important thing, I know you do not believe in all this; do you remember any stories of echizos that were used? I was told that in Izmir . . ." "Yes," the woman laughingly interrupted, "they say that it used to happen, but I got married and came here, and I don't know."

Often it was the process of questioning that was crucial for uncovering long-forgotten life experiences. Through the very act of asking questions, we jogged the memories of these old people. They pondered things they had not thought of in many years; or they thought of things in a new way, in light of the framework of our questions. Such was the process of rediscovery for Julie Alajef, originally of Rusçuk, Bulgaria, with whom we spoke in Bet Avot Bulgaria:

Isaac: I notice that you have a pendant. Did many people have amulets?

Julie: I don't have an amulet. Now that you are talking to me, I remember. And the amulet, for what was it? For the evil eye. I don't know who prepared them. My mother didn't do that. But I'll tell you something else. When a woman would give birth to a lot of children and they didn't live. It happened in our family, to a sister of mine. The older one. She would give birth, and they would die. The fourth child, my mother, it seemed that she remembered from her mother. She remembered that when they used to cut the shroud, for one year they didn't dress the child from the clothing that the mother and father would buy for the child. The undershirt would be taken from the shroud so that it would touch the body of the child. . . . . When my mother went to the cemetery and would make the shroud, she would take a piece of the material, and she would make little shirts.

Isaac: Ah, the whole shirt was from the shroud, not just a piece.

Julie: No, the whole shirt. You just hit me for a question that was interesting for me. There were very few women who did this.

This process of questioning and the resulting answers revived memories for Isaac as well. Through another's recollections, he would be taken back to his childhood in Rhodes, and he would suddenly remember something long forgotten. Mary Algrante of Izmir was recalling the use of *hova* during Passover: "Hova is an herb that we gather in a bunch and put in a vase for the night of Passover. And this is good so that no sickness would occur in the house. And this hova is also to burn as incense in the house." Isaac asked, "So how did you do it? You took it. You put it on the table for Pesach and . . ." "The night of Pesach," Mrs. Algrante corrected. "When it dries," Isaac began, and then suddenly remembered burning the dried herb. His memory was triggered by Mary Algrante's description, and by the sudden Proustian sense of recall: the smell of the hova burning.[1]

The process of recall was not one-sided. It was the interconnectedness of memory, the joint venture into the past with friends, and with Isaac and Rosemary. Interpretive anthropologist Paul Rabinow remarks on this as the dialectic process in fieldwork, a process in which both the investigator and the informant are engaged (1977, 39). In "Surviving Stories: Reflections on *Number Our Days,*" Barbara Myerhoff reflects that "neither party remains the same. A new creation is constituted when two points of view are engaged in examining one life" (1992, 231). In "A Crack in the Mirror," Myerhoff and Ruby quote the ethnographer and filmmaker Jean Rouche, who writes of this collaboration as "'shared anthropology'" (1992, 325). Myerhoff and Ruby continue, "The anthropologists and the subject of study together construct an interpretation of a cultural feature . . . that would not have come into existence naturally. The study is . . . a collusion of two viewpoints meeting in a middle terrain" (325).[2]

In our work, the responses emerged through the coming together of individuals, the blending of memories, the reemergence of their shared past. The interviews were a process of recall that involved much more than a question-and-answer format. It was an engagement in re-experiencing the past, indeed, in bringing the past into the present, of recreating it momentarily through shared experiences. The past lives again in that space created for it between those who tell their lives and those who are there to listen, to study, and to record.

Attitudes varied, however, on the worth of the venture. Some were excited to find "young" people who were interested in their traditions.[3] A few had felt rebuffed and rejected by the younger generation; they scarcely believed that we were interested in learning from them. There were others who were ambivalent about the topic of our research. They believed in certain aspects of past customs; they thought others were worthless superstitions. Still other people viewed nearly every aspect of medicines of the house as the workings of ignorance.

Bienvenida Gabay, a ninety-three-year-old woman who had been born in Edirne, Turkey, and was living in Bet Avot Leon Recanati, was one who had felt rejected by the younger generation. In fact, so convinced was she that young people did not care about the ways of the past that Isaac had a hard time convincing her of his sincere interest. She stood with the door cracked, staring out at him in disbelief when he spoke about our research topic. "The young people," Mrs. Gabay asserted, "don't give any importance to these things. They laugh at us." Because he was speaking to her with persistence in Judeo-Spanish, Mrs. Gabay invited him in and spoke with him about her knowledge of cures. She, herself, dismissed many of the simpler cures as worthless, for she was a specialist in the complex procedures of *saradura*, a cure involving seclusion of the afflicted, special diet, special formulas, and use of livianos. Mrs. Gabay punctuated her explanations with her insistence that people no longer cared about these things. She would say, "This is a thousand years old, but now it is gone," and "All is dead. There was much to explain, but with the new life, there is nothing." There was a time though, she said, when even doctors would ask for her help: "This was used by all, by young people, by everyone."

Certain individuals quite literally shifted their views about medicines of the house from one sentence to the next. This ambivalence was a fluctuation between acceptance of certain beliefs and rejection of others. Our talk with a woman in her late eighties, originally from Salonika and also residing in Bet Avot Leon Recanati, was just such a wavering between acceptance and rejection. First, she stressed that the medicines of the house worked. She spoke of her mother's various cures for a cold: the use of *ventozas* (glass cupping-jars applied to the back), alcohol rubs, castor oil, quinine, boiled *tilia* (linden tea). "And it worked," she said. For bronchitis, her mother boiled *linasa,* which were, as she said, "little black seeds, little, little." With this, her mother would apply compresses on the chest and on the back: "And thank God, it was fine. Very good, better than antibiotics, better than any pill that exists." In the next breath, responding to a question about herbs, she replied, "Mint is to eat, nothing else. Ruda [rue] was for evil eye." She continued, "A woman gave birth, there was no hospital. She gave birth at home. They would put some ruda, because you would come in, so that she would not have any evil eye. *Esto es bovedades de mujeres* [this is foolishness of women]. . . . I don't know anything about it." She added, not that convincingly to us, "I didn't see any of it." We asked her if there were protective devices used for children, as well as for newly delivered mothers; and she told us how garlic was tucked in the clothing of the baby who was to be circumcised. With no concern for contradiction, she spoke about how garlic and rue would protect against the evil eye: "Garlic is for evil eye, and ruda is for evil eye. They would put a piece of it [in the clothing] and hang it [in the house]. For fright, doctors don't know anything about fright. He is going to give you all the medicine in the world, nothing to it [it won't work]!"

At other times, a person would shift ambivalently between an acceptance and a rejection of customary practices in an attempt to distance herself from her own memories, and perhaps to correct the impression that her family might have actually followed such procedures. One woman told us of a treatment for *espanto* (fright) when one felt *desrepozo* (indisposed, not feeling well). "It happened to me every day at the same time. They took a piece of paper, put some sugar in it, they blessed it, and they placed it under my pillow. In the morning, they gave it to me to drink with a little water. This should be done at dawn. And the patient, quite often, got cured." The woman told us of another cure for someone who was ill of undetermined causes: "They went to the synagogue, *echan azeite* [they pour some oil], lit a candle, and prayed."[4] Immediately after recounting these cures to us, she added, "There were no such things done in my family, we were more open-minded."

There were those who regarded themselves as "above" these beliefs. They were more modern, or as one eighty-five-year-old woman said, "We are *liviano* [modern]. I don't believe in such things." Another woman asserted, "In my house, we didn't do such things." Asked "Why not?"

she said, "We were more educated." They were more cultivated because they were more educated: they went to school. Still another woman explained beliefs in divination and witchcraft as being *atrazamiento* (backwardness): "According to me, the way I understand it, it is backwardness. A person who is more advanced cannot believe in echizos and such things." And she added, "I don't believe in such things." When asked about the evil eye, one woman smiled somewhat nostalgically and then added quickly, "I do not know anything about it. This is stupid. I never heard of it." She concluded emphatically, "This is garbage."

For these individuals, the dividing line between themselves and those who adhered to these beliefs was class, education, place of origin, and, sometimes, political affiliation, or religious orthodoxy. Implicit in these explanations is a statement about self and other: I do not believe because I am more educated, more cultivated; by extension, those who do believe are less sophisticated, less developed, backward. This separation between "us" and "them" was stated quite explicitly and often given a locus. Two women in Bet Avot Bulgaria assured us that they, themselves, knew nothing about these practices: "Of course, you should ask the people who live in the provinces." Another identified those who lived these traditions as the ones who had resided in the Jewish inner city of Sophia, called *Los tres pozos* (The three wells). And still another at Bet Avot Bulgaria said, "I am going to take you to *las mujeres bashas de Sophia* [the lower-class women of Sophia]." While *basha* is often used in a derogatory, insulting sense (i.e., a scoundrel), here it was used to refer to the poorer, less-educated class, hence the implication of the division by class and education is clear.

Another woman, originally from Bulgaria and residing at Bet Avot Leon Recanati, also stressed the aspect of class, but added to it the importance of political affiliation. Following a question about the evil eye, she said: "Let me be frank. We in Bulgaria were not fanatics. We were patriots. We did things for the community, for the kibbutz. Zionism was important. But for these kinds of things, ah! Thank God, we were well-to-do. [My father] didn't allow us to go here and there. This way of dragging from place to place, no, that was taboo. And he saw to it that we were all well married."

When asked if there were any who practiced echizos in Bulgaria, this same woman asserted, "No, we are more modern. It is the Turks that believe in such things. Not the Bulgarians." Others made this same assertion. A woman who was originally from Salonika and resided in Bet Avot Leon Recanati stressed that the Turkish Jews knew these traditions better than did the Jews from Greece. Still another, originally from Bulgaria, emphasized, "The ones from Turkey, let me tell you, there when they say something, they grab it from the root." It was frequently someone else to whom we were directed, a person who really knew about medicines of the house. The people at Bet Avot Leon Recanati, who originated largely from Greece, and those from Bet Avot Bulgaria, largely from Bulgaria, would tell us that we needed to talk with the *Turkanos,* those from Turkey. The Turkish Jews from Istanbul would say, in turn, that the *Izmirlis* (those from Izmir) or the *Rodeslis* (those from Rhodes) knew the most. This was often emphasized while, or after, the individuals spoke with us at length about medicines of the house. The woman, originally from Bulgaria, who had told us that the Turks "grab it from the root," and that she, herself, did not believe in echizos or in telling one's fortune by reading coffee grounds, in the midst of her account had told us that a dog howling at night was a precursor of death. And in mentioning the death of her cousin's son, she spontaneously uttered the protective formula, "*Leshos de aki* [far from here]": "I have a cousin from Turkey. Leshos de aki, four or five years ago, one of her sons died, married with children. After the year, every month, she had a *meldado* [prayer service] at home. We don't do that among the Bulgarians."

Certain people felt removed from the practices associated with medicines of the house because they felt distant from preceding generations. As some told us with self-conscious laughter, these are "*kozas de muestras madres* [things of our mothers]." When asked if people in Bitola and Monastir[5] believed in medicines of the house, a woman, originally from Yugoslavia, responded, "A lot! A lot believed in it. Only the youth began not to believe." For this woman, the divide between the generations was further marked by orthodoxy. She continued, "But I remember when I was young, we were religious, my grandfather was a haham. He was not a rabbi, but he was a Jew. Very religious." In answer to our question about garlic as protection against the evil eye, Mary Algrante, daughter of a biblical scholar, said, "Eh! I'll tell you, this is something very old. In my house, I did not see it." While the use of garlic against the evil eye was "something very old," she had just a few seconds before related how rue could be used against the evil eye.

Another woman who associated these practices with the old people was adamant that the customs had nothing to do with her. Ninety-one years old, born in Vodidtsa, Bulgaria, and living at Bet Avot Bulgaria, she did not want the interview recorded because she was afraid her son might hear it and know that she had been talking about such matters. In fact, she talked very little, saying she knew of no such practices. "Esto es de las viejas," she said, meaning, "This belongs to the old people." Still, she slipped here and there, just enough to let us know that she knew more than she was willing to share. After telling us that she had performed livianos for her children, we asked, "What else did you do?" She responded, "*Lo ke azian* [that which they did]," but she caught herself, and she did not finish her sentence. Her responses to our questions ran like a litany of denial:

> Question: Anything else for the stomachaches?
> Response: No, no, I don't know anything. Even though I am so old, I'm modern.
> Question: If a person was very sick, did they change their name?
> Response: I don't know.
> Question: If a woman could not give birth, was there anything to help?
> Response: I don't know. I had two nieces who never gave birth and that was it.

"How about *prekante?*" we asked. "Ah!" she breathed, as if she recalled, and then quickly added, "I don't know!"

For some people, religious law defined what existed. For instance, Rafael Brudo of Salonika acknowledged that there were *melezinas de mujeres* (women's medicines), but for him these medicines were limited to the use of mineral waters to cure rheumatism and barrenness. He explained, "Every year I would go to take mineral waters [at Methena, Greece]. And the mineral waters there were of two types—of sulfur for those who had rheumatism, and the waters which would clean the internal organs." He had encouraged his friend, who was a rabbi, to take his wife, who could not bear children. The rabbi declined the invitation: "'If God wants my wife to give birth, she will give birth.' 'No,' I said. 'In Spanish we say, guadrate, te guadrare [protect yourself, and I will protect you]. You can't leave everything to nature.' A person did not go to the toilet in the morning. And another day, he didn't go. On the third one, he's going to take a laxative." Mr. Brudo would admit of no other medicines of the house. When asked if people might "do things at home, like call to the good angels," Mr. Brudo emphatically responded, "In Salonika, they didn't have these things. In Salonika, before the war, they tried to perform the religion, as one should." When asked if perhaps the Jews in Salonika used *bunjukas,* blue glass beads thought to have amuletic protection, Mr. Brudo responded, "We were not like the Greeks, where each believes in a different saint. We believe in one place, in a God who is in heaven. And besides, in Salonika, people had good habits."

Influenced as he was by his religious background, Rafael Brudo did not acknowledge the existence of customs and rituals that were outside

Jewish Law. If it was part of *lingua negra,* bad speech, or taboo practices, not only would he not speak about it, he would deny that it existed, both at the personal and community level: he did not know about it, nor did anyone else in Salonika, except the Greeks. He would expand only on a belief that was officially sanctioned by Judaism. For our topic of magical practices, Mr. Brudo reined us in, drawing us harshly in line with official dogma; no traipsing in the pastures of herbal cures and evil eye for him. Yet, by the religious boundedness of his responses, we learned a good deal. We could practically see the boundaries between what could be spoken about and what could not, between what was accepted belief and divinely ordained prophesy and what was not; and all this was done with calm, quiet, but firm, speech. This strictly religious view, however, was not held by many of our informants. The line between what was sanctioned by religion and what was not was much less distinct; and the judgment about magical and divinatory practices, much softer and more yielding. Still, whether the outlines of doctrinal religiosity were distinct or blurred, there was the pervasive belief in the power of speech, a belief that shaped the very words one could utter and indeed proscribed the thoughts one could think.

4 *The Power of Speech*

> Death and life are in the power of the tongue;
> And they that indulge it shall eat the fruit thereof.
> —Proverbs 18:21

In answer to her daughter's question, "Mother, is there any special time for God to listen to the blessings?" Luna Tuvi responded, "Yes, we say that in the day there is a special hour, a moment that should be propitious for us, Oh, Master of the World! That is why I tell the children to say only good things because there is a certain moment that the Lord receives the good, but evil do not utter. In that moment, the one who cannot be mentioned can grab you for the bad. This is why, evil from your mouth, you should not speak." Estrella Missistrano told us of this prohibition against speaking evil. "Only say good things, or interpret good things," she warned, "because you never know when God might be listening. If you say one wrong thing, he might be listening, and then that will come true." Rafael Brudo explicitly linked this to the sanction against *lashon arah* (evil speech): "We have something that we cannot utter, *lashon arah, lingua negra* [bad language]. That is to say, things that should not be said. . . . It is only the truth that blesses man." He continued, "In the Holy *Zohar,* it is mentioned that the person should always utter good words and good blessings, for the family and for everyone else. There's a time when God feels happy and grants it. For that reason, you don't utter bad words from the mouth."

From his childhood in Rhodes, Isaac remembers that the children were taught by their mothers to guard their tongues from speaking evil. To convey this, his elders used the formulaic phrases, "Avla bien para ki ti venga bien [Speak well so that good will come to you]"; and "Avla bueno para ke te salga bueno [Speak well so that good things will happen to you]." These were paired with other phrases that cautioned against thinking evil, "El ke mal pensa, para si se lo pensa [He who thinks evil, thinks evil thoughts of himself]," and "Ke mal tenga ken mal pensa [May evil strike the one who thinks evil]." Isaac's mother and his grandmother repeatedly cautioned his brother and him against speaking maliciously, and even against thinking bad thoughts because these would bring harm. As Isaac recalls, "We were warned not to utter even the simplest bad words, not even in jest, because any negative thought or word could be an ill-omen and could arouse the anger of the evil spirits." The boys were told, "Ke salga solo bueno di la boka [That only good should come from the mouth]." Even with this precaution, Isaac's mother would say, "I di lu bueno si tiene ki guadrar. Ken savi los ke estan sintiendo [Even from the good one must guard oneself. Who knows who is listening]." Thus perhaps the safest advice was the following: "La mijor palavra es la ke no se avla [The best word is that which is not spoken]."

Ultimately, the power of the word linked to the Divine Source, for God, in creating the world, spoke and it was good. "And God said: 'Let there be light.' And there was light. And God saw the light, that it was good" (Genesis 1:3–4). As recorded in the notes to the Hebrew Bible, "One of the names for God in later Jewish literature is 'He who spake and the world came into existence'" (Hertz 1990, 2 n. 3). This awesome link to God through the spoken word was hemmed in with prohibitions, the first of which was not to utter God's name. The Hebrew word for name, *shem*, carries with it the character and essence of that which is named. "To know the name of God is to know the divine attributes. . . . The divine name is often referred to as equivalent to the divine presence" (Birnbaum 1991, 608). In *Jewish Magic and Superstition*, Joshua Trachtenberg writes, "Of all the names employed in magic, those associated directly with the person of the deity were accorded first place in the hierarchy of magical terms. . . . Already before the beginning of our era the Tetragrammaton had become the 'Ineffable Name,' too sacred for expression, uttered only once a year [on Yom Kippur] by the High Priest" (1939, 90). Since the destruction of the Temple,[1] God's name—the four-lettered YHWH, יהוה—was never again uttered, though there were many attributes that referred to the Holy One, including *HaShem*, the Name. As Trachtenberg notes, "The Powers of Good . . . were invoked by calling upon their names, the holy Names of God and His angels" (1939, 15).[2] The power of the word formed the basis of Jewish mysticism which "involved the use of 'the Laws of Creation,' a term which was later interpreted to signify the mystical names of God and the angels" (19).

Speech was connected with breath, and thus with life and the living soul. In Genesis, God breathed life into Adam: "Then the Lord God formed man of the dust of the ground, and breathed into his nostrils the breath of life; and man became a living soul" (Genesis 2:7). According to the *Targum,* the Aramaic translation and interpretation of the five books of Moses, a living soul means "'a speaking spirit,' [that is] a personality endowed with the faculty of thinking and expressing his thoughts in speech" (Hertz 1990, 7 n. 7). Just as breath carries life, so can breath carry evil. Morris Gross writes in his article on the evolution of the Hebrew religion, "The power of magic is often believed to have resided in the breath or speech of the magician. . . . The basic idea in pronouncing spells and some other forms of magic is the power of the magician to produce results through his power of 'speech.' Cursing as an aspect of magic depends on the spoken word" (1934, 35). In the same vein, R. Campbell Thompson refers to "the Word of Power, by which the sorcerer invokes divine or supernatural aid [through] the knowledge of the name." Thompson continues, "The Word of Power consists in its simplest form of the name of some divine being . . . called in to help . . . with superhuman aid" (1971, xlvi). The spells of the magician that caused sickness, Gross notes, were believed to enter the body through the mouth (1934, 28). Thus one might be cautioned that, as the Talmud says, "'One should never open his mouth to Satan,' that is, evil talk is nothing less than an invitation to the demons" (Trachtenberg 1939, 56). Conversely, one might utter the formulaic wish, "Tu boka al sielo [May your mouth reach the heavens]," meaning, may the words of your mouth reach up to God. King David acknowledged the power of the word when he prayed, "Set a guard, O Lord, to my mouth; Keep watch at the door of my lips" (Psalms 141:3).

Like a positive and negative pairing, blessings and curses were based on similar formulas. For instance, the blessing "Di lus sielos ki li venga la bendision [May the blessing come to him/her from Heaven]," could be changed to a curse, "Di lus sielos ke li venga la maldison [May the curse come to him/her from Heaven]"; and "Il Dio ki mi ti guadri di todo mal [May God save you from all evil]," could be changed to "Il Dio ki ti lo page di negro [May God pay you abysmally]." The etymology of the words "to bless" and "to curse" shows this positive and negative pairing. *Bendezir,* to bless, derives from the Latin, *benedicere,* to speak well of someone or something. *Maldezir,* to curse, is formed from the Spanish, *mal* (bad) and *decir* (to speak), and derives from the Latin, *maledicere,* to speak evil of someone, or to slander. In describing the moral character of a person, the metaphor of speech was also used. Of her mother, Luna Tuvi said, "She was *una boka di bendision* [a mouth of blessing]"; and of her father, she said, he was *"una boka dulse* [a sweet mouth]," meaning that he always spoke well of people and was well liked for this. In a disparaging remark, we were told by several women at an old age home that another woman had *"una lingua suzia* [a dirty tongue]," a term used to denote a coarse person, often from the lower class.

For the Sephardim with whom we spoke, blessings served as protective barriers against harm. Luna Tuvi recalled her childhood memory of her mother blessing her father as he left on a trip to peddle goods in the small villages outside of their home, Chanakali, Turkey: "My mother was always blessing people. . . . To my father, she said, 'Shemuel, sano i bivo ke estes [May you have health and long life]. Patron del Mundo, guadralo de gezera, de oras malas [Master of the Universe, guard him from disaster and from bad times]. Kon bueno ke te vayas i me vengas [In good may you go and return to me]. Azlaha i beraha ke te meta el Dio Baruhu [Prosperity and blessing may the Blessed God give you].' And it was kisses and hugs for mother for all the blessings. . . . And he would leave. With these blessings he used to go away and with them he came back." From one trip, her father returned with bad news: "When he came, he was full of emotion, he did not feel like talking. 'Shemuel, why are you this way?' my mother asked. He said to her, 'We no longer have a way to make a living. I will not be able to feed you.' 'Why?' she said. 'My horse died.'" And her mother replied with protective blessings for him and for their children, "'I tu ki bivas [And may you live]. Los ijos ki bivan [May the children live].'"

Luna Tuvi was fourteen years old when this happened. She remembered going to bed that night with her four brothers and sisters, all sleeping on mattresses on the floor, with her father and her mother stretched out at their feet. Luna recalled her father's lying there and staring at the ceiling. Her mother said to him, "Shemuel, why don't you speak to me? Why are you staring at the ceiling?" He responded, "But look what is on the ceiling." With a protective statement, her mother said, "Los mijores di mozotros! Es vida i salud i todo bueno [The good among us! It is life and health and all that is good]." Luna reported, "In saying this, Eliahu ha-Navi [Elijah, the Prophet] jumped out and he appeared on the wall, just as today, I am seeing you in front of me." Elijah had a small beard; he was dressed in a Turkish fez, a robe worn by dignitaries, and slippers. Luna said, "He was an angel who came to us." She continued, "He was hoping that Father and Mother would bless him, 'Ke venga en las buenas oras, el Senyor Eliahu ha-Navi. Ke mos venga en las buenas oras [May you come to us in good times, Elijah the Prophet. May you come to us in good times].'" Elijah had come, Luna said, to help her family, but he needed a blessing in order to stay.

Unfortunately, her father fainted from emotion and shock. Luna asked us, "What could Mother do? See that her husband was dying, or receive Elijah the Prophet? She did not have the courage. She told him, 'Shemuel, Shemuel, wake up!' She is slapping him. Mother lit a small lamp. She could not receive him. They did not receive him. . . . When Elijah the Prophet noticed that mother did not receive him, [and ask him] to sit down, and that she was busy with father, taking care of him because he fainted . . . first he came and touched my head thus, and then to all the children. . . . This way he touched us. He jumped and ran away, he disappeared under the curtain, and got away through the window." Isaac queried, "How did you know that it was Elijah the Prophet? Maybe he was another spirit." Luna responded with conviction, "No, he was Elijah the Prophet because one could see that it was an angel that came. You could notice it from the headgear . . . , from the fez, from the white robe, from the slippers, and the small beard. *El Malah, Eliahu ha-Navi* [The Angel, Elijah the Prophet] came in, he appeared to us." She concluded, "Elijah the Prophet left, mad because we did not receive him, because he was not received. . . . In the morning, we got up, mother went to the chief rabbi, [who] said, 'Ah! But you did not know how to receive him. You should have told him, Vengash en las buenas oras, Eliahu ha-Navi [May you come in good times, Elijah, the Prophet]. He came to you to help because he knew what had happened to you, a sad happening that Shemuel had had. And he came to help you.'"

Luna Tuvi told us that she had learned the blessings she used for her family from her mother: "The blessings that my mother used on us, I now use on my children." She continued: "I go every morning to the mezuzah as soon as I wash myself, I wash my face, and I say, '*Dias buenos* [Good days] above all. Guadrados de hazinura i de oras malas [May we be protected from sickness and from bad times]. Amargura ke no vea por dingunos [May I not see the death of anyone]. Adelantada ke me sea Margalite [May Margalite have success]. Novia ke la veamos [May we see her engaged]. Salud buena [Good health]. Refua shelema para todos los hazinos [Cures for all those who are sick]. Il Dio ke no mos amarge por ninguna parte [May God not strike us from anywhere]. Amen.'" In sequential order, Mrs. Tuvi had asked God for a good day for all, for protection against sickness and misfortune, for safeguard against death, for success for her daughter, for the engagement of her daughter, for good health, for cures for all who are ill, and for protection against punishment from God. By thus beginning her day—with a touch of her hand to the mezuzah and a recitation of these blessings—she had grounded her pleas for God's protection at the doorpost of her house, which, of course, was where the mezuzah was affixed. She had also covered the range of requests for what Hermann Gunkel calls "the state of blessedness," which "embraces all that [one] desires or might desire, such as peace, security, sustenance, riches, victory, protection against misfortune, and sickness" (1933, 301). While Gunkel does not specifically mention it, this state of blessedness included children, their success, good fortune, and marriage, for two of Mrs. Tuvi's seven blessings were specifically uttered for her daughter, Margalite.

Blessings began the morning, as for Mrs. Tuvi, and were threaded throughout the day. When two friends met each other, their exchanges were punctuated with blessings. We were both the recipients of such blessings in our fieldwork and the observers of the exchange of blessings between friends. On two occasions, we listened as this took place in our mother's living room in Atlanta, Georgia. On September 7, 1991, Regina Arogeti, originally from Rhodes and who, in Atlanta, lived in an apartment across the hall from our mother, came for a visit. When Mrs. Arogeti finished her bowl of ice cream, she said, "Kun buenu i alegria [With prosperity and happiness]," to which our mother replied, "Helal ki ti si aga [May it become profitable to you]." (*Helal* means accepted or permitted by religion, and therefore healthy and good.) Then Mrs. Arogeti looked at Isaac and said, "Bendicha madri ki tal ijo pario [Blessed mother that gave birth to such a son]"; to which Isaac's mother replied, "Bendicha boka ki tal koza dichu [Blessed mouth that such a thing said]." Isaac's mother joked that she was going to charge for the ice cream, and Mrs. Arogeti said, "La vida ki nu ti manki [May life not be lacking for you]," meaning, may you always be full of life.

One year later, on September 26, 1992, Mrs. Arogeti and Isaac's mother had their usual evening visit. Isaac timed their conversation and counted their blessings: in 17 minutes and 20 seconds, they exchanged 27 blessings. In this instance, it was Isaac who joked with Mrs. Arogeti; and she responded, as she had a year previously, with a blessing, "Ke bivas muchos anyos [May you live many years]," thus wishing for him a long life filled with laughter and jokes.

"Blessing," Clara Farji told us, "is good." She continued, "God pays it back. In order to find rest in the world to come, one must do good." Morris Gross makes reference to this reciprocity between God and his people when he writes that the way "to assure the permanent flow of blessing was by constantly replenishing its source" (1934, 42). Thus, God blessed Israel, and God had to be blessed by his children in order for them "to maintain and enrich his power of blessing" (42). Drawing from the work of Josef Scharbert, Christopher Mitchell sees "blessing as a term of relationship." Mitchell writes, "The connotations of blessing imply that the parties involved have a certain positive relationship" (1987, 26). This blessing of God might have been as simple as "Bendicho sea tu nombre [Blessed be your name]," or "Bendicho sea el nombre dil Dio [Blessed be the name of God]"; or it may extend to general blessings of God for any propitious occurrence, such as the birth of a child or success in business, "Es de bendezir al Dio [It is to bless God]"; "Lores ke demos al Patron del mundo [May we give praise to the Master of the Universe]"; "Lores al Dio, lores al Dio sien mil vezes [Praises to God, praises to God one hundred thousand times]" (Nehama 1977, 331). As a recognition that God's will preceded everything, and that all honor belonged to God, the blessings "Primero tu, Adonai [Above all, you, Lord]," or "Primero el Dio [Above all God]," were said before an event occurred, such as the birth of a child or a wedding. For the Sephardim, all good deeds were initiated "Kon il nombri dil Dio [In the name of God]." To thank God for good fortune, one would say after an event had taken place, "Alavado sea el nombre dil Dio [Praised be the name of God]." This praise of God's name was said particularly in the mourner's Kaddish, the prayer for the dead: "May His name be magnified and made holy" (Telushkin 1991, 630). To bless God for a specific occasion, one would say, "Bendicho el Dio ke mos alkanso a esta ora [Blessed be God for bringing us to this moment]."

In addition to blessing God's holy name, the Sephardim blessed the patriarchs. To Lea Amram, in her birthplace, Kuskunjuk, Turkey, blessings were "the benedictions of Abraham, our Father, the benedictions of Jacob, our Father." This could include naming God and listing the patriarchs and other biblical characters: "Beshem Eloe Avraam, Itzhak, veYaakov, Moshe, Aron, David, uShelemo [In the name of the God of Abraham, Isaac, and Jacob, Moses, Aaron, David, and Solomon]." It could also refer to biblical events involving the patriarchs, such as, "Los kavos de Yaakov Avinu [The happy ending of Jacob, Our Father]." The latter was a reference to the pleasant culmination of Jacob's otherwise difficult life. After the reunion with his son, Joseph, he lived a happy, full life until his death. Thus, the blessing would be that a person's difficulties would end happily, as did Jacob's life. Through these repeated blessings of God and the patriarchs, the Sephardim were linking their lives with the Holy Ones. They were verbally enacting the wise counsel, "Ajuntate a los buenos i seras uno de eyos [Associate with the blessed ones, and you will be one of them]."

As well as blessing God and the patriarchs, one asked for blessings from the Holy One, the patriarchs, the angels, and from a deceased mother or father. These supplicatory blessings were plenteous and diverse. Mitchell writes, "The majority of human blessings are . . . wishes or prayers for

God to bless. They may be spoken out of friendship or fellowship, or as a prayer for someone the speaker cares about" (1987, 168). One might ask that God's help be extended to everyone present, "Il Dio ki iste kon mozotros [May God be with us]"; or to a friend, "El Sinyor del mundo ke lo abedigue [May the Master of the World help him]," "Akadosh Baruhu ke este en tu ayuda [May the Blessed One be help to you]," "El Dio ke se apiade de Luna [May the Lord have pity on Luna]." One might ask for help from Abraham, our father, "Avraam avinu ke venga en muestro ayudo [May Abraham our father come to our help/intercede for us]." By allusion, one might refer to Moses, who lived to be 120: "Ke vos envezesesh kon vuestro marido sien i veinte anyos en su kavesal [May you grow old with your husband for one hundred and twenty years, sharing his pillow]." One might also ask for God's help through the prophets: "Il Dio ke se apiade de mozotros por los neviim [May God have pity on us through the prophets]"; or any biblical personage, "Il Dio mos salve komo salvo a Itzhak del kuchio [May God save us as he saved Isaac from the knife]." If something bad had happened, one might say to a friend, "Los malahimes ke vengan en tu ayuda [May the angels come to your aid]." To a child who was injured or whose mother or father were deceased, one might say, "Andi esta tu madri/padri ke rogi por ti [Where your mother/father is, may she/he pray for you]."

To be polite, Kalina Alvas—originally from Bulgaria—told us, one should first pray for other people and then pray for oneself or for one's own people. For example, she said, one would say, "Salud i repozo para todo el mundo i el puevlo djudio [Health and peace for all the world and the Jewish people]." If one were asking God to bless one's children, the wish would first be for other children: "El Dio ke guadre a kada ijo de djudio i a los mis ijos tambien [May God protect each child of a Jew and my children also]."

Numerous blessings for good health were linked to folk beliefs, most of which had some connection with the evil eye, such as the following: "Bivas, kreskas, komo il pishkado en la agua freska [May you live and grow like the fish in freshwater]," or "Bivas, kreskas komo il pishkado en la mar [May you live and grow like the fish in the sea]." Both the fish in the freshwater and the fish in the sea are in a healthful state because they are protected from the evil eye by the presence of freshwater or saltwater. Since fish have no eyelids and thus their eyes never close, they can always ward off the evil eye; additionally, their eyes are located on both sides of their heads so they can see everything and be ever-vigilant against evil. With the general blessings, "Sanos i bivos ke estes [Healthy and living may you be]," and, "Ke tengas la kaza yena [May you have the house full]," one could ensure others that one wished them only good health and a house full of children and good fortune.

As a way of showing that one did not envy others their good fortune, one used blessings for all happy occasions. When wishing another person good luck with the birth of a child, one would say, "De ojo negro ke te guadre il Dio [May God guard you from the evil eye]," or "En vida di padre i madre ke sea [May it be with the life of the father and the mother]." One might also wish that the baby girl or boy would grow to the good fortune of marriage: "Novia ke la veamos [May we see her engaged]," or "El Dio ke mo lo deshe ver novio [May God let us see him engaged]." As the child grew older, a blessing for the anticipated wedding was ever-present: "Novio/Novia ke te veiga [May I see you engaged]." For the girl, the blessing was to see her take the ritual bath of the bride: "A los banyos de novia ke vayamos [May we go to the bridal bath]." There was also the blessing for a fruitful union: "Kon ijos i ijas ke te veamos [With sons and daughters may we see you]."

If one had spoken of misfortune or death, one would immediately say, "Leshos di muzotros ki sea [Far from us may it be]", or "Afuera di las karas [Away from our faces]." This latter blessing the Sephardim also expressed in Hebrew, "Huz min hapanim." In this way, one would ensure that the spirits would not visit misfortune or death on those present; it would be taken "away from our faces." If one had just spoken of the dead and then mentioned someone who was alive, the speaker would immediately say, "Entre los bivos [Among the living]," meaning that the one mentioned should be among the living. When our mother's friend Mary Benatar told her that she was going to visit the family of someone who had just died, our mother said to her, "Para alegrias ki salgas [May you go out (visit) for happy occasions]"; she thus wished happiness and not sadness on her friend, and she also provided a protective blessing to cushion the mention of death.

One might also wish that evil be transferred to the depths of the sea: "A la undura di la mar ki si vaiga todu il mal [To the depths of the sea may all the evil go]." One could protect those present from the ill fortune of the words already spoken by saying, "Pasado ki ti sea [May it be all over for you]," or "Para buenu ki sea [May it be for good]," or "Mas pur dingunos no [May it not occur for anyone else]." If something bad had happened to a member of the community, one might say, "Kapara ki sea para todos los djudios [May it be as a sacrifice for all the Jews]." The *kapara*, or sacrifice, derives from Abraham's intended sacrifice of Isaac and of God's substitution of the ram. This original sacrifice is acted out in the ritual fasting of Yom Kippur, and in the symbolic charred lamb shank on the Passover seder plate, as well as in the Sephardic ritual on the eve of Rosh Ashana of kapara, or the sacrifice of a rooster for a male's sins and a hen for a female's. In folk belief, kapara offered an atonement for evil or misfortune. If one broke a plate, one would yell, "Kapara!" in the hope that the spirits might take this as a sacrifice in place of some other good fortune. In any circumstance when one wished protection from God, one might say, "No kera il Dio [May it not be the wish of God]," or "El Dio ke mos aleshe de todo mal [May God keep us far from all evil]."

For greeting and leave-taking, there were also formulas for blessing and protection. To welcome a guest to one's home, one would say, "Venga en bonora [Welcome/Come in a propitious time]." The visitor would reply, "Bonora me tenga [May you also have a propitious time]." When two people took leave of each other, one might say, "*Al vermos* [Until we see each other again]"; and the other might reply, "Sano ke estes [Healthy may you be]," to which the first would reply, "Saludozo! [May you also be healthy!]" (see Shaul 1981, 32). Thus the wish that two friends might see each other again was rephrased into a wish that each person should be healthy. In the dining hall of an old age home in Israel in 1990, we overheard one woman taking leave of her brother, whom she had come to visit, and of two other older women. The visitor said, "I'll see you again." One of the other women at the table responded immediately, "Kon todos djustos! [With everyone present, alive and well!]"; and the other friend added, "En vidas de todos [With everyone alive]." Thus the two women had provided protective statements to the sister's bold declaration, "I'll see you again." The latter statement on its own, without the formulaic protection calling for everyone to be alive the next time she saw them, would have been a delicious invitation to the spirits to bring harm to this group of older people.

A Sephardic woman often greeted guests with the blessing, "May you come in sweetness and may you go in sweetness," and then put it into action by offering sweets to her guests both on their arrival and their departure. The same metaphor of sweetness was used for wishing one a safe trip: "Kaminos de leche i miel [May you have paths of milk and honey]." To one leaving on a journey, one might also say, "Kaminos buenos [Good paths]," and "Kaminos aviertos [open roads]" (Shaul 1981, 31). The following folk prayer drew all these blessings together:

Senyor del Mundo,
ke vaiga i venga,
mal ke no tenga.

Kaminos de leche i miel,
Kaminos buenos.
Ke me guadre el Dio de todo mal.

Lord of the Universe,
May I go and return,
May nothing bad happen to me.
Paths of milk and honey,
Good paths.
May the Lord guard me from all evil.

While prayers and blessings acted as barriers against harm, curses were intended to unleash the power of the spoken word in order to cause harm. Edward Westermarck commented on the malevolent intentionality of the curse: "Closely related to the evil eye and to the evil mouth . . . is the curse. It differs from them by being always an intended cause of injury, and also by the way in which the evil wish is expressed. . . . The realisation of the evil wish is brought about either directly through the mysterious power of the curse itself, or by the aid of a supernatural being invoked in it" (1968, 1:479). Westermarck's words might be summed up by the Sephardic saying, "Mas vale kayer en rio furiente ke en boka de la djente [It is better to fall into a turbulent river than into the mouth of people]."

A curse carried destructive power that, it was believed, might cause the death of the cursed one. There was an additional and even greater danger in that the curse might harm another person, rather than the one to whom it had been directed. For example, a woman might curse a neighbor in anger, but the spirits who had been aroused by such evil speech might maliciously cause the harm to fall on the children of the one who had uttered the curse, as was reflected in the saying, "Ken echa maldision, en sus ijos la topa [One who curses, in his/her children finds it]." Once the words were out of one's mouth, there was no certainty as to where the harm would be done. The evil spirits, it seems, were ready to strike with all their force and with no mercy, whether the victim be the one who was cursed, or an innocent child or adult. Eventually, however, the one who had uttered such a curse would be held accountable, for speaking evil was contrary to God's commandments. Indeed, it was believed that the curse might fall back on the one who had uttered it, as was reflected in the saying, "Ken al sielo eskupe en la kara le kae [He who spits at the sky, it falls in his face]." As Westermarck noted, "There was a belief that a curse, especially if it was undeserved, might fall back on the head of the person who uttered it" (1968, 1:491 n. 3). With remarks pertinent to the Sephardim, Morris Gross writes, "One must watch his tongue. The ancient Hebrew was fearful of the deadly weapon of the . . . curse. One must be careful of cursing since it may reflect on the person" (1934, 43 n. 1). As if confirming the ancient Hebrew belief, Clara Farji—born in Edirne, Turkey, and residing in Tel Aviv—told us in 1990, "To curse is not good. The individual who curses, curses himself. The curse comes back on him."

While the Sephardim with whom we spoke laced their utterances liberally with blessings, they vehemently denied knowing curses. In questioning one woman, Isaac said, "Now I am going to ask you"—and here he interjected a protective blessing—"afuera de las karas [away from our faces]—any *maldisiones* [curses] do you know?" The individual responded with astonishment, "Barbinan, no! [God forbid, no!]. In our family we didn't say those!" Her daughter then answered, perhaps more candidly, "My mother used to say as an attack on me, 'Enyervàda ke te veiga, no! [I should see you all nervous, no!].' That was her curse!" Her mother quickly converted this curse into a blessing: "They used to do something, and I would say, 'A Dio! Enyervada ke nu ti vea! [Oh, God! Nervous, may I not see you!]'" Even in the version given by the daughter, the mother had provided the protection of negating her wish: she had wished that she would see her children nervous, but then canceled it by ending the statement with "no!" Westermarck notes this same negation of a curse. He writes, "The curses of parents are more powerful than those of saints. Yet parents may themselves make their curse ineffective by a subsequent blessing, saying for example, . . . 'O God, don't hear us, may it be on our children only a blessing'" (1968, 1:488–89).

Moshe Shaul remarks on the negation of a curse, "There is an interesting and original aspect that characterizes the Judeo-Spanish maledictions: that is, the custom of including in these maledictions, when they were directed to a member of the family or a friend, a word that would counter the malediction, as a form of antidote against the effect that the malediction would have if it were fulfilled" (1982, 34). Shaul uses the verb *baldar* to refer to this manner of countering a curse. For example, rather than saying, "El Dio ke te mate [May God kill you]," one would say to a family member or a friend, "El Dio ke no te mate [May God not kill you]." Haim Sephiha also discusses the term *baldar*, though he gives an interpretation with which we are not entirely in accord. Sephiha suggests that the term *baldar* derives from the Hebrew, BTL, meaning "to abolish, to abrogate." He continues, "The second reason, psychological this time, is the purpose of the malediction; what does the one who curses another individual want to do? What should happen to the one who has been cursed? The one who curses wants to remove the person who has been cursed from the world or to enfeeble him, to paralyze him, to insure that he may not bring about any more harm" (1981, 45–46). We suggest that the last phrase, "to insure that he may not bring about any more harm," should refer not, as Sephiha states, to the original curse, but rather to the counter-curse voiced by the one who has been cursed, or by someone present. *Baldar* means "to repel, to render ineffectual, to nullify" (Nehama 1977, 78). We suggest that the purpose of the counter-curse is to get rid of the original malediction by transferring it to the curser or to another. For example, one might counter a curse through transferring it back to the one who uttered the curse, or to someone close to that person, with the following: "Para tus ijos ke sea [May it be for your children]"; or, through reluctance or fear of cursing another Jew, one might transfer it in a generalized way, "Para los enemigos de Israel [For the enemies of Israel]." One might also use a blessing as a baldar, or negation of the curse. For instance, in response to one who cursed with, "El Dio ke te mate [May the Lord kill you]," another could reply, "El Dio ke te de salud buena i azlaha i beraha [May God give you good health, prosperity, and blessing]."

When Isaac asked another woman about curses, she responded with smiles and chuckles, "A eya aya! [To her over there!]," meaning let the curse fall on her over there. Again, Isaac prompted the woman by asking if there were any other curses, "for instance, 'A los enemigos de Israel [To the enemies of Israel].'" Very quietly, this woman, who was originally from Turkey, said, "A los ermenis, los ermenis! [To the Armenians, to the Armenians!]." Another responded to our question about curses by shaking a finger at us and saying, "Esto no si dize! [This is not said!]"; and another, by hitting her mouth with the palm of her hand, while saying, "Dati in la boka! [Smack your mouth!]."

Some Sephardic scholars would also like to deny the prevalence of cursing among their people, especially among the upper class. Nehama, who had recorded more than 150 curses in his *Dictionnaire du Judéo-Espagnol,* wrote in explanation of one curse, "Jaram ke se te fága (Malediction), 'May all that you eat, that which you enjoy, not profit you, bring you disaster!'" Nehama then adds, "It is often said amusingly, without any true intention of cursing, of wishing misfortune" (1977, 252). In *Usos y costumbres de los Sefardíes de Salonica,* Michael Molho noted that "individuals who respected one another did not insult or blaspheme." Those who did, Molho said, were considered "low level people" (1950, 169). In his article on Judeo-Spanish curses, Moshe Shaul notes that one cannot find as many maledictions recorded for the Sephardim as for other peoples. Judiciously he observes that the subject has scarcely been studied, but he then suggests that this might reflect "quite faithfully an aspect quite characteristic of our culture. The Sephardim in fact do not curse, blaspheme, or insult other individuals with the same violence that the majority of other peoples do [who] use phrases and words that express clearly and at times brutally, that which one thinks of the person he wants to insult or that which he desires to occur to him" (1982, 33).

Certainly Shaul is correct in observing that there have been more curses collected from the Greeks and the Turks, but this does not mean that the Sephardim did not have curses in equal measure, nor that the content and intent were not equally harsh. In our own research, from both written and oral sources, we have collected more than five hundred curses. We have found that even the worst curse could be intensified: "Il Dio ki li korti las manos [May God cut off his hands]" could be rendered as "Il Dio ki li korti las manos a este ijo di un hamor [May God cut off the hands of this son of a jackass]"; and, "Il Dio ke lo siege [May God blind him]" could be expressed as "Apalpando paredes ke se vaiga [May he go groping along the walls]."

In her work on Sephardic curses, Matilda Koen-Sarano gives a refreshingly positive slant. Considering the subject from "an objective point of view, we notice that the malediction is not totally negative, because it helps us to release our tensions, to remove from us with words and not with actions, the rage that we feel against whoever has caused harm to us" (1992, 54). The maledictions take on, as Koen-Sarano says, "the force of the tradition" and provide for "us at the same time our inner equilibrium." Just as a blessing was given in God's name, so a curse called on God as well. Koen-Sarano writes, "In many maledictions, God's name is mentioned also in order to reinforce the expression and make it more efficacious and solemn, and to frighten the one who has been cursed. Thus we hear, 'El Dio ke lo ateme [May God debilitate him],' 'El Dio ke lo siege de los dos ojos [May God blind him from both eyes].' . . . But the strongest malediction, one that involves the complete family, is: 'El Dio ke te tome a ti i a tu padre, a la madre ke te pario i a la komadre ke te aresivio [May God take you and your father, and the mother who gave you birth, and the midwife who received you]'" (1992, 55).

As if negations of blessings, the curses aimed to undermine health, happiness, and good fortune. The central joys of life were under attack; indeed, life itself was the target. Isaac remembers his mother telling him about a "mean" woman who cursed a pretty young girl with the following: "Mazal basho kil Dio ti seki [Low life, may God dry you up]," meaning, may God leave you barren. One might also curse a woman with, "Il Dio ke le seke la tripa [May God dry up her stomach]," or, perhaps more cruelly, for this would ensure the death of her baby, "Kera il Dio ke se le seken los pechos [May it be the will of God for her breasts to dry up]." Isaac also recalls a Sephardic woman in Izmir, Turkey, who cursed her son-in-law for leaving her daughter: "Ke te vea largo, estirado i enkortado [May I see you elongated, stretched out, and cut to pieces]." Other maledictions involving death were the following: "El Dio ke le kite el alma i se la echi a los peros [May God remove his soul and throw it to the dogs]," or "El guerko ke venga por uno i se los yeve a todos [May the Devil come for one and take them all]." One might also curse with the anticipation of seeing the corpse laid out on the floor of the house, as is done for the dead: "En basho lo veamos, estirado de kavesa a pies [May we see him lying down from head to feet]"; or, in anticipation of seeing the body carried out of the house, feet first, for the funeral, "Kon los piezes adelantre ke lo vea salir [With his feet first, may I see him leave]." Not satisfied with death, one might say, "En jinin jinan ke se kemen sus guesos [In hell may his bones burn]." One might curse another with eternal torment: "En herem este y en niduy este, en este mundo i en el otro [May he be excommunicated, may he be damned in this life and in the other]."

There were also phrases that conveyed a blessing or a curse, depending on the intention of the one who uttered them. For instance, "Ida sin buelta [Depart without returning]" could be used as a blessing for a young bride who would join her husband in their new home. The mother expressed her hope that her daughter would stay with him happy and healthy, and that, God forbid, she would not return to her parents as a widow or a divorcée. As a curse, this same phrase meant that the individual should go away and never be seen again; and this might be finalized with "Ni eskrito, ni estampado [neither written (correspondence), nor photographed]." Other phrases that could be either blessings or curses are the following: "Il Dio te aga sigun lo ke azis por mi [May God do unto you as you do for me]"; "Mejorado ki veas [May you experience even better]"; and, "Il Dio ki ti lu pagi doble [May God pay it back double]." Parents could "disguise" their curses with what should have been blessings. An exasperated mother could say to her children, "Il Dio ki ti de ijos para bueno [May God give you children for good]," or, "Un dia tus ijos te lo van a pagar di bueno [Some day your children will pay you back in good]," which meant, they will pay you back, but good!

Just as blessings and curses gave voice to the dangerous power of the spoken word, so did swearing an oath place a person in peril. Stanley Gevirtz defines an oath as "an abbreviated, conditional self-curse," which follows the formula, "'If I do X . . . , may Y happen to me!' . . . [or] 'If I do not do X . . . may Y happen to me'" (1959, 86). In a similar vein, Westermarck says that an oath is like a curse: "It is a conditional self-imprecation, a curse by which a person calls down upon himself some evil in the event of what he says not being true" (1968, 1:492). The Sephardim would complete the sentence with "Ansi [In that manner]" or "Kil Dio . . . si . . . [May God . . . if . . .]." For instance, one might swear, "Esto ti lo vo azer ansi il Dio me deshe la vida [This I will do for you, would that God let me live]," or, "A mis ijos no vea kazar si . . . [I should not see my children married if . . .]." Reina Franco, originally from Rhodes and living in Atlanta in 1957, cautioned Isaac about taking an oath: "One never knows what might happen. These *malahimes* [angels] have ears." Here Mrs. Franco avoided causing offense by referring to the evil spirits as angels. Thus if one emphasized the truth of one's statement by saying, "Kil Dio mi mati si no dijo la verdad [May God kill me if I don't speak the truth]," the spirits might bring death to the speaker or to someone else. Often the oath was taken in the name of the sacred and was introduced by "Por," meaning, "I swear by." For example, "Por la ley di Moshe Rabenu," meant, "I swear by the Law of Moses our leader"; or it might have been taken "por la ley santa [by the holy law]." One might swear in the name of a beloved, "Por la vida de mis ijos [On the lives of my children]," or "Asi biva mi madre [Thus may my mother live]," or "Los ojos di mi kerido se siegen [May the eyes of my dear one be blinded]." Even though one was cautioned not to blaspheme, still one might swear "En il nombre del Dio [In God's name]," as if the curser were acting as an agent of God.

There were other perhaps less forthright ways of protecting oneself against the consequences of an oath. Isaac recalled people swearing, "Por estas kriaturas santas [By these holy children]," and deceiving others since they swore on children who were present but were not their own. To outsiders, one might take an oath, "Por la kavesa de mi padre [On the head of my father]," or "En vida de mis ijos [On the life of my children]," when in reality the father was dead, or there were no children. In order to avoid the danger of making a promise, one might utter the protective phrase, "Sin neder [Without promise]." As Nehama notes, when making a vow, or when asking something, especially from God, one must say, "Sin neder," which is called "tomar neder [to take *neder*], or "tomarselo de neder [to take oneself the neder]." Nehama says that this is taking "a resolution to which one gives a religious character" (1977, 381). The phrase "sin neder" was used particularly when one spoke of visiting the dead, since it was believed that the dead could hear what was said and would wait in anticipation of the promised visit.

The power of speech extended to the naming of an individual. As Joseph Lauterbach writes, "a man's name is the essence of his being"

(1932, 78). Citing Hebrew texts, Trachtenberg notes, "'a man's name is his person' and . . . 'his name is his soul'" (1939, 78). He continues, "This doctrine elevated the process of naming a child into one of major importance. The name carried with it all the associations it had accumulated in history, and stamped the character of its earlier owners upon its new bearer, so that the choice of a name was fraught with grave responsibility" (78). For the Sephardim, this "accumulated history" was also reflected in the kinship pattern of naming. In accord with the Ashkenazim, the Sephardim would not name a child after a living parent, for it was believed that the Angel of Death would deliver a death summons only to a named individual. Thus, if the Angel of Death came for Yaakov the father, he might take Yaakov the son; or if he came for Luna the mother, he might take Luna the daughter. In sharp distinction, however, with the Ashkenazim who never named a baby after someone who was alive, the Sephardim did name children after grandparents, even if they were still living. As Bienvenida Gabay explained the naming system, "The first son takes the father's father's name. If the second is a daughter, she takes the father's mother's name. If it is another son, then he takes the mother's father's name. It's one from here and one from there." Thus, the first, third, and fifth babies—that is, the odd-numbered births—received the name from the paternal side; and the second, fourth, and sixth, from the maternal. There were, however, variations according to specific families, though these variations often proved the rule. In Isaac's family, for instance, his older brother, who was the first born, was named after his mother's father, Yeoshua. This was done at the request of the paternal grandfather, Isaac Lévy, who wanted to honor the memory of his daughter-in-law's deceased father. He said, "You are an only child and might not have other children to name after your father; but I have other children who will name a child after me." Thus, when she had her second son, she named him Isaac, after the father's father.

After the birth of the fourth child, the family had the choice of continuing the naming after members of the family or of following another pattern. The names might be chosen to designate a propitious day, for example, Yomtov (Hebrew, *yom tov,* for good day), born on a holy day; or Sabbetay (Hebrew, *Shabbat*), born on the sabbath. A boy might be named Moshe or Moises if he was born on the day Moses received the Ten Commandments at Mount Sinai. The name could indicate the season of birth: Esther for girls, and Mordehai for boys, designated those born on Purim, the feast celebrating the deliverance of the Jews from the edict of King Nebuchadnezzar (605–562 B.C.E.). Nissim (Hebrew *nes,* for miracle) would be an appropriate name for a boy born in the month of Nisan, when the

Lord delivered the Hebrews from captivity in Egypt. And Matatiahu or Matatia might name those born on Hanukkah, the feast of lights, which commemorates the rededication of the Temple in Jerusalem after its defilement by Antiochus of Syria in the second century B.C.E. Jeremia would be one who was born during the first nine days of the month of Av, the period of mourning that culminates on the tenth of Av, known as Tisha be-Av, to commemorate the destruction of the Temple in Jerusalem.

While the names of males were customarily from Hebrew, those of girls were often from Spanish, though sometimes from other languages as well. The name might designate an animal or a plant: Palomba (Spanish, dove), Lea (Hebrew, gazelle), Flor (Spanish, flower), Rosa (Spanish, rose), Violeta (Spanish, violet), and Zimbul (Turkish, jasmine). A girl might be named for a precious stone or metal, all of these in Spanish: Brilante (gem), Diamante (diamond), Gioya or Goya (jewel), Oro (gold), Perla (pearl), and Zafira (sapphire). The cosmos was also an inspiration: Estrella (star), Luna (moon), Sol (sun) (all of these in Spanish). And names of regal character were chosen: Regina (Italian, queen), Reina (Spanish, queen), Malka (Hebrew, queen), Sultana (Arabic, queen). Propitious or complimentary adjectives and nouns might be used: Alegre (Spanish, happy), Bella (Italian, beautiful), Blanca (Spanish, white), Clara (Spanish, bright), Gracia (Spanish, grace), Linda (Spanish, attractive), Yafa (Hebrew, beautiful).

A name might also be chosen in advance of the birth of a child as a means to ensure fertility. For example, on the anniversary of Rabbi Shimon bar Yohay, the protector of those who suffer, a sterile woman would take an oath to dedicate the hoped-for child to his memory. The boy would be called Shimon. After a long period of infertility, a woman who gave birth to a son might name him Rahamin (Hebrew, pity or merciful), since God found favor in her and granted her wish. A name could also commemorate a propitious event. If upon the birth of a child the family experienced good fortune, a new name or an additional name might be given to the infant: Simantob (Hebrew, *siman tov,* good signal or deed), Mazalto (Hebrew, *mazal tov,* good fortune or luck), and Fortuna or Fortune (Spanish, fortune or destiny).

In certain situations, the chain of kinship through naming was deliberately broken. Bienvenida Gabay told us how she had acquired her name, which meant "welcome." Her mother had had a difficult delivery. Finally, as the baby was being born, the midwife said, "'Una ija bien venida [a welcomed daughter] is coming to us.'" The girl was supposed to have been named Rahel, after her father's mother. As she grew older and expressed a wish to have been named Rahel, she was told that she had been named Bienvenida because "your mother narrowly escaped death." Either Benvenida or Bienvenida was typically the name given to a girl who was born to a woman who had not been able to have children.

Another break with the customary naming pattern involved a woman who had the misfortune of giving birth to stillborn babies, or of losing her young children to disease. This woman would "sell" her baby at birth; the child would be named Marko for a boy, or Merkada for a girl, which signified that the child was "purchased." Thus the child did not belong to the parents who had had so much misfortune but rather to a new set of parents, often ones who had had good fortune and who had a flock of healthy children. Molho writes that customarily the one who had "bought" the newborn took it home for three days, fed it, dressed it from "head to toe," and then returned it to its birth parents. For the next three feasts of Purim, the new "parents" gave the child candy and new clothes and distributed money to the poor in honor of the child (Molho 1950, 68).

We were familiar with this custom and so when we met a woman named Merkada, we asked about the origin of her name. She replied: "I am Merkada. My mother had an older son, older than me. All the children that she gave birth [to] after that son, from the first one, died, they did not live. And four of them died. . . . Three years, four years, the children died. I am the fifth from the older one. When my mother was pregnant with me, they told her that 'When she will be born, you must sell her.' And when I was born, a young man came and bought me. He bought me . . . with sweets." This young man, a friend of the family, always gave her gifts. Had he not died young, he would have presented her with a gift on her wedding with these words, "Here is the last present that I am giving you. From now on, let your husband do everything for you." A rabbi in Salonika told us, "There were a lot of people here called Merkado before the war." He continued, "There were women who gave birth and the children would die. Then they would make a sale. They would sell the child to the neighbor, to a nephew, so that he could go on living." Another woman told us a story about her own son: "I have a son, at birth he was named Nisim. As a child he was very sick. Doctors, doctors! Meanwhile, my father-in-law told me, 'Let us sell the child.' My brother purchased him. His name from that moment on was Marko, and, blessed be the name of God, he was fine. The one who purchased him watched over him and brought him presents so that he would live a long life. When he married, then his wife purchased him." The mother recalled that the wife had to say, "'I am purchasing you from your father.'"

Since an individual's name was "the mainspring not only of a person's character, but also of his fate" (Trachtenberg 1939, 78), when a person was ill, then the name would be changed. It was believed that when one changed one's name, one changed one's fortune. Additionally, this was done to confuse the Angel of Death: when he came to take the person who was, or had been ill, that person could not be found (Elnecavé 1963, 132). One woman told us, "My sister and sister-in-law were quite sick. First it was my sister-in-law. She was called Esther. They used to go to the synagogue with oil, they opened [a religious] book . . . and the first page and first letter that appeared, that name they would give to her. And for my sister-in-law the name Vida [Life] came. From Esther to Vida." When her sister was sick, as she said, "We did the same thing to her." Typically the name change for women would be to Vida, which derived from the Spanish for life. For men, there were several names, all from Hebrew: Haim, for life; Rufuel or Rafael, from *refua,* for cure; Nissim, from *nes,* for miracles; and Rahamin, from the same Hebrew word, for mercy. A male might also have been renamed Bension, son of Zion, and thus have the protection of Zion. Additionally, since every male in the Jewish community was a son of Zion, the Angel of Death could not single out the specific individual for whom he searched. Isaac knew of a man in Rhodes who was named Moreno Biton. After his first serious illness, he was renamed, Haim Moreno Biton; and after his second illness, he was Rafael Haim Moreno Biton.

Whether one was blessing or cursing, whether naming a baby or changing one's name due to illness, the power flowed from the same source, and that was from the spoken word. The wisdom of the following formulaic phrase conveyed the sympathetic power of good speech: "Kita dulsuria para ke veas dulsuria [(Speak) sweetness so that you will see sweetness]." Thus, for the Sephardim, the proverb "Dize la boka lo ke va yevar la alma [The mouth says what will come to the soul]" represents the ultimate measure of the spoken word.

5 "Let It Go to the Garlic!"

"I remember when I was a child something very beautiful. There was a neighbor who used to call me *ojus sin kara* [eyes without face/bright eyes]. Every time she saw me, it seemed to my mother that she gave me the evil eye and I always got sick. It happened once a week, twice a week. Then they advised my mother to put in my pocket *romero* [rosemary] and *ruda* [rue], especially when this lady saw me. And it was thus. Perhaps [because of] the superstition or something like it, ever since then I never removed the rue from my pocket. And I was no longer sick."[1] In this recollection, a Sefardi man has synthesized many of the potent forces of the evil eye. As a young boy, he had been particularly vulnerable to the evil eye. The woman who praised him did so repeatedly and without a protective disclaimer, such as "*Sin ojo!* [Without evil eye!]." His mother was advised by those who knew how to guard against the evil eye: she put a piece of rosemary and a sprig of rue in his pocket. And, thus, he was protected from the woman who praised him so freely, for as Clara Farji, originally of Edirne, Turkey, pragmatically explained to us, "There are people who have the evil eye."

Zimbul Maya Suzi, born in a village near Istanbul, explained, "The first thing about *ayin arah* [evil eye], when a person doesn't feel well, he already knows that it is from the eye." Called by several names—*mal ojo, ojo malo, nazar* (Turkish), *ayin arah* (Hebrew), *ojo kui* (Judeo-Spanish, eye dark),[2] *ojo vazio* (empty/unsatisfied eye)—all of these connote the harm caused through the thought or expression of envy or greed. The one who caused the misfortune was said to *echar nazar* (Judeo-Spanish, to cast; Turkish, the evil eye), or *tomar de ojo* (to take, catch through the eye; to be jealous of the prosperity of others).

The Sephardic belief in mal ojo is part of the evil-eye complex that spans Indo-European and Semitic cultures.[3] Central to this belief is the concept that one can unintentionally or intentionally cause harm to an individual simply through thinking or expressing praise. Envy, then, is a crucial component: felt and expressed by humans, envy and greed awaken the spirits whose actions cause all manner of injury. As William Graham Sumner noted in *Folkways* (1906), "It is assumed that demons envy human success and prosperity and so inflict loss and harm on the successful" (506).

Closely related to the evil eye, though less frequently mentioned, was *la avla de la djente* (the speech of people), or *la boka del ombri* (the mouth of man), also referred to as *la boka mala* (bad mouth) and *la avla mala* (evil talk). It was through the power of speech, through the articulation of thought, that the evil eye was set in motion. As a woman from Brusa, Turkey, explained, "You say something good . . . , right away the evil eye touches him. The avla de la djente touches the baby. . . . Somebody speaks and it doesn't do good for the child. It is not that you said something bad. You said something good, but to the child [it had a bad effect]."[4] So powerful were the evil eye and evil speech that before one moved from bed in the morning, one would utter a prayer of protection. Regina Arogeti, originally from Rhodes, recited the following prayer each morning before rising: "El Dio ke mos guadre de ojo malo, de avla mala, de males demodados [May the Lord guard us from the evil eye, evil speech, and bizarre harm]." Simha Hen, from Trachia, Greece, recited a more amplified version: "El Dio ke me guadre de vizino negro, de ojo malo, de trajedia negra, de hazinura negra, de kavzos negros, de djuzgo o djuzgador negro [May God protect me from a bad neighbor, from the evil eye, from a bad tragedy, from a bad infirmity, from evil deeds, and from a bad judgment or judge]."

There were times when one was especially vulnerable to the evil eye, times of happiness and good fortune, of prosperity and fertility. At weddings, during pregnancy, at the birth of a baby, at the *brit milah* (Hebrew, covenant of circumcision), on acquiring new clothes, new furniture, a new house, in all these circumstances, the fortunate ones could be struck with disaster. As it was explained to us, there were some individuals who were more easily taken by the evil eye: "For instance, a newborn male had to be guarded carefully for eight days, from birth to circumcision, because during this time he was most exposed to the spirits." Even a passing comment by a neighbor or an envious glance by a friend or a relative would be enough to arouse the jealousy of the spirits. To protect against this, people would exclaim in formulaic response to ward off the evil eye, "*Ojo!*" meaning, "No evil eye!" and some would mimic spitting with a "Pu!" sound. As Kalina Alvas, originally of Bulgaria, explained to us, "If you see that a person is not good, that he does not say anything good, you must say, '*Sinko! Sinko!* [Five! Five!]'" This was often accompanied with the thrust of the right hand, palm up and fingers spread, and the interjection, "*Na!* [Turkish, here!] *Skata sta moutra sou* [Greek, feces in your expression/feces in your face]."[5] Symbolically, then, the protection was compounded: one would both say and show the powerful number five of the Muslim *hamsa* (hand) and would ward off the evil, simultaneously transfering it back to the guilty one, with the Greek insult of feces in the face.

If an individual has observed the good fortune of another, or has, with lack of caution, commented on that good fortune by remarking on another's good looks, success, large family, or valued possession, he or she could simultaneously show a lack of envy and protect the more fortunate friend against the evil eye by saying, "*Sin ojo!* [Without evil eye!]," "*Nazar no!* [Evil eye no!]," or "*Bendicho il Dio* [Blessed be God]." One woman explained to us, "When a neighbor came and she said something [complimentary, she added], 'Ojo malo ke no kaiga [May the evil eye not fall]'; 'Al ajo ke se le vaiga [Let it go to—be absorbed by—the garlic]'; 'Ojo malo ke no tengan [May the evil eye not strike them].' This was always the way of old ladies." One might also say, "Ke se avran los ojos [May the eyes be opened]," so that harm would not befall an individual. A more direct acknowledgment of one's own power to cause injury through praise was conveyed in the formulaic sayings, "Ke mi ojo no le aga dingun mal [May my eye not cause him/her any harm]," "Por mi ke no le kaiga mal [Because of me, no harm should befall him/her]," and "De ojo malo ke me lo guardre il Dio [May God protect him from the evil eye]."

Since the evil eye was so prevalent and pernicious, people protected themselves through various measures. Chief among these was ruda, the herb rue. Remarking on the connection between ruda, a pregnant woman, and a baby, Rosa Avzaradel said, "'Rue,' they said in Rhodes, 'goes along with the child.' When rue is planted, the seed sprouts in a month. This I did not know, it was the people who told me. The rue, one plants it as a seed, and in a month it appears, and the woman knows that she is expecting after the month. Isn't that true? That is why rue goes with the child." As one woman remarked, "Rue was the first thing. They placed a bunch of rue in the bed of the *parida* [newly delivered mother]."[6] Another woman recalled, "They would put rue on the curtains of the bed," and still another remembered that they pinned rue on the head of the new mother. Kalo Baron Levi from Gallipoli, Turkey, recalled that rue was used for babies and for paridas: "They put it next to the head, on the pillow, so that they can go to sleep. For the parida against nazar [evil eye]." For the mother, a sprig of rue was placed behind the ear. This was to protect the new mother, as one person explained, against "the people who were going to come to visit. If the baby was beautiful, and if the new mother had an easy delivery, and the neighbors were coming to visit, they would do that. So that they would not get the evil eye." When the eight-day-old baby boy is taken for the ritual circumcision, a sprig of rue was tucked into his clothes. When we asked our mother, Caden Lévy Israel, how long rue was pinned to a child's clothes, she responded, "This, one would dry, they would put a new one. Until the son was a year old. . . . This is for nazar, it's not for pleasure!"

Among the Sephardim, rue could literally be layered on other protective materials. As Inez Meloh of Edirne, Turkey, explained, "When there was a parida, they would take a sprig of rue, and they would make some sweet almond [paste], and they would put a piece [of rue] on top of it, and they would take it as a good luck sign to protect against the evil eye." It is significant that the rue, which was believed to protect the new mother, her infant, and her breast milk, was placed on top of the sugared almond, which combined the protection of sugar, to ward off evil—and particularly to protect against *espanto* (fright)—and almond, which when pressed yields a milky substance, and thus would be linked to breast milk. Isaac remembers from his childhood in Rhodes that sprigs of rue were decorated with *alvarak* [Turkish, gold leaf]. The rue was moistened with water or spittle and pressed onto a paper of gold; then the gilded sprig was placed on a dish of candies, such as marzipan. It was believed that the rue, the gold leaf, the marzipan (almond, for fertility, mixed with sugar, representing sweetness), the whiteness of the fruit (purity), and the water or spittle (the fluid of life) would protect an individual from all harm. Caden Lévy Israel, explained that the gilded sprig of rue was pinned on the child and the mother for protection from the evil eye, and Rebecca Amato Levy, in *I Remember Rhodes*, writes that it was also placed on the pillow of the newborn (1987, 10–11).[7] Here the layering of the rue and the gold leaf yielded a fragile sprig of golden beauty that was believed to distract the spirits from the new mother and from her child by both the pungent aroma of the rue and the glitter of the gold.

Besides protecting a pregnant woman against evil, rue could also be used to abort a pregnancy. As our informant told us, "Take rue and boil it. Drink a half or full glass. It is bitter, the more one drinks, the better it is to abort. It should be done two or three times, but, it may kill the mother." The genus name for rue, *Ruta,* derives from the Greek *reuo,* which means "to set free," and was connected with the herb's healing power. Aristotle noted that rue "eased the nervous indigestion suffered when eating in the presence of foreigners," and since the Greeks connected this to the evil eye brought on by eating in front of strangers, rue was regarded as an herb with powerful spiritual properties (Kowalchik and Hylton 1987, 433). There have been many medicinal uses for rue, including the treatment of heart problems, and for women, "to correct irregular menstruation, to ease the symptoms of menopause, and to induce abortion" (433).

Rue could be used in conjunction with other protective objects, such as garlic, blue beads, salt, prayer books, and gold. As Clara Danon of Zeniça, Bosnia, told us, "Rue is placed thus [pointing to the ear], garlic under the pillow so that it couldn't be seen." Caden Lévy Israel explained, "They placed rue, and [usually a bracelet] made of *bunjukas,* blue beads, on the person in order that no nazar would strike the baby." Julie Alajef of Rusçuk, Bulgaria, recalled, "Garlic they put under the pillow for the evil eye. Sometimes they would tie blue chains" by stringing garlic together with blue beads. Paolina Elazar of Sofia, Bulgaria, explained, "There was something for the evil eye. Garlic they put in the pocket, in the house, on the doors. Babies when they were born, under the pillows. And they used to put blue beads." Kalina Alvas said, "On a new baby they put a bracelet with a hamsa [hand], blue beads, a few *ujikos* [eyes (blue beads with eyes)]. They also placed a religious book [under the pillow], to keep the child safe." She added as if in affirmation, "My mother did it." As another person said, "With a piece of garlic in the pocket and blue beads pinned to the shirt, a child would be protected from the evil eye from birth until he became a big boy." The individual added, "And if the beads weren't pinned, they would make like a cord. For nazar, they did this. It's the same for boys and girls." A woman from Salonika explained that the blue beads were pinned to the left side of the baby's shirt and kept on "always, because the baby was in the stroller, the baby was *godra* [fat/beautiful], good, so that nobody should come and put the evil eye on her."

At times, the protective objects could be tied together in a little sack. One woman recalled, "Some time ago, they carried a *bulsika* [little sack] with some salt, garlic, and a blue bead." Another remembers that "with some cloves and garlic, they would put it in a little piece of cloth and sew it on top of the shirt against the evil eye." In Rhodes a blue bead was placed in between double almonds and used to ensure fertility, particularly to bring breast milk. As a *nazarlik* (protective device against nazar), people wore *bunjukas mavis* (blue beads) strung in a chain for a necklace or a bracelet. Another woman told us of the combination of protective measures used for her baby daughter: "We immediately put on her garlic with rue on glittering paper . . . [and] the blue bead, the bracelet and a *shaddai* [gold amulet with the name of God]. We want to say that the nazarlik guards the person as well as performing good deeds."

Just as the individual was protected against the evil eye, so was the house itself. As Naomi Fis of Istanbul said, "We believed in the evil eye. We used to say '*Pu, maskara!* [Pu (said in imitation of spitting), little rascal!].' Today, we make amulets of crochet, little bags. We put garlic inside, and we hang it at the entrance of the house." These crocheted containers are made of red and blue—colors that themselves are protective—and have five tiny sacks inside, each to hold a garlic clove. Thus one small object protects through colors, through garlic, and through the number five, which is symbolic of the hamsa, or the hand. Solomon Sephiha of Salonika, Greece, remarked, "There was the evil eye for some reason in the house. They used to place a horseshoe, a head of garlic, and some *nazarlik bunjuk* [evil-eye beads]." The placement was important, for as Mr. Sephiha explained, this protective bundle was hung where the eye of the passerby might fall: "And they used to put that, and they used to hang it outside the window." Isaac continued in his questioning:

> Isaac: So it wouldn't come in?
> Solomon: Well, someone would pass outside the house and see it.
> Isaac: Did they put the horseshoe and the garlic, everything together?
> Solomon: Yes, everything together. They used to put it on the balcony or in the window. All that was for evil eye.
> Isaac: When the people would pass and see it.
> Solomon and another man: Yes, of course. Everybody used to see it.
> Solomon: I used to see it. I remember when I was a child, I used to see it.

Inside the house, there were ways of protecting against the evil eye as well. As one man recalled: "For the evil eye, they used to do other things. I saw in many houses, if one had two or three rooms, and in one of those rooms there was a picture painted with the words, 'If I forget thee, Jerusalem, I will lose my right hand.' And in the other rooms, there was also a picture, smaller, but not painted, completely empty. Because they say that the evil eye should fall into that empty picture. If somebody wants to cast the evil eye, he is going to do it. So if the evil eye was already done, then let the evil eye fall into that picture."[8]

All of these protective customs had the same intent: to shield the vulnerable ones from the disastrous effects of greed or envy. At times, the shield was quite visible, as in the curtain that surrounded the bed of the newly delivered mother and her child. A woman from Izmir, Turkey, described this protection of the mother and her newborn: "What a bed it was, with its curtains and *namusias* [netting]! Everything was good. . . . The child was there all night, not left alone, with the beautiful *namusias*, hidden so that the child could not be seen."[9] Sol Azuz, from Istanbul, recounted to us: "I gave birth to a son. He was like a king. After giving birth, they didn't allow us to get up from bed. We used to hide from the neighbors, in order not to see us standing up. Because if they saw you standing up, they would start talking, '*A Dio!* [Oh, God!], you just gave birth. Are you already on your feet?' And what they said *tokava a la parida* [touched/struck the newly delivered with the evil eye]." Kalina Alvas experienced just such a result from the praise of neighbors. As she recounted:

> When I gave birth to my first child [a son], I was in bed. A husband and wife came in [to the room], sat down on the sofa, and said, "A Dio! No parese ke parites! [My God! It does not seem that you gave birth!]." Up to that point, I had been fine, dressed in red silk, in a luxurious manner. Is this a way to speak? This man burned me. At night, I could not breast-feed the child. My breasts were all bad, falling in pieces with blood. My mother held them with pillows. The doctor gave me a cream that was poisonous. He said, "You are going to wash the breasts with soap and water, and later you are going to breast-feed the baby." All of this took place because of the evil eye; it lasted three months. It used to hurt me every time that I breast-fed the child.

Mrs. Alvas concluded, "I suffered a lot because of the evil eye. I believe in it. And it is true that the evil eye exists."

To avoid such praise and the danger of the immediate strike of the evil eye, the new mother was quiescent. As Mrs. Azuz said, "She is in bed. She is not standing up, she is in bed. They can't say a word because she is in bed. We didn't move from the bed. . . . And not until all of the invited people were gone did the new mother get up from the bed." Mrs. Azuz explained that the newly delivered mother could not even be seen eating: "The tray I had here in the bed. . . . I was sitting in the bed and I was eating. Suddenly a neighbor came. My aunt came in, went and picked up the tray, so that the woman would not see that I was eating. . . . I said, 'My god, why did you pull the tray from me?' And then with her head, she made a sign to keep quiet. Until late at night, visitors were coming and I stayed without food. And I stayed without eating." Korin Madem, also from Istanbul, reiterated the points made by her friend, Sol Azuz: "It is forbidden to talk to that woman who gave birth and to tell her, 'You are already walking? You are already eating? You are already standing up? Did you already wash? Are you washing yourself?' All that is forbidden to speak." Mrs. Madem added, "And the old people say that this is nazar.

The whole family of the parida *se la komian a la parida, se la komian de nazar* [ate/devoured the newly delivered mother, tore her apart with the evil eye]. And the parida used to get sick."

In addition to being shielded by the curtains of the bed, the woman was also protected by her relatives, as Rafael Brudo recalled of the practice in Salonika: "A woman who gave birth, until the day of the *brit,* she was not left alone. People had to be with her." He added, "And the eve of the night before the brit, they gave a party. And on that night, ten men stayed home . . . for *minyan* . . . to keep an eye on the child so that no *sheddim* [spirits] would take him away."[10] Rebecca Amato Levy wrote that in Rhodes, "The father and a few male relatives stayed up all night reading from the Torah, at the same time watching over the new-born son" (1987, 11). Caden Lévy Israel also recalled the protection of the newborn in Rhodes on the night before the circumcision, "They don't leave him in the bed alone. A woman holds him in her hands to protect him from the evil eye." A woman from Izmir, Turkey, remembered the party on the night before the brit milah: "All night the parida with her mother or mother-in-law, all night, she held the child on her knees. . . . The party took place that night, all night so that the parida would not go to sleep on the child. They placed the child on the mother's knees, they did not put him in his crib. On that night, they brought a string of fish, and for the mother, a necklace of old, gold coins that they placed on the bed."[11] The mother and the baby were literally covered against the evil eye by the curtains of the bed and by the blankets. They were also *akonpanyados* (accompanied) by friends and relatives to keep the evil eye away from them. Lights were lit throughout the house to ward off spirits, and a protective sword was hung in the room where the baby and the mother were. At this crucial time, on the eve before the brit milah, when the envy of the spirits would be at its height, the new mother was not even allowed to sleep, for sleep would put her in the dangerous realm of contact with the spirits. The group of ten men had said the evening prayers in the home where she was, and they stayed on to read from the Torah; and the women relatives, including her mother and mother-in-law, were waiting on her and singing *kantes de parida* (birth songs) to keep her awake.

The same woman who recalled the beauty of the curtains and the netting surrounding the bed of the mother and child, as well as the festivities of the party on the eve before the brit milah, also remembered what happened to her on the birth of her second child:

> After three years, I gave birth to the son. To my older son. The night of the *shemira* [Hebrew, watch, party before the brit], when I was lying in

> bed, I was more modern. I was not *muy dal tiempo* [very much of the time], I was more modern. I did not let anyone cover the bed, I did not let them cover me and the child. The child was down [in the crib]. I let people pick him up. Suddenly, while I was . . . on the bed, I took out my breast to nurse the baby, a Turkish woman entered, una *vedre* [green/Muslim].[12] My milk squirted out, *ki mal ti keri* [may the evil go to the one who wishes you ill], my milk squirted out, it was all pus. The women said, "Of the evil eye [it must be]. You did not let people conceal you." You understand. This is what was said at the time. "You did not let them conceal you." Do you understand. I was more modern, and I did not let them do it. I said, "Why is the concealment necessary with the *namusias* [netting] and all that? It would make me nervous." But [I stayed] in bed, because of my mother who did not allow any other way, I was lying in bed. But to be completely covered, I could not. My mother said that day, "See what has happened to you? Look why we cover the paridas. So that people could not *echar ayin arah* [cast the evil eye]." Next day, I did not even see the brit of my son. I had a terrible fever, 40° C [104° F], burning. I did not even see the brit of my son. My sister-in-law . . . was a parida, she came and breast-fed the child, in order to take him to *la siya del Dio* [the chair of God/the chair of Elijah the Prophet]. What am I going to tell you? This [was the] way in the past.[13]

To protect her recently born baby from the evil eye, a mother would lick the forehead of the baby three times and recite the following charm:

> Te pari, te krii, el espanto i el ayin arah te kiti.
> La vaka lambe su biziriko por amar,
> i yo te lambo el espanto i ayin arah.
>
> I gave birth to you, I raised you, the fright and the evil eye I
> remove from you.
> The cow licks her calf because of love,
> and I lick [remove] your fright and evil eye.[14]

This custom was called *lanbigo*, or *lambida* (a lick of the tongue on the forehead). Certainly the cow licking her calf offered a powerful symbol for the nursing mother and child. Isaac recalls his grandmother, Sarota Amato Musafir, performing *lanbigo* for his daughter, Catherine, when she was five months old. The family was at a reception in Atlanta, Georgia, in 1964, and Isaac's baby daughter was the center of attention. Everyone picked her up; admired her curly blond hair and big, blue eyes; and complimented the parents. The baby cried incessantly. Isaac gave her a spoonful of phenobarbital, which was used at that time to settle colicky babies. She continued to cry, so someone else sprinkled a few drops of brandy on her tongue. When the baby did not cease crying, Isaac's grandmother took the baby in her arms, licked her forehead three times and spat, without saying a word. The crying stopped at once. Isaac's grandmother said, "Mi alma, ti metieron ojo [My darling, they gave you the evil eye]." Isaac remembers the younger generation attributing this cure to the effects of the phenobarbital and the brandy. His grandmother, he said, held her counsel: she knew the signs of a baby suffering from the evil eye, and she knew how to cure it.[15]

The mother's saliva could also be used to protect her breast milk from the evil eye. As one woman recounted, "When a woman gave birth and someone casts an evil eye, in order to protect the milk of the mother, one wet the finger with saliva and touched the breast, and some touched the nipple."

In some Sephardic communities, the newborn baby, whether a boy or a girl, was not left alone for forty days. From her memories as a young mother, one woman recalled, "And I used to place a religious book under [the pillow], and I went and did my work around the house. . . . And the room should not be dark, always with a light, and the book of the Torah."[16]

Gésa Róheim, an anthropologist, stresses "the oral quality of the evil eye" (1952, 217). While he situates the oral aggression with the suckling infant and sees this as "projected and personified in the hostile devouring glance of the witch-mother" (217), one might see the oral aggression at work in the room of the parida and her newborn, for as Mrs. Madem related in the interview portion above, the family used to "eat the parida." We quote her again: "The whole family of the parida *se la komian a la parida, se la komian de nazar* [ate/devoured the newly delivered mother, tore her apart with the evil eye]. And the parida used to get sick." One might expand Róheim's notion of the oral quality of the evil eye from the oral aggression associated with the experiences of birth and infancy to the spatial, sociological, and psychological plane, into the houses and the narrow streets of, in this instance, the closely intertwined Sephardic community. The relatives "ate the newly delivered mother" and so did the visiting neighbors; in the earlier account, *la vedre,* or Muslim woman, in praising the parida roused the spirits, who turned the breast milk to pus. The danger was from the people in the community, from one's own relatives and one's neighbors, and not, as Róheim suggested, from the infant at the mother's breast. The danger was admiration, envy, and greed; and the conflict grew from the necessity of interdependence. One needed the assistance of one's relatives and neighbors; but one also suffered the burden of this attention. In addition to the emotional strain that was acted out, as explained by Mrs. Madem, in the room of the parida, there was also the electric undercurrent of greed and envy of a woman's fertility, of her breast milk, of her newborn, particularly of her newborn son.

One way of protecting oneself against these intrusions—these greedy eyes—was to guard the boundaries of the house, the bedroom of the parida, and the body. As Arnold van Gennep has shown in *The Rites of Passage* (1960), it is precisely at the boundaries or at the edge where danger is most heightened, whether this be at the spiritual borders of the life crisis rituals, or at the physical borders of crossing, the doorway of the house, for example. The netting surrounding the bed of the parida and the newborn were visible boundaries, explicitly used to protect the woman at her most fertile, that is, when she has given birth to a son. The cognitive model was the parida with a newborn son being guarded for eight days prior to the brit. Other protective devices were strategically placed at the entryways. The mezuzah at the doorway was "a symbol of God's watchful care over the house and its dwellers" (Hertz 1990, 771 n. 9) and would ward off evil with its sacred script (and failing that, would be incorporated into a cure for the evil eye).[17] Garlic was hung at the door and outside the windows, and it would ward off the evil eye with its strong odor. At the doorsill of the house there was a horseshoe upon which the new mother was to step, following this advice: "Piza enriva de la nahcha ke te agas sana komo el fierro [Step on the horseshoe so that you may become as healthy (strong) as iron]." Even the light that was kept burning in the new mother's room maintained a protective boundary between day and the spirit-filled night, for spirits "shun the light" (Trachtenberg 1939, 159). And, finally, the people themselves who attended the new mother formed a protective barrier, "because demons flee when other people are present and awake" (Firestone 1962, 305).[18]

Following the anthropologist Mary Douglas's discussion of the body as a natural symbol (1966, 1973), one might even see the use of rue, garlic, rosemary, cloves, blue beads, iron, and gold as protecting the boundaries of the body. The sprig of rue was tucked behind the ear of the new mother and placed under the pillow of the newborn, where a religious book might be found as well; the clove of garlic or piece of rosemary was slipped into the shirt pocket; the golden amulet or a string of cloves was worn around the neck. One woman told us that the clove of garlic was placed "in the breast of the mother," and she further explained that the garlic was hung round the neck and between the breasts of the new mother. Rivka Sarfati used to coil her long hair into a bun, and her maternal aunt placed an iron nail inside it as protection against the evil eye. The body was protected at the head, around the neck, and at the chest. Indeed, the aperture to the body, *la boka del ombre* (mouth of man), was guarded by formulaic sayings that were believed through the power of words to ward off the evil spirits. (Conversely, part of the rationale for not speaking evil, for avoiding *lashon arah* [evil speech], had to do with the danger of allowing the evil in.) Finally, as we were told, to protect a baby from the evil eye, the mother could count the nine holes of the body, "the two eyes, two ears, two nostrils, one mouth, one *popo* [rectum] and one *pishador* [penis]," and say:

> Aki te kito el ojo malo, la ora mala i la ayin arah,
> se vaya a la profondina de la mar, i el ijo de Sarota no tenga dingun mal.

> Here I remove the evil eye, the misfortune of the moment and the evil eye,
> let it go to the depth of the sea, and the son of Sarota should not have any misfortune.

For each of these protective measures, there was either an explicit or implicit rationale for its effectiveness. The sword hanging in the room of the parida could offer the triple protection of iron, a phallic substitute for male protection, and a sharp edge to cut the danger. The folk wisdom about the protective nature of garlic, rue, rosemary, and cloves was directly connected to their strong, pungent odors. As mentioned above, garlic was believed to absorb the evil eye: "Al ajo ke se le vaiga" [Let it (the evil eye) go to the garlic]." "Evil eye will not come to rue," as Sara Nair said, "to the smell it doesn't come." *Romero* [rosemary] and cloves also had the pungent aroma to ward off the evil eye. Cloves had the additional curative property of popping when thrown in the fire and exploding away the evil eye. With its sparkle and purity, gold bedazzled the spirits, drew them to it and away from the person. Zimbul Maya Suzi wore gold earrings, which she said were "muy bueno para nazar [very good against nazar/evil eye]." As she told us, "The wife of the rabbi in Peta Tikva [Israel] used to tell me, 'Zimbul, do not remove the earrings.'" Regina Arogeti explained that in Rhodes "they attached a *dukado* [gold coin] with wax to the hair so that the people would look at the gold instead of the baby." She added, "Ansi no se echava el ojo malo [In this manner, the evil eye was not cast]." The blue of the beads was connected with the color of the sea, and, we suggest, with the curative powers of saltwater. In the *Talmud Hullin,* Rabbi Meir expounded on the significance of the color blue: "'Why is blue singled out from all the varieties of colours? Because blue resembles the colour of the sea, and the sea resembles the colour of the sky, and the sky resembles the colour of a sapphire, and a sapphire resembles the colour of the Throne of Glory'" (Epstein 1980, 177).

With a shift of perspective, we would like to move from the specific details of the evil eye among the Sephardim to an incorporation of other analytical approaches. In "Wet and Dry, the Evil Eye," Alan Dundes presents a comprehensive theoretical approach towards an understanding of the evil-eye complex. As he says, "the opposition between wet and dry is a fundamental folk idea, albeit an unconscious one, in Indo-European and Semitic worldview, a folk idea which is, metaphorically at any rate, a matter of life and death" (1981, 298). Perspicaciously, Dundes links the wet-dry opposition to the Greek humoral system and suggests that it is "much older than its articulation among the ancient Greeks [who were] concerned with humoral pathology. . . . It would appear that the formulations of humoral pathology simply formalized a folk theory already in existence" (297).

Unarguably, the wet-dry opposition was central to the Greek humoral system. In *On the Nature of Man,* Hippocrates (ca. 460–377 B.C.E.) proposed his theory of the four humors—blood, phlegm, black bile (melancholy), and yellow bile (choler)—and linked these to qualities in nature of hot and cold, wet and dry (Lloyd 1964, 92; Foster 1953, 202, 204; 1994, 5–6).[19] G. E. R. Lloyd writes, "As regards the pair dry and wet, several usages suggest that the Greeks conceived the living as 'wet' and the dead as 'dry'" (1964, 101). Richard Broxton Onians in his classic work, *The Origins of European Thought about the Body, the Mind, the Soul,* notes that liquid was equal to life (1954, 202). As Aristotle remarked, "'The living creature is by nature moist ('liquid' . . .) and warm, and to live is to be such, but old age is cold and dry and so is what had died. . . . It is inevitable that one who grows old should dry'" (Onians 1954, 215; quoting Aristotle). In the normal course of life, then, one ages, loses liquid, and dries up (Onians 1954, 214). The evil eye has the power to accelerate this process and to threaten the young and the robust with the drying of the body that comes with old age. The drying nature of the evil eye could be linked to the paired opposites in the Greek humoral system of hot and cold, since as Onians noted, drawing from a Greek source, "'Sight is an excessively hot vapour'" (1954, 76). If the hot vapor of sight were linked to the Pythagorean notion that "a ray goes forth from the eye and returns again" (76), then one might suggest that the evil eye actually carried the heat to the object of envy. Indeed, this is in accord with Foster's observations, that the heat of envy attacks the person who is envied through the evil eye (1994, 53).

Central to the understanding of the evil eye among the Sephardim is the following: "Life depends on liquid. From the concept of the 'water of life' to semen, milk, blood, bile, saliva, and the like, the consistent principle is that liquid means life while loss of liquid means death. 'Wet and Dry' as an oppositional pair means life and death. Liquids are living; drying is dying!" (Dundes 1981, 266). If one wanted confirmation of the symbolic equation between life and liquid, the Judeo-Spanish terms *bivir* (to live) and *bever* (to drink) would provide it: they are spelled exactly the same in Hebrew characters, ביב"ר, since the י (yod) represents both an "i" and an "e." In explaining why the last blessing of the funeral service was done with water, Rabbi Moise of Salonika expressed this connection between water and life: "With water you say, '*Maim haim,*' water is life. Can you live two or three days without water? You are going to die." Therefore, after a death, the rabbi explained, one says the following blessing with water for the living, "'Ke mos venga agora la vida, i ke seamos saludozos [May life come to us now and may we be healthy]."

Certainly the equation between liquid and life, and drying and death, was implicit, if not explicit, in the Sephardic evil-eye belief system. As J. E. Crombie suggested, "the element of life is sometimes believed to exist in the saliva" (1892, 252), so for the Sephardim a protective measure against evil spirits involved spitting. Trachtenberg also writes about this "most powerful liquid": "one may protect himself in unclean places, which the spirits haunt, by spitting three times, and even evil thoughts, which are the work of demons, may be dispelled in the same way" (1939, 159). Clearly the evil eye of the *vedre,* the Muslim woman, had the power to dry up liquid for the unfortunate woman whose breast milk not only dried up but turned to pus. A blessing often used by Sephardic women for children showed the equation between liquid and life: "Kreskas, kreskas, komo l'agua freska [Grow, grow, like the freshwater]," or "Kreskas, kreskas, komo l'agua koriente [Grow, grow, like the running water]." Also important here was the symbolism of fresh, running water, for Trachtenberg writes, "Running water neutralizes a magic act, and destroys the magical properties of things; it dispels mirages created by demons, and drives off the spirits themselves" (1939, 159). In referring to an old man, a woman in Izmir showed the symbolic equation between drying and age: "Seko komo la uva seka [Dry as the dry grape (raisin)]." One would also refer to the aged as *amorchado* (withered). A young person whose face was drawn with ill-health was said to have "la kara komo esponja sin agua [a face like a sponge without water]." In all of these expressions, water symbolized youth, life, and good health; and dryness, age and ill-health.

Drawing also on George Foster's theory of limited good, Dundes remarks on the "finite, limited amount of good—health [or] wealth," where a gain by one individual is a loss to another (1981, 266). The emphasis on limited good is apparent in every aspect of the evil-eye belief complex, from the care against expressing praise, to the caution at displaying one's good fortune, to the more formalized interactions between people directed towards maintaining the balance of "goods."

Among the Sephardim, one such practice shows clearly the principle of limited good, and the additional and related aspect of "the equilibrium model," in which poor or unhealthy individuals "constitute threats to persons with sufficient or abundant wealth and health" (266–67). The custom of *kambasear* involved the ritualized exchange of coins or small gifts, sometimes *alfinetes* (pins), between women of the following categories when they passed in the street: (1) two young women married in the first half of the same lunar month (and, thus, likely to be pregnant at the same time); (2) a new bride and a new mother; (3) two pregnant women; or (4) a new bride and a woman who had recently miscarried. As part of this exchange, the two women would say, "Toma tus partos i yo tomo los mios [You keep your own childbirths and I keep mine]." If this custom were not followed, the pregnant woman would miscarry or give birth to a dead baby, according to Zimbul Maya Suzi, originally of Turkey, and Benny Nahmias of Jerusalem. The first three categories clearly illustrate the concept of limited good: there is only so much pregnancy to go around, so you keep your childbirths and I'll keep mine. The last category highlights the concept of the equilibrium model, that a new bride, either just pregnant or hoping to become pregnant, would need to be protected ritually against the woman who had recently miscarried. Even the etymological derivation of the word *kambasear* illustrates this aspect of the limited nature of fertility and the need to maintain the delicate balance between health and misfortune. In our article "The Evil Eye and the Power of Speech among the Sephardim" (1987), we connect the meaning of the word *kambasear* to the Portuguese, *cambalacho*, "a deceitful and fraudulent barter, to trick." As we note, "The exchange, therefore, was carried out either to appease or to fool the spirits, who would be naturally envious of women's fertility. If the precautionary exchange did not take place, then the young woman would be *kambaseada*—that is, *asolombrada* (enshrouded/prey to an evil spirit), always open to attack" (54). We add here that the exchange was symbolically projected onto the spirit realm: it was the vexing *buenos de mozotros* (good among us/spirits) who interfered with pregnancies and caused miscarriages and not the envious thoughts of newly married Sephardic women.

The symbolic element of a woman's fertility can also be connected with the unconscious meaning of the evil eye as explained by Dundes: "In symbolic terms, a pair of eyes may be equivalent to breasts or testicles. . . . The fullness of life as exemplified by such fluids as mother's milk or semen can . . . be symbolized by an eye and accordingly threats to one's supply of such precious fluids can appropriately be manifested by the eye or eyes of others" (1981, 267). Onians identifies the liquid of life in the European worldview as "the seed, the stuff of life and strength" that issued from the eyes, particularly during times of passion (1954, 202). From the good fortune of the bride, to conception, which "goes along with the rue" and was signaled in a month, to the breast milk, the breasts themselves, to childbirth, the evil eye was intimately intertwined with, as Victor Turner phrases it, the "gross," the "frankly, even flagrantly, physiological" (1967, 28).

While Dundes focuses on the evil eye and the complex of beliefs associated with it, Mary Douglas has identified the liminal or marginal position of those imbued with the power of the evil eye. Following closely on the heels of British structural-functionalism, Douglas identifies "the well-articulated" social system with explicit powers "vested in the points of authority; where the social system is ill-articulated, I look for inarticulate powers vested in those who are a source of disorder. I am suggesting that the contrast between form and non-form accounts for the distribution of symbolic and psychic powers: external symbolism upholds the explicit social structure and internal, unformed psychic powers threaten it from the non-structure" (1966, 99). Douglas links internal, uncontrolled spiritual forces—such as the evil eye, witchcraft, and vision or prophecy—and external, controlled spiritual forces—such as spells, blessings and curses, and charms or formulas—to aspects of social structure. Douglas observes, "Where the social system requires people to hold dangerously ambiguous roles, these persons are credited with uncontrolled, unconscious, dangerous, disapproved powers—such as witchcraft and evil eye" (99). However, for the Sephardim, and we suggest for other peoples as well, the issues of spiritual health were linked much more strongly with the gendered nature of illness. What Douglas identifies as the "internal spiritual powers" were for the Sephardim closely associated with times of vulnerability that had to do with fertility, with engagements, weddings, pregnancy, birth, and brit milah. Following Douglas, van Gennep, and Turner, these are definitely times of liminal danger; they are liminal and dangerous precisely because these are the ritual and—in the instance of pregnancy and birth—the quite real markers of fertility.

When the issue of gender is added to the concerns of unconscious symbolism, social structure, and maintenance of boundaries, one finds a belief system in which women were centrally concerned with their own fertility. The elaborate protective measures against the evil eye, the divinatory rituals, and the cures for the evil eye were all intertwined with concerns about envy, about fertility, and, for women, with the production and protection of babies, particularly of baby boys. When the gendered component is added to the consideration of spiritual health, one is able to feel the pulsating power of Sephardic domesticated religion, and to trace the power to its source: to women, to their fertility, and to the health of their babies and children.

The protective measures and practices associated with mal ojo were fraught with contradictions. Domesticated religion, as Sered says, "strengthens bonds among people" (1994, 121); but we have found that the evil-eye complex sets up and maintains boundaries between people. The life of the Sephardim was grounded in intimacy; and this very intimacy was to be feared, for in the flash of the evil eye one's good fortune could crumble. Most compelling and provocative was the position of women in the evil-eye belief complex. The Sephardic women were at the center of the domesticated religion; they had the power of maintaining and perpetuating the evil-eye belief system as this pertained to women's fertility. Ultimately, their role was crucial in perpetuating a male power structure, in that their efforts to nourish women's fertility were directed towards producing male babies.

In examining the evil-eye complex of the Sephardim from a gendered perspective, one might be drawn back to the "key symbols," as Sherry Ortner (1973) designates those sacred symbols that summarize and condense meaning. These key symbols have to do with the basis of women's fertility: the fluids that give and sustain life. In the same vein, Turner discusses ritual symbols as "condensation" symbols, which, following Sapir's discussion, "allow for the ready release of emotional tension in conscious or unconscious form" (1967, 29). These condensed ritual symbols can be found at two poles: the sensory/physiological and the ideological/normative. In his essay "Symbols in Ndembu Ritual," Turner writes, "Other Ndembu symbols, at their sensory poles of meaning, represent such themes as blood, male and female genitalia, semen, urine, and feces. The same symbols, at their ideological poles of meaning, represent the unity and continuity of social groups, primary and associational, domestic, and political" (29). It is the work of ritual, and of ritual symbols, as Turner writes, "to convert the obligatory into the desirable." Ortner's "key symbol" and Turner's "dominant symbol" connect the "should" of the ethical system with the "want" of the emotions (30). Thus, the sensory/physiological pole (one might better say the "sensual pole") of evil-eye symbols is laden with the cluster of unconscious fertility symbolism so convincingly etched by Alan Dundes; and the ideological pole is crowded with the normative symbols of social interaction, undergirded as it is by the principle of limited good. As Turner emphasizes, "Norms and values, on the one hand, become saturated with emotion, while the gross and basic emotions become ennobled through contact with social values" (30).

One might add to this evil-eye brew of ritual symbolism a thought on the tension of contradiction in ritual symbolism. That the evil-eye complex sets up, and does not resolve, contradictions should not be surprising. Ritual symbolism plays with contradiction, with emotion, with that which cannot be conquered by reason. As our friend and colleague David Harris says, "The evil eye is no straight-ahead affair."

6 *Narrating Health, Marking the Social*

In their stories, the Sephardim would tell us in narrative form about what had made them ill; what had broken up families and mended them together again; about the dangers of strong emotions out of control; and of unguarded moments when one's private face was exposed to the public. In the course of telling their stories, they also explained to us the complex belief systems behind *espanto* (fright) and *echizo* (witchcraft). And by listening carefully, we could also hear how their accounts offered clues about public and private space, and the boundaries between self and other.

The two categories of illness, espanto and echizo, are linked to each other and to the evil eye by the power of emotions, and by the ineffable presence of the spirits. However, just as there was shared emotional space, there were also nuances of difference that were critical to the workings of this complex belief system. While *mal ojo* fed on greed and envy, as detailed in the foregoing chapter, a person who had cast the evil eye had not necessarily intended any harm. With echizo, the jealousy and envy were intentionally and malevolently acted out. This element of emotion out of control, of forceful hate, was emphasized repeatedly in the narratives about echizo. With espanto, the emotion was more one of embarrassment at public exposure and fear of the consequences. The narratives about espanto and echizo delineated boundaries of social space. For espanto, these boundaries were concerned with balance and control of the physical body and of the emotions in public. For echizo they had to do with the evils done by others who were unlike "us."

Our mother, Caden Lévy Israel, explained, "When someone is sick, it is that this espanto makes it. Otherwise it doesn't happen." Isaac asked, "But if someone is sick with the stomach?" His mother answered, "No matter what, it is possible that it came from the espanto." Espanto was a widespread belief in harm which results from a physical but, more important, a spiritual shock. This affliction was also found in Spain and in Spanish America, as George Foster notes: "*Strong emotional experiences* which produce physiological results characterize Hispanic America much more than Spain. Fright, commonly cited in Spain as a cause of minor disturbances such as pain in the region of the appendix, fits, fainting, and boils, is particularly thought to disturb menstruation" (1953, 211).

In "*Espanto:* A Dialogue with the Gods," Michael Tousignant writes, "The most universal trait of the belief is that *espanto* is thought to result from a magical fright" (1979, 348). Of his work in a village in Chiapas, Mexico, Tousignant notes: "The signs recognized in the patient point to a reality which is more than physical. They form the message of cosmological forces which have come to inscribe their power upon the body. . . . The signs or symptoms speak mostly of the origin and destiny of the illness, of the spirits who brought it . . . and of the mortal dangers which attend its progress. They speak of transgressed taboos, of envious neighbors, of lack of respect of dietary regulations" (347). Tousignant stresses the need to encompass both "the psycho-social aspects . . . and the symbolic discourse about illness" (347). It is precisely in their health narratives that the Sephardim represent the complex web of health, disease, and spiritual well-being or malaise.

Duka Nar of Salonika explained, "When a child is frightened, or even a grownup—a child falls down, or a grownup—they would have espanto. . . . The minute they fall down, they take fright." Espanto was the result of an accident or a shock when one became *danyada* or *danyado* (harmed), and the flow of the blood was disturbed. As Caden Lévy Israel said, "Espanto is that the blood *si albrota* [gets stirred up]." Our mother used the verb *alborotarse* to explain the state of the blood, which means "to come out of a customary calm, to startle; to adopt an irregular state" (Nehama 1977, 24). Thus, the blood of one who was frightened had been startled out of its customary calm and was in an irregular state. The aim of the cures for espanto was to remove this irregular state and to return to the state of calm.

This explanation of espanto as deriving from a disruption in the flow of the blood is precisely in accord with the discussion offered by George Foster in *Hippocrates' Latin-American Legacy: Humoral Medicine in the New World* (1994): "Strong emotional experiences such as *coraje* (anger), *susto* (fright), *celos* (jealousy), and *envidia* (envy) are thought to heat the body by producing a surge of bile (whose humoral quality is *irritante*) that overflows from the liver–gall bladder into the stomach and bloodstream. *Following such an experience the blood is often said to be 'irritated'* (i.e. extremely hot)" (52; our emphasis). As Foster explains, the concept of "irritated" blood derives from "the Hippocratian doctrine of the four 'humors,'" which included "blood, phlegm, black bile ('melancholy'), and yellow bile ('choler')" (1953, 202). In this system, good health depended on maintaining a balance between the four humors and with the elements of hot and cold, and wet and dry. In "Medicine in the Greek World, 800–50 B.C.," Vivian Nutton writes, "A common idea in the Hippocratic Corpus was that of health and illness as some form of balance and imbalance" (1995, 24). Nutton points out that, as the Hippocratic author of *On the Nature of Man* posited, "the body remained in stable balance until something, external or internal, occurred to overturn it" (24). With the blood irritated or heated by emotional experiences—and, specifically for our purposes, by espanto—then one's health was imperiled. As Foster elaborates, with humoral medicine, illnesses derive from "hot and cold insults . . . that upset the bodily temperature equilibrium that is believed to spell health. A hot insult produces a hot illness, while a cold insult produces a cold illness" (1994, 3). While there are parallels with the humoral medical system as explicated by Foster, still there are distinctions. The Sephardic folk medical system does not classify illnesses in the rigid dichotomy of hot and cold as is done in Hispanic America.

The symptoms of espanto were a general weakness of the body and the spirit. A person was said to be *agotado* (weak, depressed), *charpeado* (beaten down), *amorchado* (wilted, sad, scared), or *sikliado* (depressed, without strength). As Sara Nair of Istanbul explained, "We see that the sick person, *sikliado,* cries, can't sleep at night. . . . What does he have? . . . This person took an espanto, a *sikenti* [worry]." A person might also have a tightness of the chest. As another woman said, "If it is espanto, there is an *apretamiento del korason* [tightness in the heart, depression] for three days. The patient should not be frightened by this. After three days [of proper treatment], it passes."

For one young Sephardic woman, espanto came to her with the sudden appearance of her fiancé:

> I was approximately two or three months engaged, and Albert loved me quite a lot. And I loved him. At that time there was no telephone; he sent me a letter informing me, "Look, Luna, after two or three days I am going to visit you," from Bursa to Chanakali [Turkey]. I said, "Fine." I started to wash the windows to have the house clean because the fiancé was coming, so that he would find everything clean. My mother was preparing the best sweets. . . . While I was cleaning the glass, I . . . turned around, I find Albert in front of me. "Eh!" I said. The fright that I experienced, from that moment, I was, forgive me, throwing up, throwing up, throwing up. The fiancé was already eight days at home and I was throwing up.

For one young man, espanto came when he witnessed the knifing of his brother-in-law. Isaac recalls his mother, grandmother, and Salamon Corre, the man, himself, telling him about this event: "One day, as he was walking, he saw several men knife his brother-in-law, who was the manager of the Alhadeff Department Store in Antalya [Turkey]. Immediately, Mr. Corre was frightened and ever since then he suffered terribly. Every time that he looked out of the window of his house, he saw women [spirits], all dressed in white, floating outside, in the garden." As the effects from the espanto worsened, one might develop nervous ticks and begin sleepwalking. David Djerasi recalled such symptoms: "In Tel Aviv, when I was a child of ten, thieves entered the house with revolvers. The neighbors came, and grabbed the revolvers, and hit the men in the face, the head, the eyes." When he saw blood coming out of the eyes, David said, "Me tomo espanto [espanto took me]." His brother, Yacov, interrupted, "And David, from seeing the blood running [down the face], got frightened." This fright, David said, caused him to sleepwalk. In addition, he acquired certain nervous mannerisms: his head would jerk involuntarily from one side to another, and his eyes would momentarily shut tight. Another young boy who was taken with espanto moved "his head as if he were drunk, as if he were sick." One might also gradually lose muscular control and become paralyzed. Sol Konfino of Bitola (now Monastir, Bosnia) recalled, "My mother was frightened. I don't know what it was. And the face went to the side. The face changed and the ear became smaller." Sol Azuz remembered the progressive deterioration of her sister:

> She was working in a thread factory [in Istanbul]. She was pulling some threads, the owner of the factory saw it, he gave her a blow. . . . The spool got tangled. She wanted to find the end and was pulling the thread. He was annoyed that she was wasting the thread, he gave her a blow. My sister was near some steps, my sister. She was about to fall. When she came home, she had *gota* [a stroke] in both hands. . . . The hands were not working. We fed her. When she came from work, she could not eat.

> She was dropping the fork on the floor. "What do you have, Fortuna?" "I do not know. I do not know." Next day, the legs. The next day, the mouth. The following day, the body. Another day, the head fell like this [shows us that the head flipped down, shaking].

Another woman recalled a cousin from Bursa, Turkey, for whom espanto had potentially very serious consequences for her reputation.

> And after she got engaged, excuse me, for two months she did not have her period, while she was engaged. Everyone already had started talking about it. And they said, "This young lady, two months she didn't have it. What could have happened? Maybe she is pregnant." And the young lady would reply, "I'm not pregnant, I have no symptoms." At the time, there was not the *negreduras* [evil doings] of today. But still, everybody said, "What happened, what happened?" Finally, she told me that once upon a time she had had espanto. While walking with her fiancé to the movies, her shoe twisted her foot. And the heel broke off. From her embarrassment that this had happened in front of her fiancé, because of that she missed her periods.

Another woman went to the cemetery to visit the grave of her son who had died when he was sixteen years old. Sol Azuz recounted to us as we sat in her living room in Herzelia, Israel, in June 1990, "She fell there. Now, not too long ago. She fell. The lady was frightened. A day passed, the legs were not walking. She is going as a drunkard from side to side. She does not have any strength to stand."

For the people, these problems—the loss of muscular control, the vomiting, the emotional duress—could all be traced to the spirits; they were the cause of the problems resulting from espanto. Since there was a decided reluctance to name the spirits because this might have called them forth and given them power, we might best find the evidence for the mischievous part they played in health and disease in the specific wording of the espanto narratives. When one woman told of the *apretamiento* (tightness in the heart), she said it would pass in three days: "El apretar es ke le estan saliendo [The tightness of the chest means that they are leaving the individual]." While indirect in her reference, she clearly meant the spirits when she said that "they are leaving the body."

The texts of the prayers also evidenced this indirect reference in the respectful and formal pronoun *vos* (you), instead of the familiar *te* (you, singular). As Luna Levi said, "And then we used to ask, 'Vos esto dando dulsuria, ke me desh sultura [I am giving you sweetness in order that you can release me].'" In explanation, she adds, "From whom did we used to ask this? From the *malahimes* [angels]." Even here in her explicit reference to the spirits, Mrs. Levi avoids offense by referring to them as malahimes, or angels.

From analysis of the narratives, it seems that espanto was frequently connected with public embarrassment, whether this be falling down in the street or being struck by one's boss in the midst of a thread factory. There was danger in this self-exposure, in this loss of physical control in public places. The young woman who tripped and broke her heel in the street was doubly embarrassed before her fiancé and before everyone else who witnessed her gaucherie.

While one can take fright in the privacy of one's home, as when the fiancé came for a visit, the preponderance of examples we collected place the locus of espanto outside the home, in the streets. Fittingly, the cures might be initiated at the spot where the espanto took place, but the endpoint of the cure will be effected in the home. We suggest, then, that espanto had at least partially to do with the loss of bodily control in public space.

In his discussion of levels of organization of social space, DeWight Middleton refers to "the domains of home, neighborhood, and public space" (1986, 131). Of the household, Middleton writes, "The residence in which people sleep, eat, and relax is usually considered to be their first line of defense against the dangers and threats of the urban environment" (134). Neighborhoods, Middleton continues, have a "shared spatial identity based on common residence. Neighborhoods frequently . . . are characterized by heavy emotional investment on the part of neighbors" (136). Certainly for the Sephardim, there was a high degree of "emotional investment" (136) and thus a great emphasis on the "rules of public demeanor" (137). Public space was charged with a public opinion that weighed heavily on the individual, more heavily in small, close-knit communities than in the cavernous spaces of large population centers where, as Louis Wirth says, there is an emotional reserve and indifference that serves to immunize the urbanites "against the personal claims and expectations of others" (1964, 71).

Folk classifications for both diseases and emotions provide a social construction for behavior that does not "fit" or mesh with normative behavior. Specific categories of illness provide justifications for behavior, a way of making sense of the irrational. As George Foster writes, "The frightened individual realizes that his fright will probably lead to illness, and he will seize upon any general and slight symptoms of discomfort which he may have had for a long time as evidence that he has indeed been frightened, and will build them up to a degree where he and his family believe that medical treatment is necessary. The mere existence of a culturally recognized condition believed to result from fright produces patients who would never be produced in a culture without such definitions and expected patterns of reactions" (1953, 217).

Following Foster's analysis, espanto served as a magnet for many manifestations of upset or disease. This broadened, psychosocial perspective is reflected in Joseph Nehama's definition for espanto, which includes "phobias, nervous troubles, susceptibility to spiritual influences of which one is conscious and which are provoked by fear, by visions, by nightmares, by nervous debility" (1977, 193). Thus, one woman we interviewed described a saga of mental disturbances that had plagued her for several years and which included stays in mental institutions and treatment by medical doctors and psychiatrists. While her problems were clearly not only of long duration but also of great psychological depth, she made sense of them by using the magnet of espanto. As she explained, her problems had originated in the following way: "It was the eve of Passover, and as any woman who empties the wash water outside, I also did." She continued, "The ladies of the time told me that I had washed the house and threw a lot of water into the street. 'Maybe . . . you emptied the water in a place where they take it, and they harmed you. . . . Maybe at that time one of them was there and you poured water on them, that is something that can be seen. Something that can be known. It is possible that for this reason they harmed you. You have done something that touched them. They got hurt that something like this was done to them.'" In throwing out the wash water, the hapless woman had doused the spirits with water that was not just dirty but full of *hamez,* the flour and other leavening that each woman tries to scour from her house in order to have it kosher for Passover. She had compounded the insult with dirty water and hamez on the eve of Passover. The spirits took their revenge. In fastening on this explanation, the women had said to her, "that is something that can be seen. Something that can be known." Implicit in her recollection of what the women had said was the contrast with what was not seen and could not be known, namely, the diagnosis by the series of doctors: "And I went to many doctors, and they didn't understand it. . . . And the doctors, each one would tell me a different sickness. I went to one doctor, he told me one sickness; I went to another, and he told me another sickness; I went to another one, and another. . . . I went to a nerve doctor and he told me that I was crazy. And he put me in the sanatorium, in the hospital of the crazy people."

As a frame for her narrative of ill-health, this woman had, as if in passing, given another explanation for the possible strain she was under:

"I was about twenty-seven or twenty-eight years old when I became sick. It was about 1953. I had three children. The oldest one was seven years old. My daughter was five years old. And the young one was two and a half years old, when I became sick." In response to Isaac's question, "What was wrong with you?" she continued: "My husband was in the army. I did my *Pesah* [Passover] duties fine. . . . At night I went to sleep with the little one, and I played with him quite well in bed. After the child went to sleep, I noticed that someone was pulling my hair. I felt that they were pulling. I passed my hand over my head; I noticed that there was nothing. I said, 'I'm just imagining things.' I turned on my side in order to sleep. And suddenly I saw a hand that struck me here on the shoulder. When I turned around I saw behind my head a large hand." Thus, she was alone, with three children to care for, and her husband off in the army at a time of recurrent danger for Israeli soldiers. The pressures and demands on her must certainly have taken their emotional toll. However, her own explanation was not based on the stress and tension of her daily life. Nor, as she explained to us, was the encounter with the spirit, which took place in her bed, the cause of her espanto; rather it was the result of it. In other words, she was made vulnerable to the spirit through her careless actions, just hours before, of throwing water out the door and offending the passing spirits that she had carelessly doused.

The cause of her illness—offending the spirits with the dirty wash water—was not as central to her narrative as the intensity of the fear she had experienced when in the grip of the spirit's hand. It is here that lies the throbbing core of her narrative, the center of her emotional angst. Isaac asked, "Did you see the hand?" and she continued:

> Did I see the hand? A hand, very, very, very large. And the face of an animal. And he put his hand here *en la boka del korason* [in the mouth of the heart], and he started pulling everything out. . . . He started pulling, and he started pulling. And I noticed that I was going. . . . I just noticed that the soul was leaving me. I immediately ran away from the bed. And I ran to my mother-in-law who lived close by. I banged at the door, but I couldn't speak. My mother-in-law didn't want to open the door. She thought that it was an Arab who had come. She was afraid to open the door. . . . With a lot of courage, she opened the door. I fell down and passed out. They took me inside. Immediately the neighbors got up. They called the doctor. The doctor didn't understand a thing that I had. He gave me an injection to calm me down. I slept until morning. And I did rest. And this crisis always took me. When . . . the crisis came, I would start to shake.

Espanto provided one means of marking the social boundaries between behavior that was in control and that which was out of control.

Thus, a person was struck by espanto when losing control, either through one's own actions or when one was threatened with bodily harm or violence through the actions of others. However, to limit the consideration to social boundaries would be to overlook the emotive and sensual aspects, for espanto had to do with the grip of fear and with the expression of emotionally volatile behavior. The phrases *estar kon espanto* (to be in danger, to have a presentiment of fear) and *entrar espanto* (to be seized by fear) (Nehama 1977, 193) convey the feelings of danger and terror associated with espanto. Seized with such fear, the individual might have seemingly irrational outbursts, often in public places, and might behave in socially unacceptable ways. For instance, one young boy who had espanto used to remove his clothes in public. The woman who had thrown the wash water out on the eve of Passover described her behavior in the following way: "When the crisis would take hold of me, I ran into the street. It seemed to me that the street would cure me, and at home I would become sick. And I began to yell at everyone, 'Apiadame, apiadame, apiadame, me esto muriendo, apiadame! [Help me, help me, help me, I am dying, help me].' What could they have done. No one could have helped me." As conveyed in the narratives, young women were targets for espanto when in the company of their fiancés. For one woman, it was an attack of vomiting that stayed with her throughout her fiancé's visit; and for another it was the cessation of her menstrual cycle from her embarrassment at tripping in the street while walking with her fiancé.

Espanto, then, helps to enforce the boundaries of safety in terms of behavior in public, including proper control of the body, proper control of emotions, and proper control of sensuality. Blood and emotions are bound together in a potentially dangerous mix. In the guise of *los buenos de mozotros* (the good among us), the spirits stand ready to punish the one lacking in control; but they also stand ready to offer an excuse for behavior that is outside the norm. Just as with a little child who is learning to color in a coloring book, one cannot always stay inside the lines. Her markings are bound to jut outside the margins; her behavior will not fit. And she will tremble with fear from the blood that is stirred up inside of her, and for the emotions that show themselves so patently in her actions. The spirits, however, are not an easy out, for their hold is convincing and tenacious: they can pull so hard as to pull the soul from the body.

While espanto was brought on by an accident or a shock, echizos resulted from deliberate intent that involved the willful placement of objects with the conscious intention to bring harm to another. It might have been as simple as placing a piece of hair under the collar of someone's overcoat, or sprinkling salt at the entrance of a house, or putting a special powder in coffee. As Ida Varsano told us of her time in Sofia, Bulgaria, "How they did it, they used to put hair in the collar, in the collar of the overcoat, or someplace else. What did I tell you about the salt? Sometimes they would lift a stone under which they would place something. And the people would take it as an echizo." A woman from Tekirdash, Turkey, told how to make lovers *diskayer* (dislike each other, be repelled by the other): put a broom with hair and pins behind the door of the house. Another woman recalled her brother's apologizing to their mother: "Please forgive me, mother, I knew nothing of what was going on. It was Tia Kaloche who gave me something to drink in the coffee, and immediately I hated the family." Zimbul Maya Suzi told us of neighbor women in Peta Tikva who were jealous of her and had a *more* (Hebrew, teacher) prepare echizos against her. The women buried "papers, fingernails, hair, soap, everything to cause harm."

Often echizos were performed to break up an engagement, to curse a marriage with misfortune, or to win back an errant husband. A woman from Izmir recalled,

> I had an uncle who was quite educated. . . . This man loved a young lady and became engaged to her. There was another young lady who loved him. She loved him, but he refused. He went to Buenos Aires and the fiancée stayed here and later he sent for her. She ordered some bedspreads. The one who loved him placed some echizos in the bedspreads. How did they find out? Later, after she left and got married, while she was pregnant, she could not get up from the bed. She gave birth fine. A month passed, and she did not get up. Sick, sick, sick in the house. While she was covering herself one day, she found in the bedspread something hard. She took it out, they looked inside—fingernails, hair, nails, a bunch of things. A lot of things. They removed it all. My uncle went and threw it into the sea.

The woman was cured. However her husband, in the process of burning the echizo and throwing it into the sea, was affected: "The ashes that came to him, I do not know. He became paralyzed and he walked all his life with crutches."

In another instance of echizo, a wife successfully won back her husband from another woman. The husband was a taxi driver who had met a "Turkish lady."

> He fell in love with her and moved with her. The wife was very unhappy. She went to see someone who . . . asked her if her husband ever comes home. She said, "Sometimes to see the children." He said, "In the collar of the jacket that he wears, let someone smear some pork oil." He warned

her not to do it because he may abhor her rather than the other woman. She returned home and begged her mother to do it for her. When the husband came to see the children and give her some money for their upkeep, the mother did it with great care. A month later, the husband returned home. He said that the Turkish woman had ruined him; she had sold his taxi. The wife replied, "I will work as a servant and will buy you a new taxi."

In the following exchange, Isaac's mother, Caden, recounts how Isaac's uncle, who was a skilled furnituremaker, was invited into a home ostensibly to take the measurement of some windows in order to make furniture to fit the room; and while he was at work, he was bewitched by the client's mother, who wanted him to marry her daughter:

Isaac: Mama, do you want to tell me what happened to Uncle Isidor?

Caden: Uncle Isidor fell in love with Rika Luria[1] when he came to Rhodes from Adalia [Antalya, Turkey]. There was another woman who wanted to give him her daughter. . . . One day, the brother of this young lady invited Uncle Isidor to take the measurements of the windows in order to make furniture.

Isaac: Was the son already working with the mother or was he innocent [about her plans]?

Caden: No, no, no. He invited [Uncle Isidor] to his house. . . . No, he didn't know a thing about it. But the [mother] knew that he was going to go . . . there. In the afternoon, when she passed in front of the house, she said to the people, "To Isidor Lévy I gave something to eat. . . . He is not going to take Rika Luria." But we did not believe it. Two days later, Isidor came and he said, "Caden, I don't love Rika Luria. I am not going to be engaged to her." [I said,] "Well, Isidor, after all—" He said, "I am not going to be engaged. I am not going to be engaged." And he looked different, speaking, laughing. He was not normal. Then suddenly we realized, the people said that [the woman] must have done some kind of echizo.

In order to break the spell, Isaac's grandmother, another woman, and a man who paddled the boat took Uncle Isidor out to sea on the eve of Rosh Ashana at midnight: "They took him to the sea, they took him in a boat, they washed his face. He changed completely. But he didn't marry Rika. He didn't love her. He didn't love her, he abhorred her." Isaac asked, "But he was normal after that?"

Caden: Yes, he was fine. After he became engaged to Aunt Diana, married her, he was fine. When [the old woman] gave him something to eat, he was not normal. He didn't know what he was talking about. . . .

Isaac: Such cases occurred often in Rhodes?
Caden: I don't know. I didn't see anything else.

Another young man who had been bewitched was also taken to sea on Rosh Ashana for a cure. In Jerusalem in 1982, at the Judeo-Spanish Hour, which was hosted by Moshe Shaul, Isaac told the following story. In the midst of his account, a woman in the audience interrupted with part of the spell, and later, another person joined in with the result of the cure:

Isaac: In Rhodes, a man was going to marry a woman who had been chosen for him, but he fell in love with someone else. The mother of the first one, they used to call her *il guerko* [the devil], she took a broom, put hair—

Woman in the audience: And added pins.

Isaac: Pins. Put the whole thing behind the door. And they said that the man hated the one that he loved. And he was about to marry the other one. He started to lose his mind. He lost his mind. It was before Rosh Ashana. They put him in the boat, they took him to sea, and they washed his face. They gave something, I don't remember what. He went home and slept for twenty-four hours. When he woke up—

Another person in the audience: He recognized the one he loved.

Isaac: He recognized the one he loved.

In Izmir, we spoke with our Aunt Rachel and Uncle Yeoshua, who recalled their engagement years earlier. At first, everything was fine for the couple; but when Uncle Yeoshua, who was living in Milas, Turkey, came to visit Aunt Rachel, she was struck with nausea:

Rachel: When Uncle Yeoshua told me that he was coming to Izmir to see me, suddenly I felt stomachaches, pains, I couldn't eat. I became yellow. He used to come, I couldn't eat. When I ate, I felt like throwing up.

Yeoshua: Then we used to spend one or two days together. Then it would pass.

Rachel: But still, as long as he was there, I did not feel well. I used to call the doctor. Maybe something was wrong with my stomach. The doctor would come and say, "*Ah, Dio!* [Oh, God!] There is nothing wrong with that young lady." My grandmother would say, "What's wrong with her? . . . . The *novio* [fiancé] leaves and she eats like a human being."

Uncle Yeoshua insisted that this was because she was tormenting herself about the engagement, and he added, "I, no. I was very courageous.

And I, as I was about to leave for Milas, would say, 'Rachel, don't be afraid. Everything will pass.'" Aunt Rachel's father located a Turkish *hodja* (Muslim religious leader) who determined that she had been bewitched and who "undid this echizo." Uncle Yeoshua continued, "He didn't want to tell us anything about the echizo. From what the hodja said, he went to the place where the echizo was placed [in the cemetery], took it, and undid it." Aunt Rachel concluded, "My father came home, and he changed my name. Instead of my name, Rachel, he called me Sara. They kept calling me this for awhile. He also placed an amulet on me. And I wore this amulet until I gave birth. The amulet was prepared by the hodja." Uncle Yeoshua added, "I'm not sure, but someone in Izmir must have caused an echizo for Aunt Rachel." "*Seguro!* [Certainly!]," Aunt Rachel affirmed.

A young man was also stricken with nausea when he sat down to eat with his fiancée and her family. "It was a good family from Milas. . . . The mother always prepared good food, and when they knew we were coming, they would set the best table. And that poor man, every time he looked at the food, it looked like demons. Anything he ate, he would vomit it up. Several times in a row it would happen. He said, 'I love her. The family is good. But something has to be done.' Finally, they separated. . . . They found out that there was an echizo." The echizo had been done by a woman from Istanbul who was in love with the young man. In this case, the spell worked for he broke off the engagement with his fiancée. As we were told, "Ironically, he married the one who had made the echizo. They went to America and they are okay now, and they have a lot of children."

For another family, fighting in the home was a sign that an echizo had been done. Mary Algrante from Izmir told us about "a not too distant relative" who married and then was tormented by her mother-in-law, and consequently she "was always nervous" and fought with her husband. This, Mrs. Algrante assured us, resulted in "total unrest in the house. They lived near the sea. An aunt of hers went to the seashore, where cabins were located, and found a knot, something tied. Inside there were fingernails, hair, and rusted nails. She took the whole thing and burned it." The echizo was undone, and the fighting stopped. When asked how the aunt had found the items on the beach, Mrs. Algrante responded, "She went and searched because it was known that the mother-in-law performed echizos."

In another account, a woman who wanted the husband of another woman worked a spell on the wife in the Turkish bath. "From the moment she entered the Turkish bath, until she left, the enemy had her fingers like this [all twisted up]." The spell worked not on the wife but rather on her husband, who became *atado* (tied up, impotent). "And they all tried to find out what was the reason for the hate, until they found out the person who did that. And they went to her to beg, to give her a lot of money. And this one had the power to *dezatarlo al marido* [untie the husband]. And I heard that many men were *dezatados* [untied], and they did find the culprit, and she released them. The culprit would let her fingers go and that would untie them. And the men would regain their full force."

Another person told a story about "a handsome man" who fell in love "with an ugly Turkish-Armenian girl." "I have a friend whose older brother abhorred his girlfriend and fell in love with someone who was not Jewish, half Turkish and half Armenian. The mother of this woman, who was Armenian, performed an echizo on this young man. Truly, today he is still young, handsome, and he could have had the best, but he fell in love with someone like that. The mother of the young man wanted to know how he could fall for that Turkish-Armenian when they were so many young [Jewish] women." The mother asked for help from an *indivina* (diviner). The diviner indicated that she needed the help of a young girl "not yet thirteen years old," in other words, a girl who was not yet menstruating: "The mother took the young sister to the diviner, who went with the girl alone to a cemetery. She told her, 'All that you are going to see in this *unya* [finger nail] you are going to tell later.' The young girl was telling me the story herself. She said that she saw in the fingernail Mme. Marie, the mother of the [Turkish-Armenian] girl, who went to the grave, took some hair. She took pins, tied it all together. She saw her babbling. She didn't hear what she was saying. And she stuffed all of this inside the grave. And the diviner, when the young girl told her where the echizo was located, she . . . said, 'I now *dezati los echizos* [untied the witchcraft].' Still this young man married her, and they live now in Tel Aviv." The person relating this story explained that Mme. Marie, in working the echizo, "*le ato il mazal* [had tied up the luck] of the young man." In conclusion, she added, "And he could not see any other young lady. And he married her."

The young man in the foregoing story was not able to escape the spell cast by the Turkish-Armenian mother: he married the "half Turkish and half Armenian" daughter. However, Rosa di Bero, who was born in Rhodes and came to Seattle in 1919, told Isaac a story of a young Jewish girl who eventually was able to escape the spell of a Turkish man. "A woman worked in a house; the man [of the house] worked in the courts in the time of the Turks. He had a Turkish friend, he was black, who worked in the court with him. The maid was a beautiful lady, white as [not audible]. [The black man] fell in love with her. Whatever he tried, he did not succeed. What did he do? He made an *echizo kon un kendiziko*[2] [echizo with a little piece of candy]. 'Eat this candy,' he said, 'It is good for the health.'" When Isaac asked what the Turkish man had put in the candy, Mrs. di Bero said, "The echizo he made as a candy in order for her to eat it, and said, 'I want you to eat this candy; you are so nice. Eat this candy, you don't have to come [with me]. It does not matter.' Upon eating the candy, she said, 'Let's go.'" Mrs. di Bero continued, "The candy she ate, and she changed: Do you understand? And she went with the black man. . . . She was with him, and she got pregnant. . . . He loved her. She went. She gave birth. She was with him at home nine months. She gave birth [to a baby boy]." During the birth, "the echizo fell from inside," and she realized what had happened. Mrs. di Bero explained, "She left the baby, she left everyone. She ran away. Her husband was not even at home. . . . As soon as she got home, the family immediately hid her and sent her to America. She came here. She got married and had a family. She was very nice with her husband."

In order to protect oneself against echizos, one might use a countermeasure. For instance, one might sprinkle salt or pour urine at the entrance of one's house. Or, as one person told us, a wife might guard against the charms of another woman in the following manner: "There are people who say that in order to prevent the husband from leaving for another woman, one should take a piece of the net of fishing, and sew it in the pants." A woman from Tekirdash, Turkey, recounted how a parent might prevent a son from marrying a non-Jew: the mother made *burekas* (individual pastries) filled with feces from her son "and gave some to the young lady to eat. This was a sure way to make her hate the young man."

To counter more powerful and complicated echizos, as has been indicated in the accounts above, the stricken one must often rely on the good sense of others. A mother, father, sister-in-law, or other relative might decide that a specialist should be consulted, either a diviner or a *hodja.* Sometimes the countermeasures could be placed in the hands of a knowledgeable older woman, as in the case of Isaac's grandmother and her friend who took his Uncle Isidor to the sea on the eve of Rosh Ashana for a cure against the echizo that had rendered him temporarily fickle in love and unbalanced in his emotions.

As a countermeasure for an echizo, one might locate it and literally undo it. When something hard fell out of the bedspread, the woman "took it out, they looked inside—fingernails, hair, nails, a bunch of things." Then they burned it, and the husband "threw it into the sea." The indivina took the young, pre-pubescent girl to the cemetery to help locate the echizo so that the indivina could take apart the witchcraft. For the young Jewish girl who was seduced by the Turkish man, it was enough for her to see the echizo fall "from inside" when she gave birth. She did not need to take it apart to realize that she had been bewitched.

Echizos were often made from items that were regarded as inherently polluting. These included the leavings of the body—nail parings, hair, urine, and feces—and the taboo animal for both Muslims and Jews, the pig, for pig oil was used to turn the husband's affections away from his Turkish lover and back to his wife. At times, the same substance could be used to protect against echizos or to work echizos. Urine, salt, or hair could be hidden at the entrance of the house either to work a spell or to guard the family against harm. And at times a substance otherwise harmless, such as coffee or a specific food, was rendered dangerous through the intent to harm, with perhaps an added ingredient. The young boy hated his family because "Tia Kaloche . . . gave me something to drink in the coffee"; the woman who wanted Uncle Isidor as her son-in-law gave him "something to eat"; the Turkish man gave the young Jewish girl a piece of candy that he said was "good for the health."

The echizos of the Sephardim share in the principles of magic that James George Frazer expounded in his twelve-volume *The Golden Bough* (1890–1915). According to Frazer, magic operates on the assumption of sympathy between objects. This "sympathetic magic" manifests itself in two fundamental principles: first, the Law of Similarity, "that *like produces like*"; and second, the Law of Contact or Contagion, "that *things which have once been in contact continue ever afterwards to act on each other*" (1968, 80). The Law of Similarity is carried out by homeopathic magic; and the Law of Contact or Contagion, by contagious magic. The young fiancés who were bewitched and who no longer loved their betrothed were taken to sea at midnight on the eve of Rosh Ashana. The timing of the cure was crucial, for, following homeopathic magic, like things influence like things. The ill fortune of the old year could be washed into the sea; and the good fortune of the new year would wash over the young man who had been cleansed of the echizo. The woman who twisted her fingers in order to tie up the fertility of her victim was incorporating the principle of homeopathic magic: the husband's virility would be tied up and knotted as her fingers were.

Through the very components of many echizos, contagious magic was frequently at the core. As Frazer writes, "The most familiar example of Contagious Magic is the magical sympathy which is supposed to exist between a man and any severed portion of his person, such as his hair or nails; so that whoever gets possession of human hair or nails may work his will, at any distance, upon the person from whom they were cut" (1968, 102). In *Semitic Magic,* Thompson also remarks on this personal connection: "the magician should know something, even if only the name, of the person or demon whom he hoped to bring into subjugation. The origin of this would appear to have arisen in the beliefs about hair, rags, or nail-parings, which are collected and wrought into the charm as the connecting links between it and the victim. If these are wanting, then the name alone will be enough" (1971, l–li). As one Sephardi cautioned: "When someone cut his nails, my grandfather paid attention until even the smallest piece would be put in the *numero siete* [number seven, toilet]. It is said that if even a small piece falls down, the *sheddim* [spirits] come immediately. Also no one should step on it. A witch could take these nails and make echizos with them and cause evil to a person. . . . When someone wanted to perform an echizo, he took hair from the person . . . against whom they wanted to make an echizo." Several of the echizos referred to in the foregoing accounts incorporated fingernails and hair. In one instance, the echizo that was hidden in the bedspread was made up of "fingernails, hair, nails, a bunch of things"; and the echizo found at the seashore, which had caused fighting in the home, was made of "fingernails, hair, and rusted nails." Pregnant women were warned against stepping on fingernails, for to do so would cause them to miscarry.

In addition to contagious magic, echizos also worked on the principle of homeopathic magic. For example, one incorporated iron nails, which would pierce the relationship. The echizo hidden in the bedspread was "hard," thus rendering the young woman's pregnancy and postpartum recovery "hard"; and the echizo hidden at the seashore was tied in a knot, which tied up the love between the husband and wife. When Aunt Rachel's father changed her name—"Instead of my name, Rachel, he called me Sara"—both homeopathic and contagious magic were at work. By changing the name, it was as if she had become a new person, because the name of the person influences who that person is. The echizo that had been done to Rachel would have no effect on the new person of Sara. Additionally, the principle of contagious magic was used, because the old name, which had been in contact with the person, was discarded and it ceased to have an effect on her person.

Theodor Gaster, in his critique of Frazer, adds to the concept of contagious magic the notion of the extended self. "The self, or identity, of a person" is not only in the "physical being" but rather "embraces also everything associated with it and everything that can evoke" the presence of the person in another's mind. "Thus, the shadow, name, footprint, gait, dress, excreta, portrait, etc., of a person are just as much an essential and integral part of him as his body, the more so since they can bear evidence of him even when he is corporeally absent. . . . To bless or curse his name, for example, or to perform acts with portions of his clothing, will 'touch' him—that is, 'him' in his full, extended being—just as much as to punch him or caress him" (Gaster 1968, 118). Following Gaster, then, to change the name would be to renew the person—Rachel becomes Sara. The extension of the self and contagious magic would also be at work in the practice of washing the steps where a young man passed in order to undo his love: "When they wanted him to hate a person, for him not to marry . . . a young lady, they used to take silk cloth, they washed the steps through which the young man would pass, and he walked over them, he would hate the *novia* [fiancée]." In this echizo, the young man stepped, as it were, into a void: the space where his foot fell had been cleansed by the silk cloth. As it was empty so would his love be empty. In this instance, there is homeopathic magic (the place for his foot to fall is empty), contagious magic (there is physical contact with his body), and extended self (erasing the path of his previous footsteps to his love). Homeopathic magic, contagious magic, and the extended self combine as well in the bureka made of feces. The mother used the feces of her son—contagious magic—to form the filling of the pastry fed to the one whose love for her son she wished to destroy. The extended self was present in the bureka, and the pastry itself formed a model—homeopathic magic—of a love affair that had gone afoul.

In the narratives about echizos, there was always a sense of boundary, an implicit—and sometimes explicit—message that "we don't do that, they do!" The workers of the echizos were those not part of the social group; they were not good, well-educated, well-behaved Sephardim. They included, as we have seen from the accounts, the following: a Turkish lady—which means she was Muslim—who stole the Sephardic woman's husband, and who then drove him to financial ruin and even "sold his taxi"; the Armenian mother who worked an echizo on a young man so he would love her "half Turkish and half Armenian" daughter; the black Turk—again, this means Muslim—who put an echizo in a piece of candy in order to win the affections of a beautiful Sephardic girl. In one instance, the woman who worked the echizo to alienate a man's affections was Sephardic, but she was called *guerko* (devil) and therefore was not of the same class as Sephardim of good background.

There is a contradiction in this attribution of echizos to the Muslim, the Armenian, or "the devil." Quite obviously, a good many of the echizos were crafted and carried out by Sephardim. This is clearly apparent in the narrative accounts themselves. When Isaac asked a woman who was originally from Istanbul if any echizos had occurred in her family, she responded: "I have heard [of such things] from our grandmothers. That when they had an enemy, that they wanted for him to die, they took soap with a lot of pins, and during the day they dropped it into the well and one said, 'Asegun se derite este shavon ansina ke se dirate la persona [As this soap melts, thus this person should melt].' And it did melt. . . . And the person died." To Isaac's question, "And the Jews? Did the Jews do that?" the woman responded, "The Jews did not dare do that. But maybe there were some, it was not in my power." And she repeated, "In my power, no. In my power it was not. This we heard from the *nonas*, from our mothers." When Uncle Yeoshua ended his account about Aunt Rachel's health problems during their engagement, he said, "I'm not sure, but someone in Izmir must have caused an echizo for Aunt Rachel." Isaac asked, "Did the Jewish people make the echizos?" and Uncle Yeoshua responded quickly and emphatically, "No, the Jewish people did not make the echizos."

By excluding the Jewish people from these deliberately malevolent acts of fabricating and performing echizos, the Sephardim with whom we spoke drew the line between the social and the antisocial. They claimed that echizos were clearly outside the pale of Sephardic social life. There was this "disclaimer" of echizos, we suggest, for two reasons: (1) the Sephardim felt a need to distance themselves from the deliberate nature and evil intent of echizos; and (2) they desired to present themselves on a higher social level, for those who worked echizos were *basha*, or low class.

For those who told us of their experiences with espanto, there was no need to draw a sharp boundary. Espanto was simply a marker of that which was socially embarrassing for them at the time. Those who had suffered from espanto had been victims of the spirits' malevolence, and they had not attempted to harness the ill-will of the spirits for their own ends.

Imbalance in emotions was at the core of ill health, whether this was from the envy of the evil eye, the embarrassment of espanto, or the malevolence of echizo. To restore health, one had to strive to restore a balance both socially and spiritually. The cures, and the divinations of illness, were directed towards restoring this balance—towards exploding the envy, dissolving the espanto, and erasing the echizo. The one who was suffering was restored to health by the gentle hands of the curer, the good woman, who was knowledgeable of both the Sephardic pharmacopeia and the Sephardic universe. The social, the spiritual, and the medicinal were all blended in a healing balm that eased the sting of pain and the ache of a broken heart.

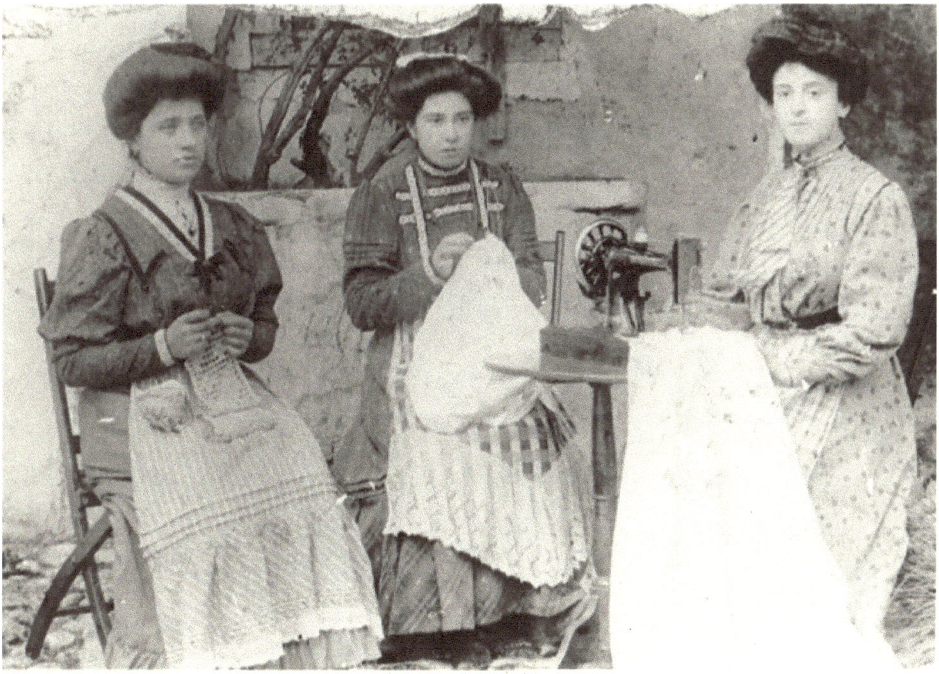

Sephardic women engaged in handcrafts, c. 1910. Lévy-Zumwalt Collection.

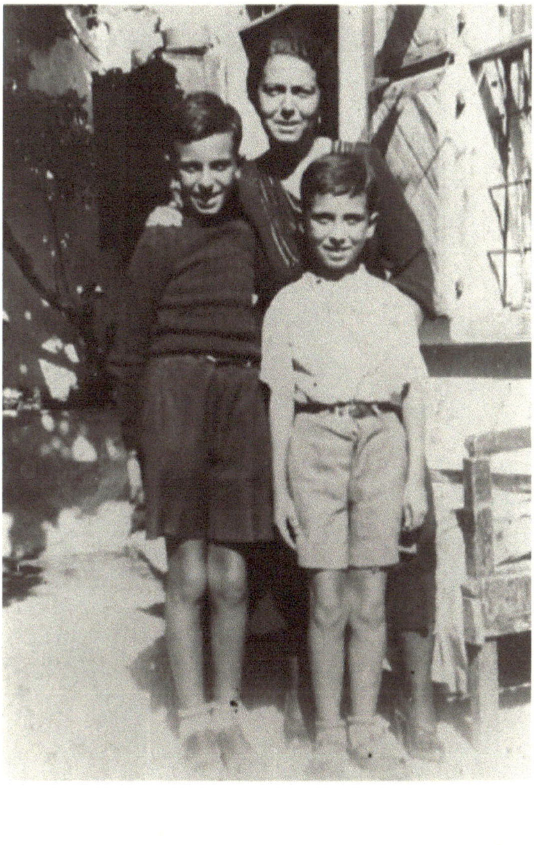

The Lévys in the patio of their home in Rhodes, 1935. Left to right: Julian, Caden, and Isaac. Lévy-Zumwalt Collection.

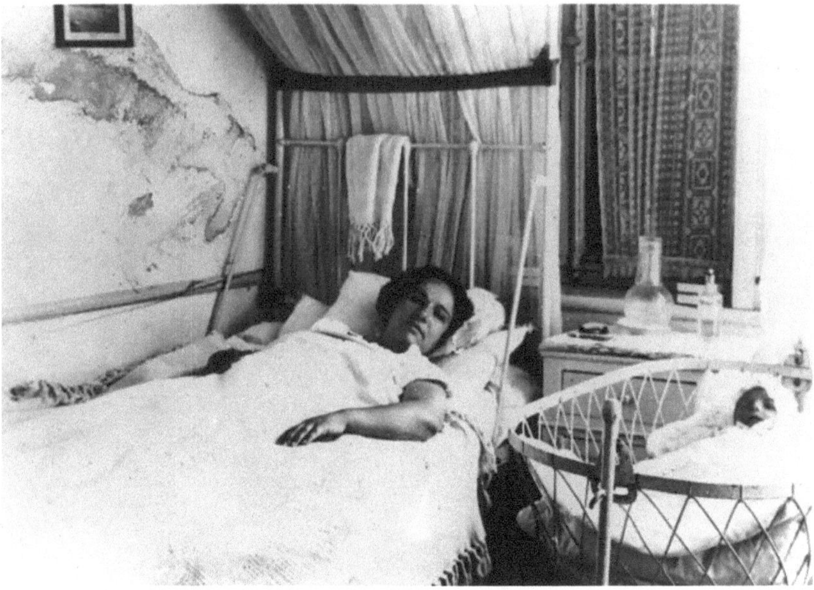

A mother and her newborn at home in Rhodes, c. 1920s. The *namusia* (netting) is tucked behind the head of the bed. Lévy-Zumwalt Collection.

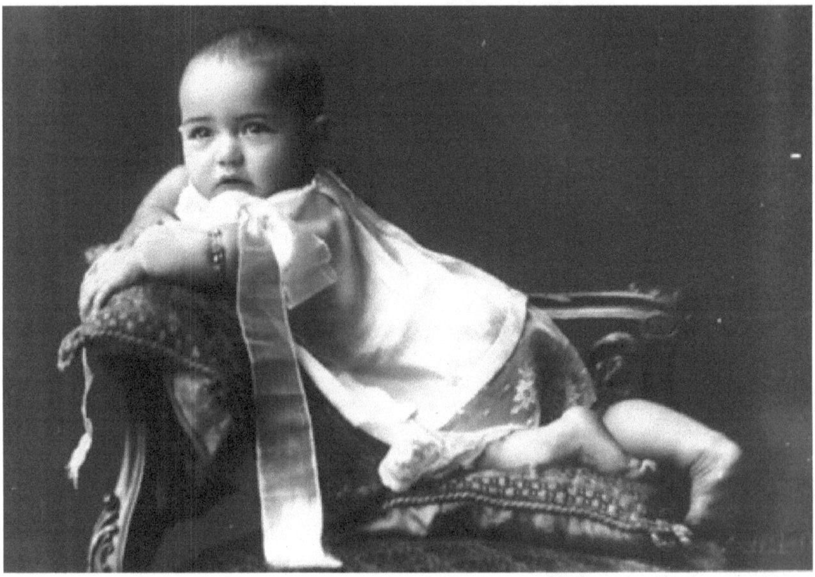

Seven-month-old baby girl, 1924, Rhodes. She wears a beaded gold bracelet on her arm. Lévy-Zumwalt Collection.

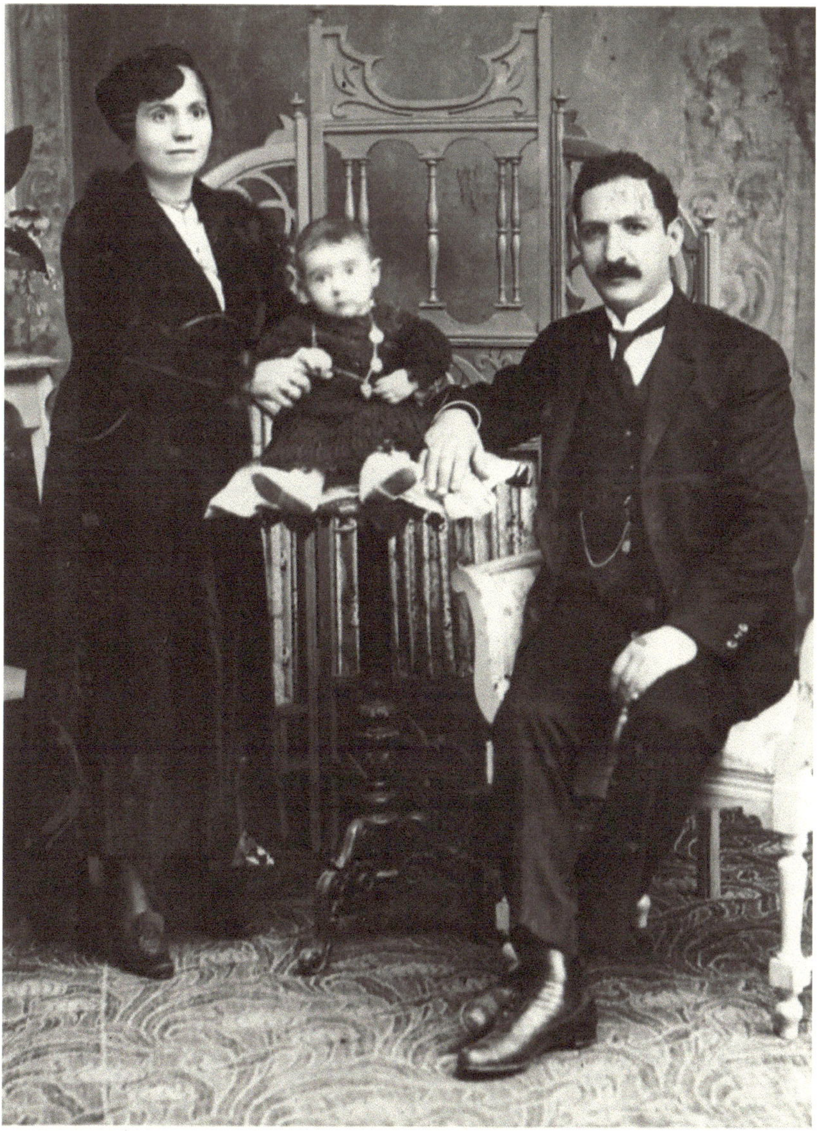

Sephardic family in Turkey; the baby wears a necklace with three gold amulets. Courtesy of Beth Hatefutsoth, Museum of the Jewish Diaspora, Tel Aviv.

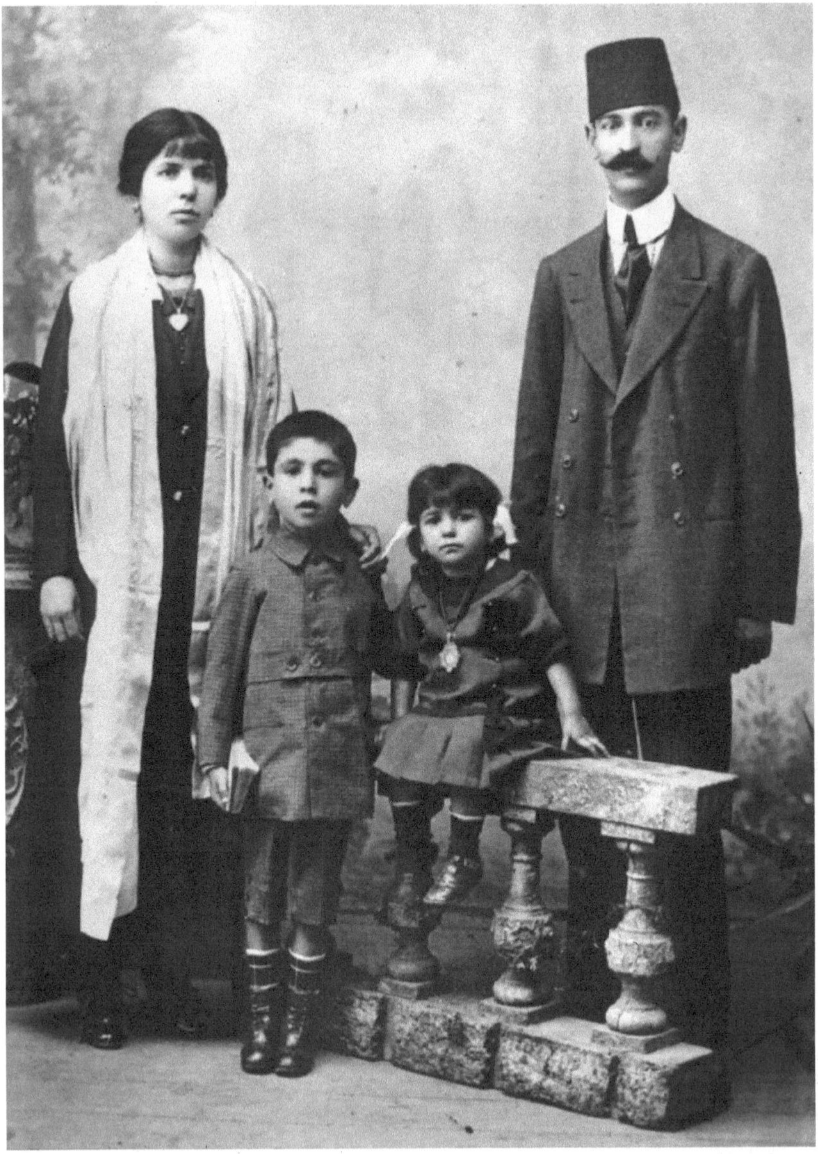

The Filosof family, Edirne, Turkey, 1922. Mr. Filosof was the director of the Jewish Community in Edirne. Mrs. Filosof and her daughter wear gold amulets. Courtesy of Beth Hatefutsoth, Museum of the Jewish Diaspora, Tel Aviv.

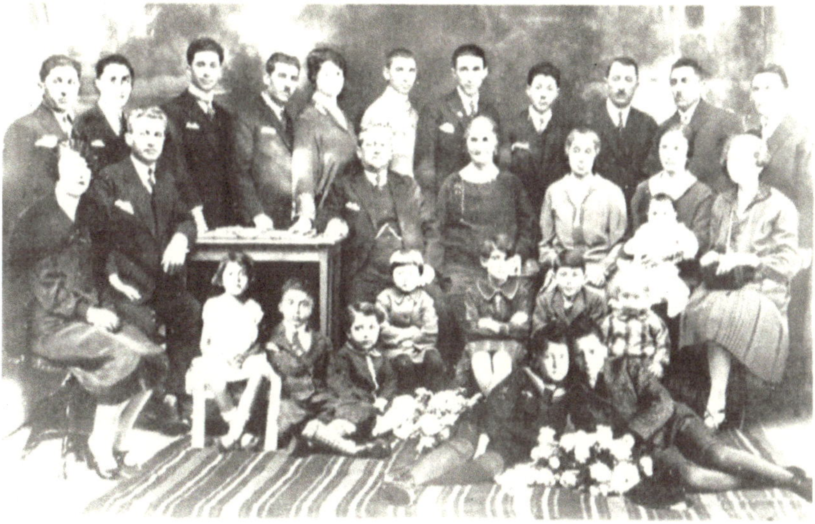

The Abravanel family, Pirot, Yugoslavia, c. 1920. Heads of garlic have been tucked behind the full blooms of the roses in the foreground to protect the family against the evil eye. Courtesy of Rachel Levy.

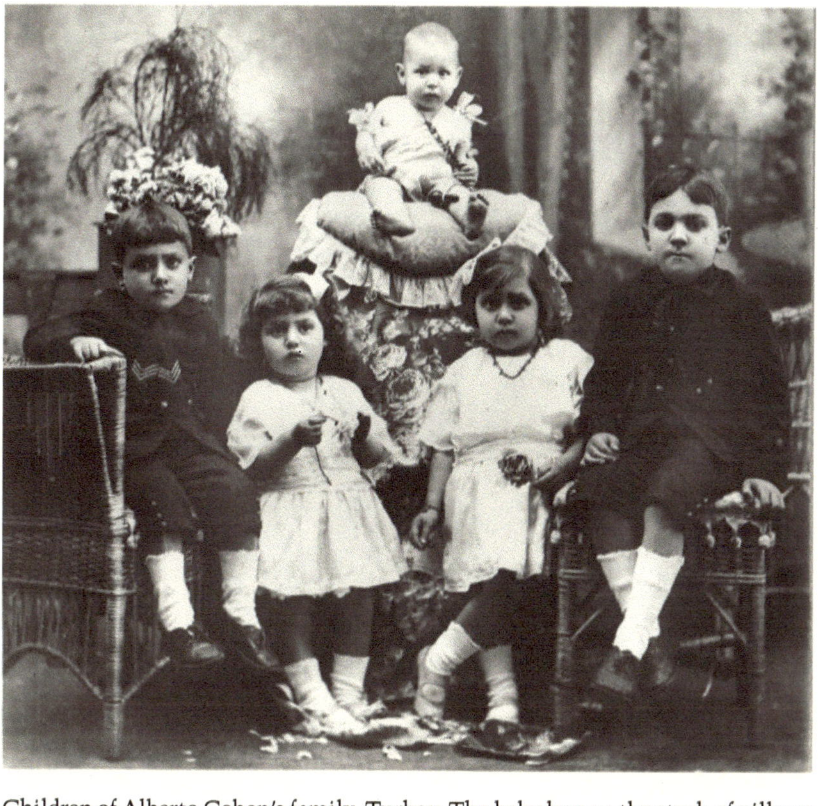

Children of Alberto Cohen's family, Turkey. The baby boy on the stack of pillows wears a garland of cloves as protection against the evil eye. Courtesy of Beth Hatefutsoth, Museum of the Jewish Diaspora, Tel Aviv.

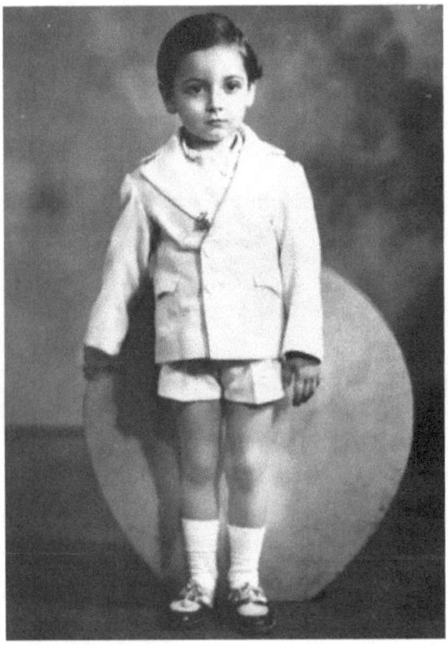

Little Sephardic boy from Rhodes with gold amulet around his neck. Lévy-Zumwalt Collection.

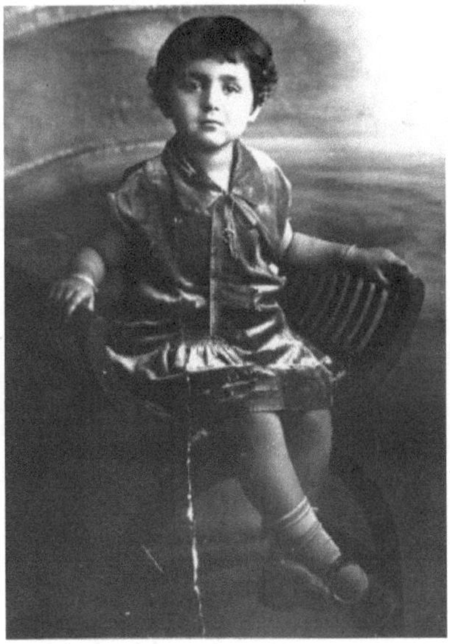

Little Sephardic girl from Rhodes with gold amulet necklace. Lévy-Zumwalt Collection.

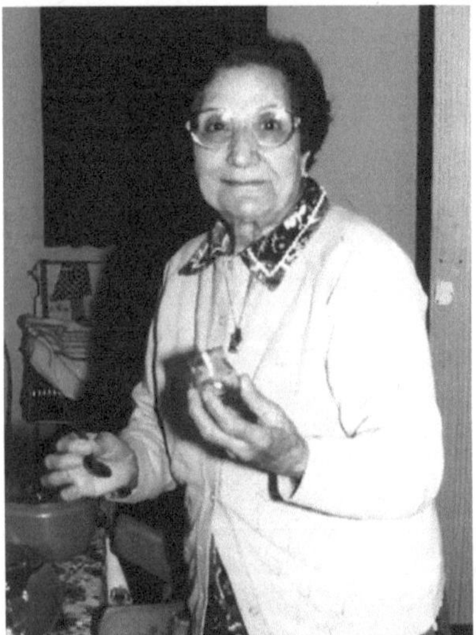

Deborah Sarfati, Bet Avot Leon Recanati, 1990. Mrs. Sarfati is holding a *ventosa* (cupping) glass in her hand. Lévy-Zumwalt Collection.

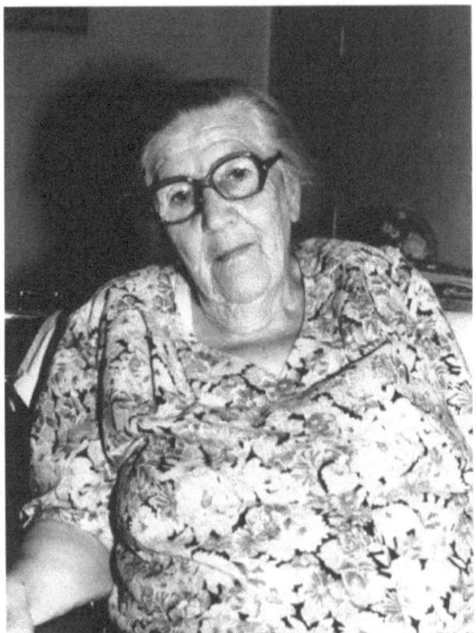

Lea Amram, a typical Sephardic grandmother who shared many remembrances with us, Bet Avot Kryat Segal, Ramat Efal, Israel, 1990. Lévy-Zumwalt Collection.

7 The Treasured Medicine and the Blessed Cure

> In the name of God, here I cut your fear. And you give two pinches of sugar. And God willing, this is the remedy.
>
> —Caden Lévy Israel

To restore health, one used a *segula,* which might be a medicinal plant, such as marjoram, garlic, rosemary, or rue, or a substance, such as salt, sugar, honey, coffee, or urine. The Judeo-Spanish meaning derived from the Hebrew, *segula,* which meant valued object, possession, treasure, or remedy. By extension for the Sephardim, a segula was a valued cure, or petition, used to restore good health to one who had been harmed.[1] To cure someone who was ill, one had to determine the cause of the problem, whether this came from the evil eye, from *espanto* or from *echizo.* For mild cases, one might know immediately the origin of the problem or one might divine the cause, for instance, by analyzing dreams or performing *livianos* (divination through the use of molten lead).

As the Sephardim told us, the cure for the evil eye was known as *azer por ayin arah* (to do, perform for evil eye), and the cure for espanto, as *azer por espanto* (to do, perform for espanto). While there was no designation for degrees of affliction for the evil eye, there was for espanto. The severity of illness could vary from a mild case, *espanto mas liviano* or *espanto un poko manko puro* (light espanto); to a more serious case, *espanto mucho* or *grande espanto* (great espanto); to *puro espanto* (pure/real espanto); to *espanto preto* (dark, awful espanto) (Nehama 1977, 193);

to the most severe, *espanto negro* (dreadful espanto). One determined the type of cure according to the severity of the espanto.

Salt could be used as a cure for the evil eye. One might throw a handful of salt into the toilet and urinate on it, while saying, "Asegun se esta dizaziendo la sal, ke se dezaga el nazar ke tengo yo enriva [As the salt is dissolving, so may the evil eye that I have on me (dissolve)]." Or, as Benny Nahmias recounted, one might put some salt in a dish and leave it outside overnight in the courtyard of the house. In the morning, the dish would be filled with water, and this would be used to wash the face of a child "from the bottom to the top, and the following words uttered: 'Ijo de Sara, sano i rezio [k'este] i ke biva [Son of Sara, may he be healthy and strong, and live (a long life)].'" The process would be repeated three times and the unused water would be scattered in the courtyard in three different directions, thus magnifying the results by the magical number three. One might also take some salt to the synagogue for a blessing and then sprinkle it in the streets, as one women explained: "They also used salt. They went to the synagogue. And then they sprinkle it in three different streets. And then the *ayin arah* is gone."

Urine was used as both a liquid of purification and of pollution. Thus, the stricken one could be bathed with urine to wash away the evil eye, and this urine could then be thrown out as a source of impurity. Lisa Dasa, who was born in Jerusalem, recalled, "A lot of us used to take urine. Among us it is called *pishu* (piss). We did not call it *urina* (urine), we called it pishu. We used to wash the child with urine. Three times the face, the legs, and the hands, and we threw it outside the door of the house." The evil eye was then transferred to the one who passed by. Mrs. Dasa continued, "The neighbor had to pass and step over the urine that we emptied in the street. But we had an idea that it was she who caused the evil eye to the child. It did not bother the neighbor because she did not know what it was. And that is the way that was." In this cure, Frazer's principle of contagious magic was employed: the harm was washed off the child into the urine, which was thrown into the street; the one who passed by "caught" the evil eye through magical contagion. Lisa Dasa apparently wished to minimize this transference of harm, since she offered the assurance that this person would not be "bothered" because she was unaware of what had been done.

Josifov Lusi of Bulgaria recalled a cure for the evil eye from her grandmother, who would take a piece of blue paper, perforate it all over, and place it on the head of the stricken one. Then she would say, "Ke se vayan todos los males [May all harm disappear]." Finally, she would light the paper. The color blue would protect against the evil eye; the holes were to puncture or break away the evil eye; and the burning of the paper would burn up the evil eye. Luzga Alsaid, originally of Filiben, Bulgaria, recalled that blue paper was used in conjunction with other remedies. One should take a small amount of dirt or small stones from the spot where the person was frightened, mix a little water, three cubes of sugar, and add a piece of blue paper, which had been perforated with small holes. For three nights, before going to sleep, one would smear some of the mixture on the face and chest of the stricken one, and say, "'Ke se vayan todos los males [May all harm go].' The last night, after smearing some, whatever is left is thrown out of the window, and, again, say, 'May all the harm go.'"

Another cure, *limpiar patines* (to wash the steps), involved washing the steps of the one who had caused the evil eye and then giving some of the dirty water to the stricken one to drink. Caden Lévy Israel explained, "They took a wet rag, something wet, they washed the steps, and from this water they gave him some to drink." The person washing the steps would say a blessing, such as "Salud para Isaac iju di Caden [Health for Isaac, son of Caden]." Our mother concluded, "They gave to drink from this water, they put the person to sleep and often he would find remedy." By washing the steps of the one who had caused the evil eye, one was symbolically undoing the contagion. In a sense, then, this was first a reversal of contagious magic—the evil eye was washed away—and then a transference of the evil eye through contagious magic: the one who gave the evil eye received it again by stepping on the contaminated urine.

One might also use *brazikas* (pieces of coal) to rid a person of the evil eye. As Nehama explains, *las brazikas* was "a remedy of a good woman against psychological troubles. . . . One rotates a metal pan with three burning coals over the head of a patient while pronouncing magical formulae" to set the spirits to flight (1977, 99). Buka Bohor, orginally of Kustendil, Bulgaria, explained that to *echar brazikas* (to cast, perform brazikas), "You would take a grill with coal, light it, and let it burn down; you would take a piece of coal and drop it into the water. And then with some formulas, such as '*Kon el nombre del Dio* [In the name of God],' you would ask for good cures, always asking for good things. And God used to help us." Deborah Sarfati recalled this custom from Salonika, "The brazikas were coal, they would light as fire. . . . When the brazikas were really hot, they would put them in a metal pot with water. They put it on top of the head, and then they would drop the coals inside. And then they would say, 'Avraam, Itzhak, Yakov,' and . . . some women knew how to pray." As the coals were dropped in the water, there would be a hissing noise, which was believed to be the sound of the evil eye being released from the body (Nehama 1977, 99).

Sugar was used extensively always to sweeten the disposition of the spirits and to lead them away from the stricken one. In her 1891 book about Jewish women in Turkey, Lucy Garnett noted the following cure: "When children are panic-stricken, sugar is strewn from their beds to a neighbouring cistern, in the hope that the demon who has caused the mischief, and who has a sweet tooth, will follow the track and tumble into the water" (67). Here the "demon" was enticed away from the child by the sugary path and was led to the cistern of the neighbors, so that the evil had been effectively transferred into a body of water belonging to someone else.

A woman from Izmir, Turkey, recalled that for espanto her mother used to take nine pinches of sugar in her hand and say, "Asukar del kuti, melezina para ti [Sugar from the can, medicine for you]." The mother would take "nine pinches, nine times," thus trebling the magical number three for both the pinches of sugar and the times it was administered.[2] Each time she would place some of the sugar in the mouth of the person with espanto. "And the rest she placed in a dish with some water and she cleaned the face with it. And this was good. This is segula [cure]."

One could cast sugar in the street, or in a body of water, preferably the sea, at any time. It was a simple, accessible cure that was believed to bring quick relief for a mild case of espanto. Immediately after a fall, one would go home, grab a little sugar, and return to the spot where the espanto took place. While casting the sugar, one might say, "Ni mal ize, ni mal ke me aga [Neither evil did I do, nor evil should he do to me]," or "Entre buena djente lo echo [Among the good people (the spirits) I throw it]," or "Milizina para tu 'spantu [Medicine for your espanto]." As Caden Lévy Israel explained, "And they would give the one with fright a little [sugar and water] to drink. And this also helped many times." Sometimes no words were uttered: "Many times they didn't say a word. They would just pour the water where the person fell. He was sitting down, he saw something, he got frightened. There, where it was, they would pour a little water with sugar. And this helped him. Many times."

If one had taken fright at the sea, one could *echar la asukar a la mar* (cast the sugar into the sea). While throwing the sugar, one would say, "Kon el nombre del Dio Santo, / melezina por espanto. / Todos los males se vayan a la ondura de la mar [In the name of the Holy God, / cure for fright. / May all evil go to the bottom of the sea]." A slightly more elaborate form of this cure was done on the eve of Rosh Ashana, the Jewish New Year. After the services and the dinner, one took the sugar from the table in the name of the sick person and gathered up the tablecloth, which had not been cleaned. The stricken one, along with the curers, went to the shore at two in the morning. Then they removed all but the underclothes of the patient, walked into the sea, and dunked him or her three times. They placed the tablecloth over the head and gave the stricken one three pinches of the sugar, each time saying, "Kon il nombri dil Dio [In the name of God]." Afterwards, they took the stricken one home to bed. As Mrs. Katz, originally of Rhodes, said, "Thank God. With the help of God, he woke up healthy."

One might revisit the spot where one had taken espanto. As it was explained to us, "At midnight, they would go to that spot. At midnight, nobody should be there, no noise. They put sugar, and they would say, 'Mal no izites, mal ke no te agan [You did not do any harm, and no harm should they do to you].' They would sprinkle sugar three times. They would go home without turning their back to the spot for about ten or fifteen steps." This was always done with someone else present, or as we were warned, "Otherwise he could be frightened all over again." Luna Levi of Bet Avot Leon Recanati provided an explanation for this cure: "I got espanto, and I suspect that I got it over here. At night, I take sugar, I mix it with water. And at midnight when everybody is already in bed, I go down and I pour this water, and I return slowly, slowly. 'Vos do dulsuria, ke me desh sultura [I give you sweetness, in order that you may release me].' I tell them that three times. I come up and I go to bed. The day passes, I am all right." Luna explained that she was giving sweetness, that is, pouring sugar and water on the spot, for "the *malahimes* [angels]." When Isaac asked, "To the *malahimes buenos o a los negros* [good or bad angels]," Luna said emphatically, "To the good ones!!! The good ones give *soltura* [release]! The evil ones do more harm."

For a cure for espanto called *asukar a la mezuza* (sugar at the mezuzah), one would put three pinches of sugar into three little packets while standing at the mezuzah, and one would say, "In il nombri dil Dio, Avraam, Itzhak, i Yaako, Moshe, Aron, David, i Shelomo [In the name of God, Abraham, Isaac, and Jacob, Moses, Aron, David, and Salomon]." As Diana Cadranel of Rhodes explained, "You are going to say this formula and going to place in each paper a pinch of sugar and you are going to close it. Afterwards, you are going to drink one before the night, the other at midnight, and the last one at dawn."

Mary Algrante from Izmir also told us about a similar cure, *kave a la mezuza* (coffee at the mezuzah). She said, "If the person was frightened, it is a segula [cure]." As Mary explained the procedure, "They mixed the coffee, nine pinches, and nine of sugar. Nine of coffee and nine of sugar, and they *meldavan* [prayed] under the mezuzah. What is *meldar*? To read, to pray to God to be the medicine, to cure each person, daughter of such a person, and they gave it to her in three installments. [First] *de prima noche* [early evening] . . . three pinches. *A media noche* [at midnight], three, and *a la madrugada* [at dawn], three." Another person explained, "When somebody was without any strength or didn't feel well, they would go to the mezuzah. They used to use [sugar or coffee], and say, 'Kon il nombre dil Dio, Avraam, Itzhak, i Yakov. No izites mal a dingunos, ke no te agan mal [In the name of God, Abraham, Isaac, and Jacob. You did no evil to any one, may no one do evil to you].' Then they would give them three pinches of sugar, . . . put it under the pillow. Then he would sleep." Whether sugar or coffee was used, it was important that the cure be effected in silence. As we were told, "Without talking, he would go to sleep, the other [pinch of sugar or coffee was given] at midnight, and the third just before the sun came up. . . . But always without talking."

Lea Amram from Turkey told us that kave a la mezuza, or asukar a la mezuza, was "performed for three nights." The woman performing the cure, whom Lea referred to as "the mother," would take three little glasses of water, put coffee or sugar in them, and place a religious book over them. She would give the person a little to drink in the evening, at eleven, twelve, and one, under the mezuzah, and she would say, "Esto te da la refua, la shehina, la melezina [This gives you health, divine presence, medicine]." A similar cure for espanto was done using sugar cubes. As Paolina Elazar from Bulgaria explained, one would take four or five cubes of sugar under the pillow: "We used to take the sugar cube in the mouth, three times you did that. We did that three times during the night, three nights in a row. It would pass."

For some people, there were special days for performing kave a la mezuza. Sol Azuz of Istanbul said that it was done on Monday and Thursday, "the days of the Sefer," by which she meant the days on which the Torah was read in the synagogue. Sol explained, "I used to take some coffee in my hand, in my fingers, and I went to the mezuzah, and said, 'Ke me de la refua, la melezina [May he give me the healing, the medicine],' and then I took it on Monday night." Luna Ganon said that kave a la mezuza must be performed "on Friday, twelve o'clock noon." She continued, "One takes a new bag of coffee, and the patient must open it under the mezuzah. And take three *prezikas* [pinches], and put them in the mouth without sugar. And she should say to herself, 'Refua shelema para tal i tal [health for so-and-so].' That's it!" Estrella Missistrano warned that kave a la mezuza should not be performed when "la luna esta kresiente [the moon is growing]," which would be during the first fifteen days of the lunar month, or the problem, like the moon, would grow larger. During the second half of the lunar month, it could be performed on *erev* (the night before) Thursday, Friday, or Saturday, but only with the precaution that the person not be left alone for nine days, or the stricken one might be *solombrada* (open for attack by the spirits).

Isaac's grandmother, Sarota Amato Musafir, told of still another form of kave a la mezuza for espanto. A man would take sugar packets to the synagogue for *arvit* (evening service). He should not talk with anyone but return home with the sugar packets, which he placed "under the pillow in the name of the person who was sick. . . . If you want, take it in one night, three different times. Or if you want to, one every night for three nights." Estrella Missistrano recounted a variation of this cure in which three packets of sugar were placed randomly in different sections of a religious book. "Around five o'clock in the morning, just as the sun appears, take one envelope and place the contents in a glass of water, drink it, and go back to sleep. Do this for three mornings when the sun shows up, that is, when the *hodja* [Muslim religious leader] calls the faithful to prayer. 'Kon el nombre del Patron del Mundo, esto ke me sea mi melezina [In the name of God, Master of the World, may this be my cure].'"

In the cure of *al sereno* (night dew), one would put a few drops of water with sugar, sweet wine, honey, or marjoram in a glass outside the window and then at dawn give this to the sick person to drink. Nehama explains that *agua al sereno* (water of the night dew) was formed from the condensation of night air, "to which popular medicine attributes magical curative virtues" (1977, 508). Interestingly, as reported by George Foster, this same cure was present in Spain where, unlike for the Sephardim in our study, it was specifically connected with the hot/cold dichotomy of humoral medicine: "In Spain, many remedies are left *al sereno,* in the open air at night to gather the night's cold" (1953, 211). The same Spanish influence was present in Hispanic America, where it was believed that "night air cools the body, as does *el sereno,* . . . an icy mist that falls at night, manifesting itself in the form of morning dew" (Foster 1994, 25).

One woman used sugar first to sweeten the spot where the espanto had taken place and then to sweeten the water to be placed in the night air. As Inez Meloh explained, "We used to take a little sugar, we used to sprinkle it on the place [where we had taken fright]. We would gather the sugar, and put it al sereno on the windowsill at night. And in the early morning, we poured it carefully into the glass and gave it to drink." Sol Azuz told us her cure for espanto: "Even today I do it. Even now. We take three *filjanikos* [demitasses] of coffee, small ones, we put some water and a little sugar in each coffee cup. And at five o'clock in the morning we placed them in the windowsill, covered with a clean cloth, after one hour we drink it with blessings. . . . At six, one of them. At seven another one. At eight, another. Also, one massages [the body] with the water . . . each hour, wherever it hurts, in the head, the arms, the hands." Sol explained that each time, one recited a blessing: "Dame la refua. No vos ize dingun danyo. Ni mal vos ize, ni mal vos azeresh [Give me the cure. I did not cause you any harm. Neither harm I did to you, nor you shall do any harm to me]. Dame la refua . . . shelema i kitamelo esto de endriva. [Give me . . . speedy cure and remove this from me]. Kon salud [with health]." Estrella Missistrano told us of a similar cure for espanto, which involved placing a glass outside the window at night. "One night with sugar and water and at the dawn, drink it. On the second night, use *asukar kande* [rock sugar], and drink it at dawn. On the third night use *sharope kolorado con agua* [colored sugar candy] and water. Again, eat it." Each time the stricken one would say, "Entre buena djente me lo bevo [Among good people (spirits) I drink it]," or "Entre los buenos de mozotros me lo bevo [Among the good among us (spirits) I drink it]."

Our mother, Caden Lévy Israel, told of the cure where sweet wine was used: "A little wine is taken and placed *al sirenu* [outside in the night air]. It is placed *pur la numbradia* [in the name of] a person who is sick. They place a black-handled knife on top of . . . the glass." The most propitious time for this was on Rosh Hodesh (the first of the lunar month). The wine was left outside all night long. Our mother concluded, "In the morning, quite early, this wine is given to drink . . . [with the words] 'Kun il nombri dil Dio, salud para Sarota, ija di Clara [In the name of God, health for Sarota, daughter of Clara].' That is all."

Sara Nair of Istanbul told how honey was placed al sereno: "We see that the sick person . . . cries, can't sleep at night. . . . What does he have? . . . . This person took an espanto (fright), a *sikenti* (worry). I'm going to do something for him. I place for him three small glasses of honey in the window, *al aver* (in the outside air). In the morning, al sereno [in the dew], I give it to him to drink. Three mornings in a row." Sara explained that there are "many cures inside the honey. There is something of every kind of flower inside." On the third morning after drinking the honey at dawn, the sick person is given a bath. She continued, "All the glasses are washed and from the water you make a sweet drink. And then we pour it behind him, and I tell him, 'Do not look back. Don't turn your face back. I'm pouring out all the evils behind you.' Behind the body, I pour out all the evils and tell them, 'Get out.' We dress him, and that's it."

Another woman explained the use of marjoram for "espanto un poko manko puro [espanto a little less (than) pure; espanto that is not grave]": "Marjoram is a kind of herb that has a nice, sweet smell. [It] was put three nights al sereno. You put it in the window [with some water] after the sun went down, and you remove it before the sun came up in the morning." A little was given to the sick person to drink. The woman cautioned, "And at the same time, there shouldn't be any smell. And there shouldn't be any contact with people that they didn't know with whom they had been in contact."

Certain cures were performed at *kuatro kaminos* (four roads, an intersection). A woman from Istanbul recalled a cure that had been used for her when she was suffering from *granos* (boils): "I was full of granos . . . all over. . . . Doctors, one to another. [The boils] didn't want to be cured. Somebody said, take a few bonbons. . . . Go to *kuatro kalejas* [four streets, an intersection]. Where there are one, two, three, four. Place yourself in the middle, and throw [the bonbons] over your shoulder. Without turning your head [say], 'Komo no veo estos bonbones, ke no vea estos granos [As I do not see these bonbons, I should not see these granos].' . . . I am throwing these bonbons. I am going, I am going, I am going, I am walking." In this manner she continued until she reached home. As she recalled, "Hardly two or three days passed, until the boils slowly, slowly started disappearing."

Bela Meshula, originally of Turkey, also told of the cure of kuatro kaminos for the evil eye. Her baby son was so sick that he could not eat. He vomited constantly, and he never slept: "One day, a lady told me . . . 'Bela, Hanum, this is no life. Four of us women are going to do something. . . . We are going to lay him down in kuatro kaminos. From this child we are going to *kitar el ojo* [remove the evil eye.] We are going to bring him in the middle of four roads.' At night, [Madame Sinyora] came over, she gathered four women, and they came . . . at midnight. I placed the child inside a clean sheet, with new clothing; I changed him completely. I was told, "He must be clean." She said, 'Bela. We are taking him. Bless him and do not cry.' And they took the child to kuatro kaminos." Two women took him to the place of the four roads and handed him to the other two women. "And after twelve o'clock at night, . . . they picked up the child and brought him to my house." She was warned by the women, "'It must be absolutely quiet! You are not going to scream or yell. And between husband and wife, no argument should occur.'" Bela concluded, "And in this manner, I picked up the child, put him to bed." In the morning the child woke up "hungry for food."

There was a special cure, which was performed by three women at Friday noon, for a child who had fear of walking. The participants formed a line, with the first carrying a pitcher of water; the second, two knives; and the third, the baby. They started from an interior room of the house, passed through three doorways, with the third one being the front door. One woman carried a pitcher of water; at each step she would pour a few drops on the floor and say, "Aki ti lavu il mal [Here I wash the harm from you]." The second woman, with the knives in hand, followed her. As she walked, she struck the knives together and said, "Aki ti kortu il mal [Here I cut the harm from you]." Behind these two came the woman with the child. With her arms bent at the elbows and extending forward as if for a chair, she held the seated child, who was also facing forward. All three women and the child kissed the mezuzah (by first touching it with the fingers of the right hand and then kissing the fingers) as they exit the doorway to the house. On crossing this last threshold, the woman with the pitcher poured all the water out and said, "Kon il nombri dil Dio, aki ti lavi todu il mal [In the name of God, here I washed all the evil]." On stepping out of the house, the woman with the knives struck the knives with a sharp jerk of her hands and said, "Kon il nombri dil Dio, aki ti kiti todu il mal [In the name of God, here I removed all the harm from you]." The child was put to bed and allowed to sleep quietly until about three o'clock. Then the women would pick up the child and put her on her feet. Usually the little one fell once or twice, but as we were told, by the third time, the child would walk. As our mother said in recounting this cure, "En primeru il Dio, es sigula [God willing, this is the remedy]."

While our mother did not specify a particular color for the knives (in fact, when Isaac asked, "What color knives?" she responded, "It doesn't matter"), other people stipulated that black-handled knives be used. One person from Turkey stressed that one needed to take four black-handled knives to the intersection of four streets on a Friday night, and that this had to be done for three Shabbats. As Rita Mipussi relates,

> My second son was four years old, and he never spoke. He would go to the store [and say like a chicken], "Ko, ko, ko, ko, ko; ko, ko, ko, ko, ko." One day he went to the butcher. My older one, who spoke beautifully, I was telling him, "Jako, go to the butcher, buy sausage." As soon as I spoke to the older one, the younger one left. He is telling the butcher, "Ma, ma, ma, ma, ma, momo, momo, mo." The butcher asked me, "What's wrong with your son?" I said, "I don't know, he's not speaking." "If I teach you something, are you going to do it?" the butcher said. I said, "Why shouldn't I do it? I'll do it." "You are going to go on the night of Shabbat [Friday night]. [Place yourself] between four streets, you will take four knives, and you will take your son also." Look, look, I am full of goose bumps! "You should take your son also. You will take him to the street. You should cut the streets with the knives. And from there, three Shabbat nights in a row, you are going to go to a house [where they say] kiddush [and] do everything that is proper. The first bite of hamotsi [bread

which has been blessed], you are going to give to your son to eat." . . . . I took the knife from my house, I took four knives. Knives like swords, they have to be. Because it is the butcher who told me that. He gave me knives like swords. I took my son, I went to the right. As I am cutting, I am saying, "Segun se apartan estas kalejas, asina ke le mande el dio la avla a mi ijo [As these streets are divided, may God give speech to my son]." And I turned back. As I am turning back, again I went to the right. Only to the right. I came back that way, only cutting to the right. Again I went to the right to my house. This is the way I was instructed to do. And truly, the first thing we did was the knives, after the three nights, and at the end of the month, my son began to talk. He started talking as if he descended from the heavens.

At the end of Rita Mipussi's account, Isaac checked again about the color of the knives by asking, "The handles were black, or of any color?" Rita responded, "Kacha preta, kacha preta [black handles, black handles]. Because they were the knives of the butcher." Presumably, the butcher would have particularly sharp knives that would be effective for cutting the evil. In addition, he would be a kosher butcher, and therefore he would be particularly holy. Thus, by extension, black-handled knives, often used in magical cures, would be efficacious for such a cure, since they would cut through the spiritual force, whether this was at the intersection of four streets on three Shabbats for the unfortunate child who had been struck dumb, or at three doorways at noon on Friday for the child who could not walk.

There was another cure, simpler and more direct, for the child who was late in talking. One might take a living fish and let it bite the tongue of the child. As one woman said, "Si azian buenus [They were cured]." Isaac remembers his grandfather, after whom he was named, telling of this cure being done to him in Antalya, Turkey, when he was seven years old (circa 1875). A Turk suggested that his parents take a living fish and have it bite his tongue. They did it, and he started to speak.

As a cure for serious cases of espanto—when one was "*agotado* [weak, depressed], *charpeado* [beaten down], like insane"—the Sephardim in Istanbul used to consult a hodja for the cure of the *foyas* (graves). Sol Azuz recounted, "And there was a hodja, one of them, theirs, like our *haham* [Jewish religious leader]. The one who was quite, quite frightened was taken at night, at midnight." There, at the cemetery, three graves were prepared. The hodja stood outside: "And he would read, read, and read. And then he would make him go inside the grave, a little, and then to the other, and then to the other. To the three of them. And this was done at two or three in the morning. . . . They would go two or three times, and that sick person was cured." Korin Madem told of her cousin who had been struck with espanto at his *brit milah,* and the subsequent performance of the cure of the graves: "The rabbis and the people came in from the *Bet ahaim* [house of life, euphemism for cemetery]. From the Bet ahaim, they came in to perform the brit to the child. . . . They performed the brit. That night he got sick. He was sick! It was finished. Charpeado entero [Beaten down entirely]! He is not eating anything. Well, several entire months. Finally, to the graves! They put him three times in the graves. . . . With the hodjas. And with the women who took him. My aunt took him, took the grandchild." To emphasize the effectiveness of the cure, Korin concluded, "And the child became well. And now he is married, and he has six children."

In Rhodes and Izmir, if a person had taken fright, or if she was anxious and depressed and showing the signs of espanto, her friends could secretly give her *mumia tapada* (covered, secret mummy) mixed with sugar or some other sweet. Sara Nair, an expert in Sephardic curing, noted, "Mumia is used in Izmir. Only there it is given. In Istanbul there is none." Isaac quickly added, "In Rhodes there was mumia." And Sara agreed, "In Rhodes there is. And still there is in Izmir." She continued, "This is . . . like an amulet. Like a thing that is not found in the world. This is for a sick person for whom there is no other cure left." As noted earlier, mumia could be made from the bones of the dead or from the dried foreskin of the circumcision, and it was obtained "from special women who sell it." As one man explained, "The best one is not from the bones of the dead, the best one is when the brit milah is done to the baby, from the foreskin of the circumcision. When it is dry, dry, dry, they mash it, and this mumia is better because it is a blessed mumia." Another person explained its origin, "It seems that they took it from the body of an old, old dead person"; and another, "They say that the people who go to the mountains and are lost, the sun dries them and they become bones; this is the mummy." Our Aunt Rachel explained that mumia came from the desiccated bones of animals: "You know, they used to take some bones, animal bones. They put them on the fire, and then mash them down into powder. And that is used for mumia." Then she added, "But I have the real mumia. That is the one that dries up in the desert. The animals who die in the desert, and the sun disintegrates them. The big things that they are, they shrink smaller and smaller, and the bones are taken. They are mashed, and that's mumia."

Raphael Patai explains the historical origin and use of mumia. Initially the powder was made from minerals, called bitumen, whose potency was believed to vary according to its place of origin. That mined from the Dead Sea, designated *bitumen judaicum,* was believed to be especially powerful. The Arabs derived the term, bitumen, from the material "used by the ancient Egyptians to embalm the dead, although this material was in reality not bitumen but resin" (1964, 8). With fanciful interpretation added to mistaken assumption, the powder came to be called mumia, since bitumen was associated with Egyptian embalming, and the bodies, themselves, were mumias. During the Middle Ages, both Arab and Jewish physicians recommended the use of "*mumia,* i.e., bitumen, as a drug for many and varied ailments" (8). The Jews of Alexandria, in the twelfth century, were employed to break up the "embalmed bodies of ancient Egyptians in order to obtain what they believed was bitumen, but what in reality was resin. . . . In the course of time, the belief developed that *mumia* was efficacious only if it was taken from an embalmed human body" (8). In an 1870 account about the Sephardim, Moshe Reischer wrote: "The Sephardim make to this day a remedy, mumia, which is prepared from the ground dry bones of dead people found in the desert in the sand. . . . And the Sephardim, when they have a patient sick for many days, God forbid, take it and grind it well and put a certain amount of it into honey-water which the patient drinks from time to time during three nights. Before he drinks it, they wash him and clothe him into a white robe, and lay him on a bed covered with a white sheet" (Patai 1964, 9).[3]

Whatever its origin, mumia was regarded as a powerful medicine. When Rosa Avzaradel asked Isaac if he knew what mumia was, he responded, "I have some at home." Mrs. Avzaradel exclaimed in amazement, "You have some at home?" Isaac replied, "Someone gave me a little amount." She continued, "This is not found at all. This is better than diamonds. Keep it [well]. This is a diamond. It is not found easily. This is a medicine truly blessed. It is blessed."

Mumia, we were told, should be given in secret. It should be given in the early morning, preferably on the days that the Sefer was read, or on the eve of Rosh hodesh (the new month). As Zimbul Maya Suzi counseled, "If someone is sick in bed, and he does not want to undergo an *aldurko puro* (ritual cure by enclosure), that is to say a very powerful cure, then you do the mumia. You don't say anything to the sick person. You take a pinch of mumia, put it in the cold food, and give it to the person to eat. Everyone in the room remains silent." Isaac's grandmother, Sarota Musafir, did not stress special times for administering mumia: "Mumia you give any time. But the person who is to take it shouldn't know anything about it, mumia tapada. You give a pinch of it in cold food or drink, not in hot. In cold [food or drink], three times, one after the other. And this is good." Isaac's grandmother indicated that one might whisper, "Kon il nombre dil Dio [In the name of God]," or "Salud para Sarota, ija di Clara [Health for Sarota, daughter of Clara]."

Once mumia was administered, the person had to follow a special diet. As our mother explained, "And in a case like that he wasn't supposed to eat a meal with onion, fish, or garlic." Bienvenida Gabay, originally of Edirne, Turkey, offered the same cautionary advice, "The sick person must not eat garlic, onions, anything fried, salted fish, or anything with a strong odor." Mrs. Gabay continued, "Three days later you must tell the person that you have done it. If the problem was espanto, she should feel better in three days. But for nine days, she shouldn't eat any of the above foods. You tell her after three days so that she can be careful about avoiding these foods." Zimbul Maya Suzi suggested that the stricken one should stay inside: "It's better when the patient is home and doesn't go in and out. Why? Because whoever takes care of him or her knows about the mumia and does not give the patient any food, such as garlic, onion, salted fish, or fresh fish, anything with a strong odor. It is better if the patient does not know anything about it and does not leave the house for forty nights." When we asked why one should stay inside at night, Zimbul replied, "Because during the night, *eyos salen* [they (referring to the spirits) go out]. . . . If the patient goes out and takes fright again it will be worse."

At times the cures did not work. Then one had to check further as to what had caused the illness. This could be done through *avrir goral* (to open destiny) and *avrir serko* (to open the circle, tell one's fortune). As Rosa Avzaradel explained, "The Turks would tell the fortune. *Goral* is to divine. . . . They would open a book and read, from the Koran." Our mother told us that there were "special people who knew to avrir goral. . . . They would investigate with a book, they read, they knew what it was all about, and they explained." One woman had consulted a haham (religious leader) in order for him to divine the cause of her illness. In answer to the question, "How did he do it?" she responded, "With a book . . . a religious one. . . . He opened the book and he placed my name, the name of my mother also in the book on a small piece of paper." She continued, "He opened it and he looked. He looked for the letters which connect with his book, the book of law. Now he called me Sol. He saw 'S.' What does it mean? This [letter] what is it? He was quite, quite, quite knowledgeable. Quite knowledgeable. He understood. . . . He told me everything that I had seen."

Caden Lévy Israel tells of a time in Rhodes when Isaac's older brother, Julian (then called Yeoshua), was ill. In this complex account, there is a combination of divination of the cause of illness, the use of an amulet to restore health, a deceased rabbi speaking to the mother in a dream, a cure for espanto that involved immersion in the sea on the eve of Rosh Ashana, and administering a drink of mumia and sugar. Since Isaac had been a participant in these events, his questions become themselves a recollection of time past:

> Isaac: Tell me what happened to Julian, when he was quite sick, before going to Athens.
>
> Caden: One day you came and told me that Julian was walking in the street and [suddenly] he stopped and that a car was going to hit him. Afterwards, watching him two, three times, we noticed that his eyes did some kind of movements and that way, he stopped talking and walking, but he did eat.
>
> Isaac: As if he were paralyzed.
>
> Caden: Yes. As if paralyzed. He stood there on his feet.
>
> Isaac: He had been sick seven or eight months.
>
> Caden: Seven or eight months, yes. We visited many doctors and he did not see any improvement. We had no remedy. Until I had a dream. Harbi [Rabbi] Ruben Israel came to me in a dream and told me to take care of Julian. Then I remembered that we had a friend, the wife of Harbi Ruben [the chief rabbi whose downstairs apartment we rented]. She was in Egypt.

Isaac's mother wrote to Mme. Zafira, the rabbi's widow, and asked her to contact a man named Habif, who was from Izmir, and who "*avria goral* [told fortunes]." Isaac's mother continued: "He was a haham [Sephardic, rabbi/holy man]. Habif they called him. I wrote Mme. Zafira if she could go to him to *avrir un serko* [open, tell one's fortune]. I sent a piece of the clothing that Julian wore, for the sweat." After a period of two or three weeks, Isaac's mother received a letter from Mme. Zafira saying that they had read Julian's fortune and that he had been "frightened in a certain spot." Habif sent a *nuska,* a Turkish amulet, for Julian. Isaac's mother related, "He said to place it on the head, under the hat, and to keep it for a week. But Julian, being a child, would take it and throw it, he could not keep it." Isaac's mother had a second dream about Rabbi Israel of Rhodes in which he told her, "'Try to help your child, otherwise we are going to lose him, daughter of mine help him. . . . Take care of him.'" Following the suggestion of the local physician, Dr. Bruneti, she took Julian to Athens for treatment: "Three doctors checked him up. He had a worm moving in the intestines. They gave some medicines to help him. I was there two weeks. I came back to Rhodes again. I spent no matter what; we did not see any benefit." Then she dreamed again of the rabbi, who said, "'Daughter of mine, Rosh Ashana is approaching. Do for him whatever you can on Rosh Ashana.'" Isaac's mother awoke in the morning crying and told her mother of her dream. She continued, "We called an old woman . . . , Mazalto Chamal. . . . She came home the evening of Rosh Ashana. She prepared some packets of sugar and mumia. Three of them. She placed them under the pillow of Julian. . . . At midnight, the lady came, she took Julian and me, we went to the seashore, La Puerta di la Mar [the gate to the sea]. She undressed Julian. . . . She walked him into the water. . . . She gave him the three packets [to drink, mixed with water]. She immersed him twice in the water. She immersed him and pulled him out. . . . She immersed him one more time in the water and afterwards I took him home and she said to me, 'Put him to sleep.' Julian hardly ever slept before. But we put him in bed and he slept until noon. And this was the cure." Isaac's mother reiterated, "This was the cure for the fright. The mumia was the cure. After I spent [so much] with doctors, with everything. This was the cure."

In another divinatory practice, called livianos, as noted earlier, one would melt lead, pour it into a pan of cold water, and then divine the source of the illness through the shapes, or *estampas*, formed by the lead.[4] The best time for this was early on Monday or Thursday morning before the Sefer Torah was read; it could never be performed on Shabbat. One woman claimed that livianos were "the cure for everything." She continued, "This is one of the most important things that one can do. The livianos are the best, that is why they are called livianos (light). The livianos are better than any other thing." Julie Alajef, originally of Bulgaria, said, "My mother would also *echar livianos* (perform livianos). . . . She had a special spoon. In a pot she would put a little ruda, small pieces of moistened bread and water. The lead, she would put it in the spoon and on top of the fire. The lead would melt, and they covered the patient with something white [as protection], and took the melted lead and *patliava* [it would burst]." Kalina Alvas, also originally of Bulgaria, explained, "It is lead that is melted. Take a large spoon and melt the lead. Then they would place a sheet over us so that the lead would not splash us. Then they would pour the lead in a basin of water [which was placed over our head]. The melted lead would form shapes. Sometimes the figure of dogs or horses, or snakes would appear. According to the shape, they said what had frightened the person." Ida Varsano explained, "And the figure that would form, the shape that would form, they would begin to say, 'This has the shape of a wolf, and he was frightened because of that. . . . That was an animal, it looks like a bear, it looks like a horse.' And in this manner, every single animal would have its interpretation for the fright." Mrs. Alvas recalled when she took fright and livianos was performed for her: "When I was twenty-six years old, I was in a village of Bulgaria. Some young men were with us. One of the young nephews said, 'Aunty, let us go to the tree of the tourists.' At first I did not want to go, but I went. Halfway up, I felt badly, 'Here the snakes are going to eat me. Why I am staying here? It is high.' From this spot, I saw way down, how the villagers were working the wheat fields with their horses going round and round. I fainted, and they took me home. My mother called an old lady and she echar livianos. The phssshhh [the noise of the hot lead dropped into the cold water], they saw that the lead made the shape of a snake and of horses. They gave me to drink the same water." For Mrs. Alvas, the liviano did not work. As she said, "It didn't do me any good."

For some, livianos provided the diagnosis and the cure for the illness. When Rivka Sarfati was fourteen or fifteen years old, she had trouble with her eyes. When the livianos was performed, they found out that she suffered from the evil eye because of a young man. As she explained, "Once we knew that my problem was due to the evil eye, everything ended up well." Another woman told of how she had performed livianos for a friend's daughter, "She was not quite normal. 'As a mizva [good deed],' I said, 'I have to save this child.' I took her home. She was sixteen years old. She was quite nervous to the point of being insane. I took her home and I did livianos." As she poured the melted lead in the water, she uttered the following prayer: "Ruler of the world, anyone who has caused the evil eye, anyone who has spoken evil, let him be present here." She continued, "I did this three days in a row. We then uncovered it and found inside the water a small head of someone who had turned entirely to ashes. Yes, ashes, because they cast the evil eye on her because she was very smart and quite advanced in school. This caused her problems." She told the young girl, "You must not eat onions, fish, and such things for eight days, not even see them." She concluded, "And she became a good woman, and got married, had children, and the mother could not find how to repay me."

There were those who performed livianos with a more elaborated flourish. As Zimbul Maya Suzi explained it, one should put a handful of sugar, marjoram, and rue in a handkerchief, place this under the pillow, and sleep on it for one night. In the morning, one would hold *kurshum* [lead] in a spoon over a hot fire until it had melted. Put the sugar, marjoram, and rue in a pan of cold water, and add nine pieces of bread: "When the lead is melted, cover the patient with a sheet, take the large kettle and place it over the head. Then pour the lead into the water. If the patient has been stricken with evil eye, the lead explodes. If it becomes fine, it indicates that there was *avla mala* [evil speech]. If the lead is grasped by the rue, it means that there was *mal ojo.* If it is grasped by the marjoram, that the patient is *sikliado* [oppressed, with anxiety]. If it is grasped by the bread, it means that someone is devouring the patient as the bread is devoured." After this, the lead was removed from the water and melted again in the spoon. In a molten state, it was held three times over the head; three times, over the heart; and three times over the knees. "Finally, the lead is melted once more, but this time it is not put in the kettle, but between the feet, on the ground. There whatever frightened the person will be formed."

Bienvenida Gabay also performed an elaborated livianos, which was then followed by certain precautions: "The livianos has to be done all in one day. Then for nine days, the patient cannot eat onions, garlic, fish, fried food, food with strong odors, salted fish. Usually they eat sweets, halva, or pasta. It's better if you do not leave the house at night. During the day you may because there are always people around. At night, you don't know what is outside which might cause harm. It is better if you don't, but if you have to, you may go out with someone else." Another woman explained, "When I am finished doing [the livianos], which I have done three, nine times, I wash the face with this water, and what is left, I placed under the head of the bed for nine days. Afterwards, I place the water in a clean pot, that is, not unkosher. And after the nine days, we throw it in the sea, in a river, or in a body of water."

Sugar, honey, and sweets formed a central ingredient in the cures of the Sephardim. Whether in taking pinches of sugar under the mezuzah, or sipping the sugared water placed al sereno, or casting sweets at the four corners of the street, or throwing sugar and sweets into the foyas, the person effecting the cure and the person being cured were sweetening both themselves and the spirits. This was a literal acting out of a metaphor: sugar and honey, the essence of sweetness, were consumed by the stricken person and were offered to the spirits. This ritual action was underlined in the spoken ritual as well, for as one blessing went, "Vos esto dando dulsuria, ke me desh sultura [I am giving you sweetness, in order that you can release me]." In the cure of the foyas, Sol Azuz and Korin Madem explained that the hodja threw sugar and sweets into the graves in order to sweeten the *buenos de mozotros* (good among us).

The use of sugar as a symbolic cure for spiritual ills is linked historically to the works of Arab writers in the tenth and fourteenth centuries, in which, as Sidney Mintz notes, "sugar figures as one of the most important medicinal ingredients" (1985, 97). While there was but "meager reference to sugar in Greek texts" (96), the Arab-Islamic physicians introduced a plethora of sugar cures through their Latin translations of

Arabic texts, particularly "through the traditions of the School of Salernum (Salerno) via Spain, especially in the period 1000–1300 A.D., and through the Byzantine Empire" (98). Mintz continues, "Scholars like the Persian Avicenna (ibn-Sina, 980–1037)—known for his assertion . . . 'As far as I am concerned, sweetmeats are (always) good!'—who wrote the *Canon medicinae Avicennae* . . . remained authoritative in the practice of European medicine until nearly the seventeenth century" (98).[5]

Water and salt were also core ingredients for effecting cures. Water washed and purified the stricken one from all evil; and salt purified and preserved her in good health. Additionally the location for the cure was also crucial. In *Semitic Magic*, Thompson writes, "When a man has fallen sick of a headache, the Assyrian magician takes water from two streams, at the spot where they run into one another, which, like the cross-roads, is always a place for magic" (1971, li). In like manner, the Sephardic curer sweetened the four crossroads and symbolically "cut" the illness in the same manner as the streets were divided.

According to Trachtenberg, "Astrological considerations loomed large in determining" (1939, 114) when something was to be done. The emphasis was often on performing the cure during specific times of the lunar month. Thus if one wanted to increase one's fortune, the magical performance would be effected on Rosh Hodesh, as the moon began to increase in size, or if one chose, at any time during the first half of the month. If one wished to diminish one's illness, the cure was scheduled for the second half of the lunar month when the moon was diminishing in size. There were also propitious times during the week, when the Torah was taken out of the ark to be read in the synagogue; and propitious times during the year, often on the eve of Rosh Ashana. One of the most crucial and consistent aspects of timing had to do with nightfall. As Trachtenberg wrote, "The commonest specification was that the magical act be performed before sunrise, for the rising sun vitiates magic and drives the spirits into their hiding-places" (114). Firestone writes about the time of cure for espanto: "This is done two or three days before *Rosh Hodesh* [the new lunar month], but it is preferable to perform it on a Friday night, just before Shabbath begins, four or five days before *Rosh Hodesh. Rosh Hodesh* is the beginning of the lunar month" (1962, 306).

Threefold repetition was crucial for the success of a cure. An action, a blessing, and the cure itself were done three times, and even three times three. Trachtenberg comments, "Three is the favored mystical number of all times. . . . The number three occurs more often in magical texts than any other. Actions and incantations were to be performed three hours before sunrise, or three days before the new moon, or three days in succession; preparatory rites were to last three days; the magical act comprised three stages, or required three objects . . . incantations were most often to be recited three times. The number three came to be recognized as a mark of magic, so that 'anything that is repeated three times is magical' was a frequently quoted rule" (1939, 119). In his article "The Sephardic Community of Los Angeles," Stephen Stern quotes an elderly informant who remarked on the importance of the number three: "'The Turks have a saying, *Yauch, yauch,* either three or nothing. I moved into this house two years ago. In three months the woman dies next door. In six months the woman on the other side died. I wanted to get out of here. My wife was sick. Sure enough she died, and was the third'" (1980, 150).[6]

The ritual power of pollution, as discussed by Mary Douglas in *Purity and Danger,* adhered to the stricken one. To be cured, she had to be set apart, if just for a time; and the evil causing her illness had to be cast out through magical transference. Often this was to a body of water that would absorb the evil and by association would purify the stricken one. Through its transparency, water was, after all, a symbol of purity (Budge 1930, 445). The transference could also be made to salt, which, as a symbol of incorruption, could absorb and then repel the evil. The stricken one urinated on the salt and transferred the illness to the salt, which dissolved in magical duplication to the dissolving evil. Infrequently, the transference was to an individual, as in the case of the person who was bathed in urine, and the urine was then splashed into the street where the unsuspecting neighbor, who after all had caused the evil eye, would step. When sweetened water and simple blessings were not enough to cure the sick one, and when reading the shapes of molten lead did not reveal the cause of the illness, then one turned to the *maestras* (the specialists) of the more complex cures.

8 Prekante: *A Ritual Prayer for Curing*

Pur un kaminiku pasi,
Kun un viezijiku 'skontri.
Ali vedri vistia,
Tres yavizikas tenia en su mano,
Una d'avrir, una di sirar, una di kitar todu il mal.
Ben pura Yusef, ben pura adalai.

As I walked along a narrow street,
I met an old man.
In resplendent green, he was dressed,
Three keys he had in his hand,
One to open, one to close, and one to remove all harm.
May the sacrifice of Joseph, Lord, be accepted instead of
mine.

Whether in simple verse for minor ills or in elaborate verses for serious illnesses, the *prekante* was used as a curative rite in earnest supplication for the recovery of an individual. As a ritual prayer for the release of "all the evil eye, all evil talk, all types of harm," its main purpose was to cast off the demons that had invaded the body as a result of *espanto* or *mal ojo.* In all instances, the harm had already taken place and the stricken one's health was in danger. Thus, these formulas that came to the people from generations past were a source of relief from the injury caused by the evil spirits.

The origin of the term *prekante* traces a path the Sephardim followed in their exile from the Iberian Peninsula, and that was the one leading from Portugal. While the term *precantar* cannot be found in medieval

Spanish literary works or dictionaries,[1] it does appear in Portuguese dictionaries, with the following meaning: to conjure an evil act, to prevent witchcraft through the recitation of magical formulas, almost always as rhymed verses. A *precantador* is defined as a sorcerer, a priest, or a magician who chants a magical formula in order to remove evil spells. The connotation in Portuguese is the same as in Latin, where *precantrix* means "enchantress" or "sorcerer." The Portuguese *precantar* is equivalent to the Latin *praecno* and *praecanto,* "to foretell," "to predict," "to anticipate," that is, "to destroy in advance the power of an enchantment." Thus the term *prekante* must have been in circulation in the Iberian Peninsula prior to the expulsion of the Jews in 1492, and the Sephardim who emigrated from Portugal in the early sixteenth century must have introduced the word to their coreligionists of the Ottoman Empire. We suggest that the Latin, medieval Spanish, and Portuguese terms lost the original meanings for the Spanish Jews: *prekante* no longer referred to bewitchment, *praecantrix* to witch, or *praecno* to predict. Instead, *prekante* connoted a ritual curing through prayer that was conducted by the *prekantadora,* who was a specialist and a healer of bounteous goodwill.

Encarnación Marín Padilla provides a link to Spain for the Sephardic prekante in his article entitled, "Relations between Jews and Converts during the Second Half of the Fifteenth Century in Aragon: Sicknesses and Deaths." From his research in the archives of the Inquisition, Padilla concludes that the converts made recourse to Jewish practitioners of "magical formulas and superstitious ceremonies" for curing their ills, including those resulting from the evil eye (1983, 258). While Samuel Armistead also points to connections between the Sephardic prekantes and the Hispanic charms, he thrusts even deeper into the past for the roots of the practice: "The charm against the evil eye, despite its distinctively Jewish invocations of God, the Patriarchs, and Miriam the prophetess, is closely related to ancient Pan-European folk-charms and folk-beliefs" (1992, 371).

The tie to Spain is here also through the verb *encantar.*[2] In *Diccionario crítico etimológico castellano e hispánico,* Juan Corominas glosses *encantar,* as used by Juan Ruiz in the *Libro de buen amor,* to mean *hechizar* (to bewitch). Commenting on a series of terms derived from *encantar,* Corominas and Pascual remark that these "can be explained by the formulas, sung or recited, by the sorcerers" (1980).[3] Another term used in medieval and present-day Spain, and sometimes by the Sephardim, is *ensalmo.* According to *Diccionario de la lengua española* (1970), the term refers to "a superstitious process of curing by means of prayers and the empirical application of various medicines." On the other hand, *Vocabulario de romance en latín* (1973) defines it as "exorcism." As with *encantar, ensalmo* denotes "enchantment" and the use of spells and charms. For the Sephardim, *ensalmo* meant "to cure," whether by means of a petition, such as a prekante, or by providing a home remedy, such as an ointment. The Sephardic meaning of *ensalmo* corresponds to that given by Covarrubias in *Tesoro de la lengua castellana o española* (1977), "A certain method of curing by means of prayers, at times by themselves, and at times using jointly some remedies." This latter definition, by extension, would be accurate for *prekante.*

The ritual verse of the Sephardic prekantes shared both theme and content with that of the Christian ensalmos of Spain and Portugal. Victor Lis Quibén (1980) and Francisco Rodrígues Marín (1927) trace the thematic parallels between the prekantes and the ensalmos of the traveling supernatural figure who meets an old man or woman on the road, the reference to the three keys, and the transference of the harm. Additionally these authors show the shared formulaic verses for framing the cure in God's name and for removing the evil and casting it into the sea. In the Sephardic ritual, prayer and supplication were always made in the name of God, the patriarchs, and biblical personages, as is evident in the opening verse to the *prekante de chefalo:*

Beshem Eloe, Avraam, Itzhak i Yakov,	In the name of God, Abraham, Isaac and Jacob,
Moshe veAaron, David i Shelomo,	Moses and Aaron, David and Solomon,
i Sinyor di Eliau ha-Navi, zihur letov.	and Elijah the Prophet, may he be remembered for good.

The Christian ensalmo usually ends with a recognition of, and a request for, God's mercy and the Virgin Mary's favor. In the prologue of Lis Quibén's text, F. Bouza Brey states that many of the magical formulas located in Galicia are of "ancient roots" (1980, x):

Con gracia de Dios	With God's favor
e da Virxen Maria,	and that of the Virgin Mary,
un Padre Nuestro	[Recite] one Our Father
e-un Ave María.	and one Holy Mary.
	(Lis Quibén 1980, 119)[4]

In both the Spanish ensalmo and the Sephardic prekante, the evil was removed from the body and thrown to "the depths of the sea" with precisely the same wording:

Saca todo o mal que no
corpén tén.
[Remove all evil so that this
body may not experience it.]
(Lis Quibén 1980, 281)

Kita todo el mal i ke este kuerpo
no tenga dingun mal.
[Remove all evil and that this
body may not experience any.]

Que se vaia o fondo do mar,
donde non sinta galos cantar,
nin campanas tocar
[Let it go to the bottom of the
sea,
where no roosters can be heard
to crow,
nor bells ring.] (170)

Ke se vaiga a la profundina de la
mar,
ni andi gayo kanta, ni pero yama
[mauya].
[Let it go to the bottom of the
sea,
where no rooster crows, no dog
barks.]

Often in published works, the term *prekante* has not been translated at all. When translated, it has been rendered as "incantation," more often than not, giving the Latin or Portuguese meaning of "enchantment" and "bewitchment." The term "imprecation," that is, the act of praying for evil or invoking a curse, has also been suggested as a possible translation. However, the Judeo-Spanish prekante had nothing to do with invoking a malediction or destroying in advance the power of an enchantment since the harm had already been done to the stricken one. The prekante also did not refer to witchcraft or to hypnotizing and magnetizing a subject, either human or spirit. The Sephardic women who performed prekantes had no intention of insulting the spirits by attempting to trick or enchant them. For fear of the wrath of the spirits, the prekantadoras rarely commanded the demons but rather begged for their help. They knew, as Trachtenberg observed, that "magical action was not one to be entered upon lightly. It was a dangerous adventure which might recoil disastrously upon the unwary practitioner" (1939, 114). Always cognizant of the power of the spirits, the Sephardic curers were respectful towards *los buenos de mozotros* (the good among us). They genuinely pleaded on behalf of the patient for forgiveness from the spirits.

At times, those writing about prekante associate it with the undertakings of a superstitious woman or even of a witch.[5] Referring to Sephardic diviners "who exorcized the evil spirits," José M. Estrugo begins, "Había 'aprecantadoras' (vide 'encantamientos,' en libros antiguos)," which translates as, "There were women performers of *prekantes* (see 'enchantments,' in old books)" (1958, 58). While not offering a definition, Michael Molho describes the woman who performed prekante as "generally, an old hunchbacked woman who mumbles with her toothless mouth the magic formulas" (1950, 277). We take vigorous exception with the foregoing representation of the curers. From our personal experience and research, we know with certainty that the prekantadora, the performer of the prekantes, was a highly respected member of the community. Rebecca Amato Levy, originally from Rhodes and now living in Los Angeles, told us, "These ladies were saints, they were sought for their knowledge and their dedication to the welfare of the community." Izahar Avzaradel, also from Rhodes, told us of his grandmother, Mazaltov de Yakov Israel, who performed prekantes. She was "a saintly woman. No matter whether it was a Jew, a Greek, a Turk, she greeted everybody. She blessed them, 'May you have a good day, good health, long life, and everything.'" Izahar assured us that she was in demand by everyone for her expertise in the ritual, and for good reason: "My grandmother Mazaltov would *prekantar* [whoever came to her for help], and 99 percent of them would be cured." Isaac's great-great aunt, Dolsa Musafir, who was in her late nineties when we spoke with her in her home in Izmir in 1990, also referred to the prekantadoras with respect, "Only benedictions came out of their mouths. Their hands were to cure the sick, to save lives."

The Sephardim whom we interviewed referred to the act of performing the prekante by several different terms. The verbs *aprekantar* or *prekantar* were the most straightforward and quite simply meant "to perform the prekante." As David Bunis informed us, this same term, with a variation in spelling, appeared in an 1898 article published in Izmir: "The author, Yosef Bakish, told of an agitated father who brought his son to the teacher of the elementary school for a 'treatment,' called *pregantar.* The teacher recited a long prayer in order to cure the child of an illness which had prevented him from attending class on that particular day."[6] The phrase *pasar la mano* (to pass the hand) emphasized the manner in which the prekante was enacted: the person reciting the ritual verses would pass, or circle the hand over different parts of the body, usually the head, the chest, and shoulders. This same term, *pasar la mano,* had been in use in sixteenth-century Spain. As Padilla recounts, the woman convert Antona Ferrer "used to pass the hand from the face down and would spit" (Padilla 1983, 259).[7] Finally, the Sephardim also used the general terms *echar por nazar* and *azer por ayin arah* (to perform for the evil eye), or simply *azer* (to do).

As with all medicines of the house, a crucial aspect of the prekante was its immediate availability. A mother or grandmother could perform the prekante whenever a person did not feel well simply by taking a handful of sugar, salt, or cloves and passing it in circles over the head, and sometimes in front of the face and around the shoulders and chest, while repeating a verbal formula. For the evil eye or espanto, one could burn cloves in a procedure called *klavos a la lumbre* (cloves in the fire). Clara Farzi told us that, as a child, she was constantly stricken by the evil eye; "My mother always kept cloves handy. When I returned home, my head would drop as if I were sick. This was due to the evil eye. My mother would take some cloves, a handful. First she would recite over my head, 'Aprekanto, aprekanto a mi ija. Ni mal azi, ni mal ke no le agan. Kon estos klavos ke tope la melezina [I recite the ritual formula, I recite the ritual formula to my daughter. She does not cause any harm, nor harm should be done to her. With these cloves, may she find the remedy].'" Clara's mother would burn the cloves in a large spoon with hot coals and have her daughter smell the aroma. Then she would take the cloves as they exploded and say, "As these cloves are exploding, let the eyes of whoever has seen her [given her the evil eye] explode with them." Finally, her mother would put the cloves in water and give her some to drink.

The popping sounds of the burning cloves signaled the release of the evil spirits. As Zimbul Maya Suzi of Celebria, near Istanbul, explained, one could select an uneven number of cloves, preferably thirteen, all of which must have "the little heads on them"; then one could thread them onto a pin and put them in the fire. One gave the name of the person and as the cloves exploded away the evil eye, one said, "Here I remove from you the *ojo malo* [Spanish, evil eye], the evil speech, and the *ayin arah* [Hebrew, evil eye] that you may not experience any evil." One might also say, while casting the cloves into the fire, "I vow to you and implore you by the Wailing Wall that such a woman should not experience any harm."[8] Still another woman told of a similar cure in which she first held five cloves in her palm and "passed the hand" in a circular motion over the head of the stricken one while repeating the following prekante three times: "Here I take/remove the evil eye, all manner of evil, [and I cast it to] the depths of the sea, and my daughter should have no harm." The woman added, "Then you throw them to burn in the fire, over coal. And they would go 'Chak, chak, chak!' In the fire, the coal was hot ashes, that is where we used to throw it. We didn't throw them into the fire itself, but onto the hot ashes. And it began to jump. That's it!"[9]

Salt was used in prekante for the symbolism of purification and of dissolving all evil. Estrella Missistrano, from Bat Yam, Israel, told of her grandmother's cure for espanto: "We were young, four sisters and one brother. We lived in Orta Köy [Istanbul]. A Shabbat evening, the work was completed, and we were going to sit down when an earthquake started, a strong one. Our house had three wooden floors, a beautiful one. It seemed that it was going to break. From fear, the young ones fainted. Our grandmother who lived with us squeezed two lemons in a dish and added a little spoon of salt." She went to each child in turn, pressed to the soft palate a lemon peel that she had moistened with the salt and lemon juice, and said, "Vos vo salar i desalar del espanto ke tomatesh [I will salt and desalt you from the fear that you have taken]," and then added the formulaic verse for the prekante, "I remove your fright, I remove the evil, so that you may not experience any evil."

In some cases, the prekantadora substituted one ingredient for another or combined several in her performance. In the following instance, a lady from Istanbul made use of sugar, saliva, a candle, and cloves. When asked if she held something in her hand when performing a prekante, she replied, "Sugar. With sugar. I did everything with sugar in my hand. I gave the patient three pinches of sugar in the mouth and I licked the forehead. I licked the forehead with my tongue and after that I took five or six cloves and I stuck them on a pin. On this side [pointing to her left] I had a candle. I lit it and said, 'In your name, since you gave him the evil eye.' If the cloves exploded, it meant that it was true. Now, such a person saw her. Ah! It is already passing, tak, one exploded, and they exploded until they were all gone." Vera Mizan, who was born in Istanbul, said that the sick one would then say, "'Grandmother, I am already fine, Grandmother, I am fine.'"

A major component of Sephardic ritual prayers was the naming of the one being cured and the mother of that person (Schiffman and Swartz 1992, 13). Trachtenberg refers to this as "a curious feature of the spell"[10] and traces its origin: "In the Talmud, we read that 'all incantations are in the name of the mother,' and Talmudic incantations followed this rule, despite the general principle that the people are to be identified as children of the father rather than the mother. . . . This practice has been excused on the ground that *pater incertus, mater certa* [father uncertain, mother certain]" (1939, 115–16). While the prayer was always personalized, some women would avoid mentioning the name of the stricken one out of fear that the spirits, once cognizant of who had insulted them, would attack the person mercilessly. They considered it prudent to refer to the infirm by the indirect object, *le* (to him/her) or *te* or *vos* (to you), or by other means of identification, such as "I mi ija [And my daughter]," "A mi ija [To my daughter]," "En tu nombre" or "En nombre tuyo [In your name]," "Ke tala senyora [That such lady]," and "Fulana, ija de fulana [So-and-so, daughter of so-and-so]."[11] Isaac, however, recalls that the prekantadora did identify the stricken one by name, as, for instance, "Isaac, ijo de Caden [Isaac, son of Caden]," "Lea, ija de Rahel [Lea, daughter of Rachel]," or "Lora, ija de Matilda [Lora, daughter of Matilda]."

The power of the spoken word was encapsulated in the manner in which the prekante was learned and performed. Many of the Sephardim with whom we spoke insisted that the prekante lost its effectiveness if it was written down. One woman recounted that the one she had was useless because it was written; she added, "they say that the prekante is no good unless it is stolen."[12] In his review of *Sefer refuot* (The book of cures), a book published originally in Judeo-Spanish in Izmir in 1878, Moshe Shaul remarked, "Our mothers and grandmothers, who best knew these *prekantes* and used them in ceremonies destined 'to repel the evil eye,' were so convinced of the peril of uttering these *prekantes* outside of the ceremonies, that they obstinately refused to teach them to other individuals, even when it had to do with their own daughters and friends. The only method to learn a *prekante,* they said, is for one to 'steal' it, or to try to listen and memorize it, when they were reciting a ceremony against the evil eye" (1986, 44–47).

For a woman who wanted to "steal" a prekante, the challenge was in being able to follow the words, since the prekantadora often uttered the verses "in a low voice, almost hard to hear" (Koen-Sarano 1989, 44). Trachtenberg remarks on this "frequent injunction," that "incantations were not to be uttered above a whisper" (1939, 114–15). Bohora Biton, originally from Rhodes, told how she had learned several prekantes: Tia Jamila la Almileha had recited them aloud to enable her to learn them by memory, since "es mas saludozo [it is more beneficial]" than having it written. The *prekante de kulivreta* (prekante of the serpent) was so important to Mrs. Biton that she was even able to recite the genealogy, as it were, of this ritual verse: it had been given to her "by Mr. Yako Mayo, the son of Dona di Nisim Mayo, from Megri, Turkey."[13] Because this particular prekante was known by so few people and was in danger of being lost, Mrs. Biton said that she had "reluctantly" given it to Albert Hemsi in the 1920s. Her reluctance had nothing to do with passing on the prekante—this she willingly did—but rather with the manner in which she did so. She gave it to Mr. Hemsi "in writing because he did not know Judeo-Spanish."[14] While she had saved the words of the prekante in this written form, its power might either have been diminished or lost through committing it to paper.

The Sephardic prekantes composed of elaborate verses were divided into four types: (1) *prekante de ojo malo,* or *ayin arah* (prekante against the evil eye); (2) *prekante de chefalo* (prekante against mental anguish); (3) *prekante de pelo* (prekante against engorged breasts); and (4) *prekante de kulivreta* (prekante of the serpent). There is some evidence that the prekantes had been composed and even performed by rabbis centuries ago (Benbassa-Dudonney 1982, 28) and then had passed into the women's domain. In our interview at the old age home in Izmir, Turkey, in March 1990, Mary Algrante also remarked on the rabbis' involvement in certain cures against the evil eye. She said, "There are some ayin arah that they *meldan.*" Algrante used the Judeo-Spanish verb *meldar,* which translates "to read," "to recite," or "to pray." When this was done for a sick person (*meldar a un hazino*), Nehama provides the following definition: "to exorcize someone, to expel the evil spirits that possess him, by reciting mystical prayers, magical formulae, practices performed by a cabalist, a wonder-worker, a magician" (1977, 355). Whether performed by a rabbi or a prekantadora, the ritual prayer spoken aloud, albeit in a whisper, was intended to drive out the evil spirits.

The prekante was to be performed preferably at the beginning of the Hebrew month, when the moon was growing fuller, not at the end of the month, when it was diminishing. A particularly propitious time was at Rosh Ashana, the Jewish New Year, when both the year and the moon promised new and full growth. The most appropriate days for reciting the ritual verses were Monday and Thursday, when the Torah was read. For an extremely dangerous circumstance, one could recite a prekante on Saturday, though this was highly unusual. If the prekante was performed on Saturday or on a holy day, then the prekantadora would "sweeten" the ritual by using sugar in place of salt. As Rachel Musafir told Isaac in 1968, "During the week, you put salt in the palm of your hand. On Saturday, you put sugar."

To perform the prekante, the specialist and the stricken one usually went to the sea. As we were told, "The sea is deep and can endure everything." In Ashdod, Israel, in 1990, Dora Shemaria of Rhodes told us, "When I was a child, I was very nervous and very sickly, and my mother said that it would be better if she performed a prekante on me. And an elderly woman, the sister of Simha Tarica, took me to the seashore, and she began with a fistful of salt in her hand, to *pasar* [pass, perform the ritual]." This gesture of placing the hand over the sick person was, Samuel Armistead writes, "like Miriam the prophetess [who] places her hand over the sick and performs cures and gives the medicine." He records this initial verse of a prekante:

Con el nombre del Dio, Abraam, Itshak, Yakov, Aarón, David, Šelomó: Yo meto la mano . . .	In the name of God, Abraham, Isaac, Jacob, Aaron, David, Solomon: I put in my hand . . .

Como la señora de Miriám a-nevía	Like Miriam the prophetess,
que sanava y melezinava	who performed cures and gave medicine
y todo el mal eya quitava	and took away all the sickness
y a la fondina de la mar lo echava,	and threw it into the depths of the sea,
ansí yo quito el mal de fulana,	so I take away the sickness of so-and-so,
hija de sistrana.	daughter of such-and-such. (1992, 371)

In the event that one could not go to the sea, then the prekante could be performed at the spot where the injury had taken place, or at the home of the sick one. Salt and water could then provide a substitute for the sea. Bohora Biton remarked, "If there is no sea, the salt is put in a basin with water. . . . And this water is thrown into a ditch that will go to the sea."

The prekante against the evil eye was the one most frequently used. Matilda Koen-Sarano notes that at the first sign of illness from the evil eye, "the grandmother who knew how to perform for the evil eye was already prepared with the assistance of a *prekante*" (1989, 43–44). Perhaps because the prekante against the evil eye was so popular, there was also an early historical record of it. Samuel Elazar remarks that it was published circa 1720 in a medical book in Bosnia-Herzegovina. Entitled *Prekante de ojo malo,* the book was, as Elazar says, "written in Ladino and in square Hebrew characters" (1987, 248). In an article on the evil eye, Esther Benbassa-Dudonney observes that there was the "'*Aprekante,*' a prayer written in the seventeenth century by Rabbi Yosef Azulay"; she notes that Hayim Palache (1788–1868?), the Great Rabbi of Izmir, added certain details to the verses (1982, 28).

As Mary Algrante told us, "When you already had used many medicines and there was no relief, and nothing happened, they used to say, 'It may be that someone caused him the evil eye.' And then they performed it," the prekante de ojo malo. With salt or sugar in her palm, the prekantadora would "pass her hand in a circle over the head, shoulders, and chest of the patient."[15]

Isaac's grandmother, Sarota Amato Musafir, gave him the following prekante against the evil eye in 1965:

Pur un kaminiku pasi,	As I walked along a narrow street
kun un vizijiku 'skuntri	I met an elderly man.
Ali vedri vistia.	In resplendent green he was dressed.

Tres yavizikas tinia en su manu,
una d'avrir, otra di sirar,
i una di kitar todu mal.
Pur ayi paso Eliau ha-Navi, zahot litov.

Dishu, "Andi vas a ir?"
"Andi Itzhak, iju di Caden,
a darli dulor di kavesa,
a rumperli sus guesus,
surverli su sangri,
surverli su sangri,
a mashkarli su karni,
kurtarli sus fuersas,
darli apretamientu di kurason."
"Ti juru i ti kunjuru k'ayi vaigas,
dingun mal nu li agas.
Li kitis todu il mal, toda l'ayin arah,
toda l'avla mala, toda l'angusia di kurason,
si la echis a la undura di la mar,
k'en el kuerpu d'Itzhak nu tenga dingun mal."
Ben pura Yusef, ben pura adalain.
Komu las muntanyas nu si vienin abrasar,
ni l'agua di la mar si vieni a mizurar,
k'in esti kuerpu nu va tiner dingun mal.
Ben pura Yusef, ben pura adalain.
Sez di goy, si va kimar komu il tizon,
sez di ave muda, Kadosh Baruhu ste en su ayuda,
sez di ombri, piedra il nombri,
sez di muchacha, piedra la sensia.

Three keys he had in his hand,
one to open, one to close,
and one to remove all harm.
Through there passed Elijah the Prophet, may he be remembered for good.
He said, "Where are you going?"
"Over to Isaac, son of Caden,
to give him headache,
to break his bones,
to suck his blood,
to suck his blood,
to chew his flesh,
to cut his strength,
to cause him anguish."

"I pray and implore you, to go there,
and no harm you cause him.
Remove from him all the suffering, all evil eye,
all the evil talk, all the anguish of the heart,
and cast it to the depth of the sea,
so that the body of Isaac may have no harm."
May the sacrifice of Joseph, Lord, be accepted instead of mine.
As the mountains cannot embrace themselves,
nor the water of the sea can be measured,
this body will not experience any harm.
May the sacrifice of Joseph, Lord, be accepted instead of mine.
If it is from a gentile, he is going to burn as cinder;
if from a mute bird, may the Blessed come to its aid;
if from a man, let him lose his name [lineage];
if from a maiden, may she lose her reason.

Ti juru i ti kunjuru k'ayi vaigas,
dingun mal nu li agas,
li kitis todu il mal, toda l'ayin arah,
toda l'avla mala, toda l'angusia di kurason,
si la echis a la undura di la mar,
k'en el kuerpu d'Itzhak nu tenga dingun mal.
Ben pura Yusef, ben pura adalain.
Komu las muntanyas nu si vienin abrasar,
ni l'agua di la mar si vieni a mizurar,
k'in esti kuerpu nu va tiner dingun mal.
Ben pura Yusef, ben pura adalain.

I pray and implore you, to go there,
and cause him no harm,
remove from him all suffering, all the evil eye,
all the evil talk, all the anguish of the heart,
and cast it to the depth of the sea,
so that the body of Isaac may have no harm.
May the sacrifice of Joseph, Lord, be accepted instead of mine.
As the mountains cannot embrace themselves,
nor the water of the sea can be measured,
this body will not experience any harm.
May the sacrifice of Joseph, Lord, be accepted instead of mine.

If the prekantadora or the stricken one yawned during the recitation of the ritual verse, it meant that the spirits were leaving the body, and that the pain and illness would leave with them. At the end of the verse, the prekantadora mixed the salt or sugar with water; and as it dissolved, so did the evil dissolve. As she washed the face of the individual, the curer would say, "I wash off all the harm"; and then she would toss the water into the sea, while saying, "I cast all the harm to the sea."

The second type of ritual verse, the prekante de chefalo, was seldom performed. Isaac's mother explained that it was used for a person "who was, God forbid, dizzy and confused"; and Bohora Biton said it was used for someone who was "charpeado di la kavesa [deranged]." Suffering either from evil eye or witchcraft, the individual was tormented with mental anguish or with drastic fluctuations of mood. As Mrs. Biton explained, the stricken one was a person "who had little strength, who was sick, who did not get well easily. [The practitioners] did that while he was sick, real sick. Ah! They used to be tired of going to the doctor, doctor, doctor. Well, a prekante de chefalo. A prekante de chefalo. To the seashore. To the sea. They would perform the ritual twice, three times, at the sea. Performed it with salt in the hand." As important as going to the sea was for most cures, for the prekante de chefalo it was requisite; otherwise the cure would not be effective. Mrs. Biton concluded, "And it worked." Rebecca Levy told how the prekante de chefalo was performed:

"It was used in the morning. The patient was not to have had any food before the prekante. The process: A fistful of salt is passed over the body, a few inches over the body, never touching the body. While doing this, recite the prekante. Then put the salt into a bowl of water and wash the exposed parts of the body with the saltwater—the face, arms, hands, and legs."[16] The person performing this prekante would slash through the air with a black-handled knife while reciting the verses, "Ti kortu la kavesa, ti kortu lus rinyonis, ti kortu il kurason [I cut your head, I cut your kidneys, I cut your heart]." For those listening, this part of the prekante inspired dread. On any other occasion, such words would be greeted by protective phrases, such as "*Haz vehalila!* [God forbid!]," or "*leshos de mozotros* [far from us]."

The dramatic enactment of slashing the air and calling out "I cut your head" might well be connected with the derivation of the name for this prekante. As Rebecca Levy remarked, "*chefalo* comes from the Greek word for head, *kefalo* [*kefale*]." Michael Toumazou suggests that *chefalo* derives from the Greek word *kethalós*, mullet, a fish that lives in very dirty waters; by extension, the word connotes "a big, thick-headed fellow." As an example, he quoted the following Greek proverb: "The donkey called the rooster a *kethalas*, empty headed." Beki Bardavid suggests that *chefalo* might "be the fish *kefal*, as we say in Turkish." She continues, "In *de kefalo* [head of a mullet], referring to a muddle-headed individual, to someone who has nothing in the head. Since the mullet has an empty head, there is nothing in it to suck [used to denote a tasty food] as compared to the head of other fish that are savory and are eaten."[17] Whether the term derived from *kefale* (head), *kéfalos* (mullet), or *kefálas* (muddle-head), all have the same root and refer to the head, where, according to the practitioners, the illness derived.

Bohora Biton recited the following prekante de chefalo to Isaac in 1965:

Beshem Eloe, Avraam, Itzhak i Yakov,	In the name of God, Abraham, Isaac and Jacob,
Moshe veAaron, David i Shelomo,	Moses and Aaron, David and Solomon,
i Sinyor di Eliau ha-Navi, zihur letov.	and Elijah the Prophet, may he be remembered for good.
Andandu pur un kaminu inkuntri kun mansevu,	While walking along a street I encountered a young man,
di fieru vistia i di muera [maya] kalsava.	dressed in iron and wearing iron shoes.
Li dishi, "Andi vas?"	I said to him, "Where are you going?"

"Andi fulana, ija di fulana,	"Over to so-and-so, daughter of so-and-so,
a raerli su[s] guesu[s],	to shred her bones,
a kumerli su karni."	to chew her flesh."
Li dishi, "Stringa esta vena [vela].	I told him, "Raise the sail.
Ki pasi la vela.	Let the sail navigate.
Todu il mal lu echu a la mar.	All evil I cast to the sea,
La mar es ancha i todu lu puedi reivar,	The sea is vast and can endure everything,
lu puedi reivar i simportar,	it can endure and tolerate it,
i [esta] vela puedi navigar.	and this sail is able to navigate.
Salud i refua.	Health and cure [for the patient].
Chiflu [in]chifladu,	You, crazy muddle-head,
ti kortu la kavesa,	I cut your head,
ti kortu il kurason,	I cut your heart out,
ti kortu lus rinyonis,	I cut your kidneys,
ti echu a la profundida di la mar,	I cast you to the bottom of the sea,
la mar es ancha i onda,	the sea is vast and deep,
lu puedi reivar i simportar.	it can endure and tolerate it.
Esti kuerpu es kuerpu di asar vada [basar vadam],	This body is a body of flesh and blood,
ki nu lu puedi reivar i simportar."	and cannot endure and tolerate it."

The third type of prekante, the prekante de pelo, was used exclusively for women who had engorged breasts and who thus could not feed their infants. The sickness involved an infection and an obstruction of the mammary glands of a nursing mother. As a category of illness for the Sephardim, *pelo* must have dated back to medieval Spain, for in *Diccionario de Autoridades* it is defined as the following: "a disease that strikes women in the breasts, caused by the coagulation of the milk which becomes toxic and harmful. . . . There develops in the breasts of women inflammations, abscesses, cancers, and other diseases that have to do with the state of the milk or its production, as well as the lack of it, the abundance or coagulation, which one calls *pelo* (1979, 196)."[18] The *Cassell's New Latin Dictionary* defines *pello* as "to strike, to drive away, to dislodge" (Simpson 1959). Salvatore Battaglia writes that in Italian, *pello* denotes the following: "to straighten the hair: in symbolic context to indicate the reaction caused by a strong fright, by a great fear or emotion" (1984). In his 1516 dictionary, Antonio de Nebrija defines *pello* as "cosa redonda," "globus," "sphaera," all of which refer to a rounded object, possibly the breast of a woman, from which the Judeo-Spanish, *pelo*, may have been derived (1973). Thus, the prekante de pelo joined together the fright and emotion as conveyed in the Italian *pello*, with the act of driving away or repelling the spirits as denoted in the Latin *pello*, with the Spanish symbolism of *pelo* for breast.

Bohora Biton described the affliction as follows: "The breast would go down, it would swell, it became like this [she gestured with her hand that the breast was swollen], and the breast got sick at times. . . . It turned the breast red. Fever used to come to that person. It used to come to us. I had it, but, it should have happened to the one who wished me evil, never that bad. . . . And they took . . . a black comb. They circled the breast while reciting [the prekante]." Another woman told of her experience during one of her pregnancies, "My breasts would fill, but they would become like a cyst." Other people who were listening to this woman's recollections, exclaimed, "Ki li kayo il pelo [The *pelo* fell on her]." In her community, one who was afflicted in this way would buy "a small matchbox filled with ointment" from a woman who specialized in making it. As this woman recalled, she would rub the ointment in slowly on the breast and the pus would come out. Bohora Biton remembered the use of ointment for this ailment in Rhodes: "Tia Ester la Tarica used to prepare a salve for the sick breasts, for every type of thing. We only had to call, 'Mana Ester!,' and she would rub [the breast] two or three times, and [with an affirmative tone] they were cured." Mrs. Biton explained that the content of the ointment was wax, *mumia* (the dried and powdered foreskin of the circumcision), and *sharlagan* (oil of sesame). Caden Lévy Israel recalls the consequences for the nursing women who suffered from the malady: "They could not feed their children. Their breasts were inflamed, hard with abscesses. They could not produce any milk and the children cried."

This condition, known as "kaer el pelo a la mujer," "abashar el pelo," or "dar pelo en el pecho," may have been the result of the evil eye given by a woman who could not give birth herself, or by a woman whose child was not so beautiful and healthy as that of the nursing mother. This envy of other women would have provoked the jealousy of the spirits, particularly of Lilith, who was always in search of newborns. Additionally, should a nursing mother chance to smell the aroma of enticing foods and not be offered a taste, she would have been stricken by the *pelo*. In this instance, it would have been her own longing, or envy, which would have made her vulnerable for the evil spirits.

We collected the following prekante de pelo from Caden Lévy Israel, Sarota Musafir, and Bohora Biton:

Beshem El hay vekayham,
Eloe Avraam, Itzhak, veYaakov,
Moshe, Aron, David, uShelomo.
Kaminando por un monte,
m'enkontri kon un lonso:
un palmo era su boy,
un palmo era su kavesa,
un palmo era su frente,
un palmo era su oreja,
un palmo era su ojo,
un palmo era su naris,
un palmo era su boka,
un palmo era su brasu,
un palmo era su pie.
Li dishu, "Di mi vus riyitish i burla mi izitish?"
Dishu, "Nu vus abashare pelu [*sic*] para ke lechesh a vuestras kriaturas."
Pur un kaminiku pasi,
kun un vieju m'inkuntri.
Pur ayi pasarun tres muchachas vestidas di vedri,
Di el si sunrierun, i burla li izieron.
Lis rispundio il vieju:
"Di mi vos riyitish i burla mi izitish?
Pelo vus abashara para ke no
alechesh a vuestras kriaturas.
Vuestrus peshus vus si sikaran
I vuestras kriaturas al ambri muriran."
Li disheron, "Li juru [juramos] i li kunjuru [-ramos]
ki muzotras di el nu mus riyimus ni mus sunriyimus.
Rogamos Beshem El hay vekayham,

In the name of the Living and Eternal God,
the God of Abraham, Isaac, and Jacob,
Moses, Aaron, David, and Solomon.
While walking on a mountain,
I met a bear:
a palm was his height,
a palm was his head,
a palm was his forehead,
a palm was his ear,
a palm was his eye,
a palm was his nose,
a palm was his mouth,
a palm was his arm,
a palm was his foot.
He said to her, "Did you laugh at me and ridicule me?"
He said, "I will not cause you *pelu* [*sic*] in order for you to breast feed your children."
As I walked along a narrow street,
I met an old man.
Three young ladies passed dressed in green,
They laughed at him, and they ridiculed him.
The old man replied to them:
"You laughed at me and ridiculed me?
Pelo will strike you so that you may
not breast-feed your children.
Your breasts would dry up
and your children will die of hunger."
They told him, "I [we] pledge and affirm to you[19]
that we did not laugh nor smile (scorn) [you].
We pray in the name of the Living and Eternal God,

Eloe Avraam, Itzhak, veYaakov,
Moshe, Aron, David, uShelomo,
Ki juresh ki nu mus abashi pelu [*sic*]."
Pur ayi paso Eliau ha-Navi, zahor litov.

I al vieju li dimando, "Purke avlas?"
Dishu, "Di mi si sunrierun."
Disherun las muchachas, "Ni mus riyimus,
ni pur el nunka mus burlimos."
Eliau ha-Navi li dishu al viejo,
"Ti rogu ki ayi yiras,
dingun mal nu lis aras,
siempri en sus favores avlaras."
Ben pura Yusef, ben pur adalain,
Ben pura Yusef, ben pur adalain,
Ben pura Yusef, ben pur adalain.
[Eliau ha-Navi asegura a las muchachas]
"I vuestrus pechus siempri komo il agua di la mar kuriran."
[Eliau ha-Navi avla al viejo]

Ya vus dishi, "Sus pechus komu rius kuriran,
a sus kriaturas mantiniran,
i en estus kuerpus nu van a tiner dingun mal."
Sez di mansevu, si dirita komu il sevu,
sez di mujer, piedra il saver,

sez di goy, si kemi komu il tizon,

the God of Abraham, Isaac, and Jacob,
Moses, Aaron, David, and Solomon.
Do swear that *pelo* will not strike us."
Through there passed Elijah the Prophet, may he be remembered for good.
And he asked him, "Why do you speak thus?"
He replied, "They laughed at me."
The young ladies said, "We did not laugh
nor have ever ridiculed you."

Elijah the Prophet said to the old man,
"I pray for you to go there,
and cause no harm to them,
always in their favor you shall speak."
Ben porat Yosef, ben porat 'ale 'ayin.
Ben porat Yosef, ben porat 'ale 'ayin.
Ben porat Yosef, ben porat 'ale 'ayin.
[Elijah assures the young ladies]

"And your breasts will always run as the water of the sea."

[Elijah again speaks to the old man]
I already told you, "Their breast will run as the rivers,
their children they will feed,
and these bodies will not experience any harm."
If it is [originates] from a young man, may he melt as the wax,
if from a woman, let her lose her judgment,
if from a gentile, let him burn as cinder,

sez di ave muda, Kadosh Baruhu, este en su ayuda.	if from a mute bird, may the Blessed One come to its aid.
Komo las olas di la mar nu si vienin a kuntar,	As the waves of the sea cannot bring themselves to be counted,
estus kuerpus nu van a tiner dingun mal.	these bodies will not experience any harm.
Ben pura Yusef, ben pur adalain.	Ben porat Yosef, ben porat 'ale 'ayin.
[El viejo al fin se kree de las chikas]	[The old man finally believed the young ladies.]
"Mas pelo no ternash,	"*Pelo* will not strike you,
fulana ija di fulana,	So-and-so, daughter of so-and-so,
para ke alechesh a vuestras kriaturas kon alegria."	so that you may breast-feed your children with joy."

Although well known in the Balkans, Turkey, and the Dodecanese Islands, the prekante de kulivreta (prekante of the serpent) was not readily used due to the violent wording of the text. As Shelomo Reuven, originally from Salonika, Greece, told Isaac in Tel Aviv in 1982, there was a great uneasiness among Sephardim even to speak of snakes. Perhaps this was associated, as Nehama notes, with the fear of the "jerem del kulevro [the excommunication, the anathema of the serpent]" (1977). Indeed, even the prekantadoras felt some anxiety when speaking of the kulivreta, and those listening were uneasy. Isaac remembers one woman exclaiming in alarm when another began reciting the prekante, "Esto no! Leshos de moz! Esto no! [This no! Away from us! This no!]."

In his article entitled "Folk Medicine of the Sephardic Jews in Bosnia," Samuel Elazar writes that the ritual is used for someone who suffers "with fever, chills, and fever blisters" (1966, 163).[20] According to Zoran Kuzmanovich, Elazar discusses "an invocation against a particular type of fever that produces snake-like welts, blisters, or patches of redness that resemble little snakes."[21] There is a record of this infirmity in Spain during both the medieval and the classical period. In 1611, Sebastián de Covarrubias Orozco defines *Culebrilla* as "a certain intracutaneous disease in the form of eczema that usually tends to appear on the chin."[22] The *Diccionario de la lengua española* states that the disorder "receives its nomenclature due to the undulating [serpentine] arrangement of the line of vesicles that distinguishes the ailment" (1970). In his article on popular medicine in Galicia, Victor Lis Quibén discusses ritual verses from Pondevedra that were used to treat an inflammatory disease of the skin.[23] In similar fashion to the Sephardic prekante de kulivreta, the Galician ensalmo was called *Aire de culebra* (Air of the snake). Both were used to treat a disease of the skin.

The Sephardic prekantadora performed the ritual three times, while holding a black-handled knife in her hand and symbolically cutting the disease with it. At the same time, she passed her hand over the stricken one's body. At the conclusion of the ritual she dissolved in the water the salt that she had been holding in her palm, and she washed the face, arms, and legs of the stricken one. The Spanish curer also recited the verses three times, though sometimes she recited them nine times, thus trebling the ritual number three. She held a knife in her hand and made the sign of the cross on the upper body of the patient, while uttering the following verse, which was addressed to the snake:

Te corto el Cobro,	I cut your safety,
te corto el sollo,	I cut your breath,
te corto todo.	I cut everything.
Aquí te estendo,	Here I stretch you down,
aquí te seco,	here I dry you up,
e-aquí te prendo.	and here I restrain you.
	(Lis Quibén 1980, 48)

The Sephardic prekante de kulivreta followed essentially the same wording:

Ti kurtare la rais,	I will cut your root,
ti kurtare il kuerpu,	I will cut your body,
ti dizminuzare lus miembrus,	I will wither the extremities of your body,
ti ichare a lus montis.	I will scatter you throughout the mountains.

As Marie Biton, originally from Rhodes, explained to Isaac in 1965 in Atlanta, Georgia, *kulivreta* was a disease "with redness of the face. *Leshos de mozotros* [Away from us], with some form of skin disease, at times with high fever." The stricken one was placed in a room and isolated from everyone, save for the curers and close relatives; she followed a special diet by avoiding fish and salted foods until the cure was effected. Mrs. Biton continued, "The sick one was covered with something red, with a red cloth or red towel. A black knife was used. The woman cut across the blemish with the knife." The ritual verse was repeated three times. Samuel Elazar explains the procedure as follows: "Against the snake fever, one behaves in the following fashion: with a knife one goes across the snake fever scar and says, 'Walking along a road I met a living snake with legs. I caught it without hands, I cut its throat without a knife, and I swallowed it without a palate. May I prosper and grow as I speak the truth,' and after that one throws the knife on the ground" (1966, 163).

In most cases, the prekante de kulivreta was used when no positive response was obtained from the use of herbal cures, the recitation of minor ritual prayers, or the performance of the prekante against the evil eye. When all of these failed, the prekantadora resorted to the stern, frightening, even aggressive language of the prekante de kulivreta, such as this one collected from Bohora Biton:

Kun il nombri dil Dio alto,	In the name of God up high,
kulivreta maldicha, ondi fuetis venida?	cursed snake, where did you come from?
Ti kurtare la rais,	I will cut your root,
ti kurtare il kuerpu,	I will cut your body,
ti dizminuzare lus miembrus,	I will wither the extremities of your body,
ti ichare a lus montis,	I will scatter you throughout the mountains,
ni andi gayo kanta, ni pero yama [mauya],	where no rooster crows nor dog barks,
ni padri a su iju yama.	nor father calls his son.
Andi pur un kaminiku,	I walked along a narrow street,
inkuntri kun un kulivriku,	I met a snake,
sin manus lu mati,	without hands I killed it,
sin kurer lu alkansi,	without running I reached it,
sin dientis lu almashki,	without teeth I chewed it,
sin paladar lu ingluti,	without palate I swallowed it,
sin garon lu kumi.	without a throat I ate it.
Tantu kreska kuantu k'es virdad.	So much may I grow as it is the truth.
Era la nochi kuandu intrarias, ti 'stirarias,	It was the night that you entered; you stretched out,
ti arelumbratesh vos kon mozotros, Amen.	you rejoiced with us, Amen.
Todu il mal a la profundida di la mar lo tinemos ki ichar,	All harm to the bottom of the sea we must cast,
al pishkadu di la mar ke lo puedi reivar.	to the fish of the sea that can endure it.
Dingun [iju d']Israel nu tenga dingun mal,	No member of Israel should have any harm,
ni chiku ni grandi nu tenga dingun mal.	neither young or adult should have any harm.
Kon fuersa d'il Patron, Amen,	With the power of God, Amen,
Refua shelema si topara [para] fulanu iju di fulanu.	a cure will be found [for] so-and-so, child of so-and-so.

In the standard format of the prekante there were three interlocutors: (1) the prekantadora, who recounted the conversation that usually took place between (2) an old man on his way to cause harm and (3) a divine figure, who, in turn, begged him to restore the stricken one to full health. In all save the prekante de kulivreta, the person identified as "I," who was the prekantadora, was walking along a narrow street when she suddenly encountered an old man, or sometimes a young man (prekante de chefalo), and once, on a mountain, a bear (prekante de pelo). The mysterious and magical nature of this malevolent figure was heightened by his enigmatic identity. Nothing was known about him, but much was known about his apparel—he was dressed in green, or he was wearing iron clothes and was shod in iron shoes, or he was carrying three keys. Even more was known about the gruesome details of what he intended to do to the victim—he would "break his bones, . . . suck his blood, . . . [and] chew his flesh." Only in the prekante de pelo did the evil one also tell why he was intent on causing harm. Because the three girls had laughed at him, he would dry up their breast milk and cause their babies to die. The Lord, Elijah the Prophet, Abraham, Isaac, and Joseph, and other biblical personages, all were named and thus provided their holy protection.

The persona of the prekantadora was the one who cajoled or forcefully threatened the evil one, and who promised that all evil would be cast to the bottom of the sea. Mary Algrante preferred to use a positive approach; as she said, "One speaks well so that the outcome will be good." In her version of the prekante de ayin arah even the old man spoke nicely; he was going "'To Mary, the daughter of so-and-so, to bring her perfect health for all her afflictions wherever they strike.'" Even the "I" voice of Mary Algrante's prekante offered no threats; rather she prayed to him "by the heavens and the earth, by the tablets of the law [Ten Commandments], by the seventy Sanhedrim, who are seated at the entrance of Heaven."

En kaminando por un kaminiko,	While walking along a narrow street,
enkontri un viejiziko,	I met an old man,
de fiero kalsava,	wearing iron shoes,
de fiero vistiya.	dressed in iron.
Le demandi, "Onde vas ir?"	I asked him, "Where are you going?"
Me respondio, "Andi Mary, ija di tala persona.	He replied, "To Mary, the daughter of so-and-so.
A yervarle salud kumplida	To bring her perfect health
para todos sus males,	for all her afflictions,
en kualker lugar ke le van."	wherever they strike."
Te juro, te konjuro,	I pray and implore you,
por los sielos, por la tierra,	by the heavens and by the earth,

por las tavlas de la ley,	by the tablets of the law,
por los *Shevim* Sanedrim,	by the seventy Sanhedrim,
ke estan sentados en la demiza de ganeder	who are seated at the entrance of Heaven
rogando por la salud de tala persona,	praying for the health of such a person,
ija de tala persona.	daughter of such a person.
Ben parat Yosef, ben parat al ayin.	May the sacrifice of Joseph, Lord, be accepted instead of mine.
Yo te meto la mano,	I place my hand on you,
el Dio de Avraam te meta la refua komplida.	may the God of Abraham accord you perfect health.[24]

In another version, by Rachel Musafir, the old man was also of kindly intent: "As I walked along a narrow street, I met an old man wearing green shoes. I asked him, 'Where are you going, sir?' He replied, 'To the Blessed Creator, Who comforts all harm . . . and gives the cure.'" In other versions of the prekante de ayin arah, this voice prayed and implored that the old man cause no harm, but rather that he remove "all the suffering, all evil eye, all the evil talk, all the anguish of the heart." In the prekante de ayin arah and the prekante de pelo, the voice threatened, but even this was indirect, for the old man was not accused of doing evil. The one who was causing the evil was threatened, but unnamed: "If it is from a gentile, he will burn as cinder . . . if from a man, let him lose his name [lineage]; if from a maiden, may she lose her reason (prekante de ayin arah)." Still another version eliminated even the indirect threat: "Si es ombre, ke *no* piedra el nombre, si es mujer ke *no* piedra el saver [If it is a man, may he not lose his name, if it is a woman, may she not lose her knowledge]." In the prekante de pelo, "the three girls dressed in green" and Elijah the Prophet prayed to the old man to cause no harm; no threat was made to counter the old man's threats that "*Pelo* will strike you so that you may not breast-fed your children. Your breasts will dry up and your children will die of hunger." In the other categories of prekante, the threats were direct and violent. In the prekante de chefalo, the voice addressed, in this instance, the young man and detailed his punishment: "I cut your head, I cut your heart out, I cut your kidneys." In the prekante de kulivreta, the "I" voice did not even pause to ask the "cursed snake" about its intentions. There was only a question posed, "Where did you come from?" Then came the series of threats: "I will cut your root, I will cut your body, I will wither the extremities of your body, I will scatter you throughout the mountains where no rooster crows, no dog barks, no father calls his son."

This mysterious old man, who might he be? According to Rabbi Yossi Y. Groner, he could be the old foolish king (*meleh zaken u hasil* in Hebrew) who either causes harm himself or tries to get others to inflict it. This personage is identified with *yetser ha-ra,* the evil inclination that an individual is born with, according to an ancient rabbinic notion.[25] Clearly drawing from the less threatening and more benevolent versions of prekantes, Matilda Koen-Sarano (1983, 1989)[26] and Gad Nassi (Shaul 1993, 49)[27] identify the old man as the protective figure of Elijah the Prophet (Eliahu ha-Navi) or Joseph the Righteous (Yossef ha-Sadik), who directly intervened on behalf of the stricken one. Alan Corré posits, "The man is undoubtedly Elijah the prophet who is referred to in Arab folklore as *al-hidra*—the green man."[28] Nassi's text has an idiosyncratic addition. Joseph and an old man, familiar characters in prekantes, came to remove all harm from none other than Alexander the Great and his entourage. Still, that prekante concluded with the basic formulas, "I swear to you and implore you by all types of vows, to go there and all types of harm you remove from him." In a prekante recorded by Abraham Galanté in French, the "I" voice of the prekantadora met two figures "while strolling": Joseph, who portrayed the old man, and a young man who carried three golden keys, the third of which would remove the evil eye:

> In the name of the God of Abraham, Isaac, Jacob, David and Solomon, I place my hand and God the *haslaha* (success). While strolling, I met a little old man dressed in iron and wearing iron shoes. His name was Yossef ha-Sadik ([Galanté's endnote 1 states] At times . . . , instead of Yossef ha-Sadik, one says Eliaou ha-navi). Where are you going? To so-and-so, son of such-and-such, or to so-and-so, daughter of such and such. [Joseph does not seem to enumerate the reasons for his journey.] As one cannot count the stars, measure the sea, make the mountains embrace one another, in the same manner (one wishes) that this son or that this daughter have no harm. If (the evil eye) comes from a widow, may she lose her sight; if from a young lady, may she lose her honor; if from a young man, may he melt as wax; if from a married woman, may she lose her reputation; if from a *goya* (a non-Jewish woman), may she dissolve as the salt; if from a mute bird, may the God of Abraham come to its assistance. While strolling, I met a young man, who had three golden keys in his hand. With one, he opened; with the other, he closed; and with the other one, he removed the evil eye (and said): I remove from you the *aynarah* (*ayin ara,* evil eye). I remove from you the evil speech (that others have said against the sick person), and all kinds of ills, and all of it I cast to the depth of the sea, (so that) this son or this daughter would not have [suffer] any harm. May the evil eye go there where one eats eggs without salt. *Ben porat Yossef, ben porat 'ale 'ayin* (1935, 119).[29]

In Palache's *Refuah beHaim* (Shaul 1980, 47) and Elnecavé's "Folklore de los sefardíes de Turquía" (1963), Lilith, the nemesis of mothers and their newborn babies, took the place of the old man. Elnecavé gives the following "magical formula" to drive away Lilith and her band: "In the name of the God of Israel, Great and Reverend! Elijah met along a road the witch Lilith and all her company. He asked her: 'Where are you going, cursed of impure breath [spirit], with all your company also cursed as you are?' She replied, 'Sir Elijah, I am going to the house of the new mother in order to bring her the mortal sleep, to carry off the newly born, drink her blood, suck the marrow of her bones, and leave behind only her cadaver'" (131). Elnecavé says that Elijah warned Lilith about excommunication. Out of fear, she promised in God's name not to cause any harm to the mother and child. She then named all those in her company and handed to Elijah an amulet for him to hang in the house of the mother, assuring him that the mother and the child would be protected until the end of their lives (131).

According to Samuel Armistead, "The idea of a supernatural or divine apotropaic figure traveling or being met along a road as part of his curative mission is prominent in many folk-charms. Spanish texts continue to represent a meeting with the curing agent while on a journey" (1992, 371). Indeed, in the Spanish and Portuguese ensalmo, the traveler, Christ, and, infrequently, the Virgin, while walking along a path, encounter an old man, represented by St. Peter or St. Paul. (In some cases he is identified as St. John, St. Bartolomeu, St. Julian, St. Barbara, St. Lucy, or even Jacob.) The traveler usually inquires from those he or she meets, "Where are you coming from?" "Where are you going?" or "What is happening there?" The following two examples were from the region of Pontevedra, Spain, and both were used to treat skin diseases:

San Xacobo,	Saint Jacob,
San Xacobar,	Saint Jacob,
¿A ónde vás?	Where are you going?
—A-o mote Calvar	—To Calvary
—¿Qué vas buscar?	—What are you looking for?
—Follas de xar.	—Tea leaves.
—¿Pra qué?	—What for?
—Pra esta *Decipela* cortar.	—To cut the *erycipelas.*
Con el poder de Dios	With God's power
e da Virgen Maria,	and the Virgin Mary,
un Padre Nuestro	an "Our Father,"
e-unha Ave María.	and a "Hail, Mary."
	(Lis Quibén 1980, 48)

Lis Quibén classifies the following ensalmo also as *Aire de culebra* (Air of the snake). Unlike the Sephardic ritual in which the prekantadora touches the different parts of the body with the black-handled knife while reciting the prekante, the Spanish curer, depending on the region, lightly taps the different parts of the body with three twigs of fennel, anise, or parsley (46). While reciting the proper verses, she blesses the patient by making the sign of the cross all over the body, from head to toe, and then in reverse.

Tres homes santos;
se levantaron,
se vestieron,
con Jesucristo encontraron.
Jesucristo lles preguntóu:
—¿Homes santos, a-ónde ides?
—Imos a Monte Calvario,
a buscar folla da fístola,
pra *Decipelas, Urceras e Fistolas*
e *Fogo Salvaxe.*

Pra que esta enfermedad
non corra, nin labre.

Three holy men
got up,
dressed themselves,
they met Jesus.
Jesus asked them:
—Holy men, where are you going?
—We are going to Calvary
to search a leaf to cure "fistula,"
for *erycipelas, ulcers, fistulas*
and *inflamatory disease of the skin.*
So that this disease
does not expand nor run rampant. (140)

Both the peninsular ensalmo and the Sephardic *prekante kontra el ojo malo* (or ayin arah) have the motif of the three keys. In "The three keys and the eggs without salt: Hispano Christian and Sephardic versions of two traditional magic *ensalmos,*" José Manuel Pedrosa includes the following verses, which he collected in 1989 from a ninety-five-year-old woman who lived in Salamanca, Spain.[30] This passage is reminiscent of the Sephardic prekante kontra el ojo malo:

—¿De quién es este niño?
—Es de María.
—¿Dónde está María?
—Sentadita al sol,
lavando sus pechos
con agua de loor.
Tiene tres llaves:
con una cierra,
con otra abre,
con otra dice
el Ave María y la Salve.

—Whose child is this?
—It is Mary's.
—Where is Mary?
—Sitting under the sun
washing her breasts
with blessed water.
She has three keys:
with one she closes,
with another she opens,
with another she says
the Hail Mary and the "Salve." (2000, 113)

In the Sephardic prekante, the opening verse set the scene: "As I was walking along a narrow street, I met an old man, in resplendent green he was dressed, three keys he had in his hand—one to open, one to close, and one to remove all harm." While the meaning behind the third key is clear—it removes all harm—hardly any of the Sephardim could tell us the meaning of the first two keys. According to Midrash Rabbah, "God holds three keys in His hands over which no creature, not even angel or Seraph, has any control" (Rabbinowitz 1983, 137). With these keys, God opens the graves of the dead for resurrection, the womb of the barren woman for fertility, and the celestial reservoirs for rain:

> R. Menahema said in R. Bibi's name: Three keys are in the hands of the Holy One, blessed be He: the keys of burial [i.e., resurrection], rain, and the womb. The key of burial: Behold, "I will open your graves" [Ezekiel 37:12–13]. The key of rain: "The Lord will open unto thee His good treasure, the heaven, to give the rain in its season" [Deuteronomy 28:12]. The key of the womb: "And the Lord saw that Leah was hated, and he opened her womb" [Genesis 29:31]. Some add, the key of sustenance too, because it says, "Thou openest Thy hand, and satisfiest every living thing with favour" [Psalms 145:16]. According to Rashi of the Sanhedrin (passage 113a),
>
>> Three keys were not transmitted in the hand of a messenger. Over the treasure of the Holy One, Blessed is He, there are keys, and He transmitted them to the hand of appointed messengers. But He has three keys in his hand over which he did not appoint a messenger. And the Holy One, Blessed is He, said to Elijah, "I have held back those three keys since Creation and have not appointed a messenger over them except you whom I have made the appointed one over one of them. And now that you will ask for the second key they will say, two are in the hand of the student and one is in the hand of the Master."[31]

Four keys are mentioned in several Talmudic tales and rabbinic literature. For instance, the amulet TS K1.168 (lines 85–88) "mentions the 'four keys' given to the angels by God—'The Key of sustenance, the Key of birth, the Key of rain, the Key of graves.'" According to Schiffman and Swartz, "This device is available to the magician who invoked . . . them" (1992, 24, 158).[32]

In keeping with the Talmudic, rabbinic, and Midrashic literature, in some versions of the prekante de ojo malo, the old man was Elijah. For these versions, there was a comfortable fit: God had appointed Elijah to receive one of the keys in order to assist his people in time of need. In other versions, the old man dressed in green with the three keys in his hand in no way resembled Elijah. Instead, he was of *yetser ha-ra,* of evil inclination; he was on his way to cause grievous harm to the stricken one. Rabbi Kosovske queries, "Can the old man be God? If so, does he come to test or reprove an individual and, while walking along a path, he encounters Elijah, Joseph, Miriam, or an angel, who sways him to change his mind and bring forth the cure to the patient?"

When asked the purpose of the keys, Caden Lévy Israel explained: "Una es di avlar, una d'iskuchar, i una di kitar todu il mal [One is to speak, one to listen, and one to remove all the evil eye]." After some reflection she added, "The first is when one is sick, one [the specialist] speaks to him to make him relax. The second, to find out what is wrong, and thus close off the body from the sickness. The third to remove the evil eye." Recently, we once again asked Isaac's mother to explain the three keys. She took some time and then said, "The first key was to unlock one's *mazal* (destiny); the second to close one's *mazal;* and the third, to remove the evil eye." If one follows this line of thought, then all of life is in the hand of God, who can reward or punish by opening or closing one's destiny.

Mention of the first two keys was also found in the special *Shema,* "Las kuatro kantonadas [The four corners]," which the Sephardic women recited in Judeo-Spanish before going to sleep. The last two verses were a plea to God to keep them safe during sleep:

Con las yaves de los *mallakim*	With the keys of the angels
Estamos arrecomendados,	we are entrusted [to God].
El que mo la serre,	May He close it for us,
El que mo la avra.	may He open it for us.
	(Molho 1950, 163)

The theme of the keys was also found in the Sephardic formulaic phrases: "Kon su yave piadoza mos venga a salvar [With his merciful key may he deliver us]," and "La seradura ke se avra para bueno [May the padlock open for good]."

In "The Magical Transfer of Disease," Wayland D. Hand discusses how people free themselves by shifting a malady to another person, to animals or plants, and to various kinds of objects (1980, 17). In both the Sephardic prekante and the Spanish ensalmo, the patient was released from suffering because the torment of evil thoughts and deeds was transferred away from the individual, most frequently, to a body of water. In *Semitic Magic,* Thompson writes of an ancient Assyrian spell that washed the evil away into the water: "May all that is evil . . . (be carried off) with the water of his body and the washings of his hands, and may the river carry it away down-stream." Thompson continues, "The explanation of the phrase 'perform the Incantation of Eridu,' which is so often prescribed, must be some simple ceremony of this kind, for Eridu is the home of Ea, the sea-god. . . . In this same text mention is made of an 'Incantation of the Deep,' which is probably a purification of a similar kind" (1971, lii). The Assyrian hymn to the Euphrates ends, "Within thee, Ea, the King of the Deep, created his dwelling" (liv). Thus, the home of Ea, the sea god, was the Euphrates, which for the Hebrews of Babylonia was regarded as sacred and was referred to as "the River" (liii).

During the performance of the prekante, the transference was ritually enacted. While most women would take a fistful of salt before initiating the ritual, Rebecca Levy and Izahar Avzaradel, both from the island of Rhodes, would summon the patient: "Dame un punyadu di sal [Give me a fistful of salt]." Then they would show the salt in their palm and ask, "What is this?" The response was, quite simply, "Salt." To some, the salt ensured that both the specialist and the patient would be protected against the evil eye. At that moment, the prekante began. At the conclusion, the salt was placed in a basin of water and the prekantadora said, "As this salt dissolves in the water, may all harm dissolve." When the ritual was performed with cloves instead of salt, then the cloves burned away the evil. As they burned, the prekantadora would take a whiff of the aroma, which represented the departure of the evil spirits, and then she would transfer the harm to whoever had caused it: "Komo se estan apatladiando los klavos, / Ke se patladee los ojos del ke la miro kon eyos [As these cloves are exploding, / Let the eyes of whoever has seen her explode with them]." However, the preferred method was to shift the evil to any body of water: a toilet bowl, a basin of water, a river, or the sea. As Isaac's grandmother said, "Nothing is like the sea." Then she quoted the two most common verses of a prekante: "La mar es ancha i todu lu puedi reivar, lu puedi reivar i simportar [The sea is vast and can endure everything, it can endure and tolerate it]." Bohora Biton, in the prekante de kulivreta, also emphasized the importance of the sea and the fish that live within: "Todu il mal a la profundida di la mar lo tinemos ki ichar, / al pishkadu di la mar ke lo puedi reivar. / Dingun [iju d']Israel nu tenga dingun mal. [All harm to the bottom of the sea we must cast, to the fish of the sea that can endure it. / No member of Israel should have any harm]."[33]

Representing spiritual redemption, fertility, and rebirth, the waters of the sea dissolved the harm brought about by the spirits and cleansed the body from all evil. Harold Bayley observes that "water, whether in the form of sea, river, fountain, well, rain, or dew, has universally been employed as a symbol of cleansing, refreshing, and invigorating qualities of spirit" (1992, 243). As the prekante emphasized, the deep and vast sea could withstand one's suffering. Additionally, the ever-watchful fish—whose eyes, like God's, were never shut—were protected by the waters of the sea and could also absorb the harm. The symbolism of the fish extended to the Jewish people, for "Jacob blessed Joseph's two sons, and all their descendants, by comparing them to fish" (Frankel and Teutsch 1992, 255).

In addition to the water and the fish in the sea, salt was deemed effective for countering all manner of spells. As a symbol of purity and preservation, it has been a source of life and of protection. According to the Kabbalists, "It drives off the spirits" because the numerical equivalent for the Hebrew letters spelling "salt" are "the mathematical equivalent of three YHVHs" (Trachtenberg 1939, 160). The absence of the "salt of life" was death, and thus the custom at the meal following Sephardic funerals of eating a whole egg without salt. As Rabbi Samuel Benaroya explained, offering the complete egg without salt was "a sign of life now missing."[34] For both the Sephardim and the Ashkenazim, the roundness of the egg represented "the continuous nature of life" (Donin 1972, 302), and the "endless circle" of life and death (Greenberg 1983, 293). On occasions other than a funeral, a Sephardi, after peeling a hard-boiled egg, would cut it in half to "separate" or "cut" the connection with death, and would sprinkle it with salt to give the symbolic protection of life and preservation. Thus, the closing line in the prekante recorded by Galanté, "May the evil eye go there where one eats eggs without salt," banished the evil and, by association, the malevolent one to the land of the dead (1935, 119). This same concept is reflected in the Sephardic proverb, "Andi ki vaya il mal? Andi komen gueṿos sin sal [Where should the evil go? Where one eats an egg without salt]," that is, to the land of the dead, where the evil should not cause any harm (Lévy 1969, 117). Pedrosa, in "Las tres llaves y los huevos sin sal" (1998, 162–64), has identified the following Sephardic formula in several ensalmos from Spanish golden age manuscripts: "Aya vayas mal donde komen guevo sin sal [There go evil where one eats eggs without salt]." Pedrosa was able to locate, almost verbatim, the same formula in several medieval compilations of proverbs: "Alla vayas mal: do comen el hueuo sin sal," "Allá vaia el mal, donde komen el guevo sin sal" (1998, 163).

Words and symbols are put into action in performance. Thus, as Victor Lis Quibén remarked in his study of the Galician ensalmo, "Pay attention not to what is said, but how it is said, not to what is done, but how it is done" (1980, 100). So also for the prekantadora, the "enactment" of the words and the symbols was crucial, and it was individualized. Here was the personal rendition of verses, the variation of wording from one performance to the next, and the interpretation of Hebrew phrases by women who often had no knowledge of the language. Where we might have remarked on the omission of words, or on incorrect pronunciation, the women who taught us the prekantes never perceived any inconsistency. For them, there was no concern with a rigid adherence to textual format or to a standard "accepted" pronunciation. Our mother, Caden Lévy Israel, assured us of this: the exact words were not important. Instead the women were concerned with the essentials, that the cure was being done in God's name, that there was sincerity of belief, and that their own prekantes, with their regional and individualistic interpretations, would bring relief.

Still, variation and personal interpretation existed within a shared structure that marked the verse as part of a prekante. For instance, Lea Amram, originally from Istanbul, gave us the following example of a common format: "Te kito el ojo malo, la avla mala, l'ayinarah, i todo el mal, / Ke se vaya al fondo de la mar, / Ke Lea, ija de Rahel, ke no tenga dingun mal [I remove from you the evil eye, the evil speech, the ayin arah, and all harm, / Let it go to the bottom of the sea, / And Lea, daughter of Rachel, may not have any harm]." After reciting this, Mrs. Amram immediately repeated it to make sure we had been able to record it properly. However, she changed the last line from "ke no tenga dingun mal [may she not have any harm]," to "ke no tenga ni sar ni mal [may she not have any fright nor any harm]." In her view, she had given us the exact same line. Thus, it was quite common for the wording to vary according to the person uttering the prekante, even within immediate repetition.

For the women who recited the prekantes, the phrases in Hebrew were powerful because they were in God's language. With but little knowledge of Hebrew, the women did not understand the meaning of the Hebrew verses. For instance, the original Hebrew from Genesis 49:22, "Ben porat Yosef, ben porat 'ale 'ayin [Joseph is a fruitful bough, a fruitful bough by a spring],"[35] was given the following renditions: Ben pura Yosef, ben pura adalai; Ben pura Yusef, ben pura adalain; Ben para Yusef, ben para adalaid; Ben para Yosef, ben para elal [or helal]; Ben para Yosef, ben para ilai; Ben purat Yosef, ben para alaila; and Ben porat Yusef, ben para layla. When asked for her interpretation of the phrase, one woman said it meant, "May the sacrifice of Joseph, Lord, be accepted instead of mine." Most others said simply that the words were holy and were not meant to be understood by the average person. Thus, the concern of the women was not with the actual meaning, but rather with the inclusion of the phrase, because it was holy and it had power. In accord with this view, Thompson writes in *Semitic Magic,* "Treasures are kept locked by means of sacred words" (1971, xlix).

When Isaac's great aunt Rachel gave him the following prekante, he immediately suspected from the opening Hebraic phrase, "El rahum vehanum," and from its general tone that it had been taken from a written amulet:

El rahum vehanum.
Dio piadazo i graziozu,
Grande de folores,
Para munchos azez bueno,
Te apiadas di todo el puevlo,
I todu el bueno azez al mundo.
Rogu ki agas bueno,
Ki milizines a _______ [a tal i tal].
Lishuateha kiviti Adonai,
A Tu salvasion espero Adonai.
Kiviti Adonai Lushateha,
Adonai lishuateha kiviti.

God, merciful and compassionate.
God, merciful and compassionate,
Great in wrath,
For many you do good,
You take pity on all the people,
And you do good to all the world.

I beg you to do good,
To cure _______ [so-and-so].

For your salvation I hope, Lord,
For your salvation I hope, Lord.
I hope, Lord, for your salvation,
Lord, for your salvation I hope.[36]

Two days after he had collected this prekante, his great aunt handed him some written prayers and a long list of proverbs that she had copied years earlier from the oral tradition. Among the material, he found this specific prekante, which was inscribed with the Star of David at the beginning, as was standard with many Jewish amulets. His great aunt recalled that her father, a student of the Bible, had written it years earlier for a member of the family who had suffered from headaches, lack of appetite, and fatigue, all symptoms of the evil eye. It was written on a piece of paper, folded, sealed in a leather pouch, and worn on a leather thong around the neck. When Isaac asked Aunt Rachel how the written amulet had passed into oral tradition, she replied, "Lo sentieron [They heard it]." Through repetition, the women of Izmir included the text of the amulet in their repertoire of prekantes. From his experience of working with the Sephardim for over forty years, Isaac views this transmission of a written amulet to a spoken verse for curing as unique. The composer of the amulet, Isaac's great-great uncle, took the first verse, "El rahum vehanun," from Exodus 34:6. These words, "God, merciful and compassionate," are the first of the thirteen Attributes of God. According to Rabbi Howard Kosovske, the ninth, eleventh, and twelfth verses are permutations of the three words of the text from Genesis 49:18. These borrowings from the Bible and the writings of the rabbis were common in the composition of Jewish amulets.

When Isaac asked his great aunt to define *folores* as it appears in line three of the prekante, "Grande de folores," she said "bondades," or "goodness," since the Sephardic woman envisioned a God of "piadades," of mercy, and not of wrath, as the term "folor" denotes in Judeo-Spanish. Isaac later realized that the composer of the amulet had intended to convey both God's mercy and his wrath (Psalms 86:15). Additionally, in the penultimate line, "Kiviti Adonai Lushateha," Isaac's aunt said "lushateha," and not the Hebrew pronunciation of *lishuateha,* which she had rendered correctly in adjacent lines. Such inconsistencies in definitions, mispronunciations, even incorrect spellings, may have been due to an earlier error of a scribe in copying the original amulet, or to a misunderstanding of the term by the one reciting the verse, a misunderstanding that was then passed into oral tradition. These frequent inconsistencies, substitutions, misspellings, and mispronunciations were not only common from one country to another, and from city to city, but also within one community, as well as within renditions given by one individual. Often they occurred within the same prekante or ballad, tale, or proverb. For the people, these permutations were simply not perceived as inconsistencies; they were accepted as the correct rendition.

In addition to the challenges of working with intricate verses that have been orally transmitted, we have encountered the difficulty of deciphering verses recorded by others in published form. For example, Isaac could not make sense of an old prekante from Bosnia, as it was published by Samuel Elazar (1987, 247–48), until he checked several Judeo-Spanish dictionaries, and a Hebrew-Turkish one as well. Isaac even had to pronounce some of the phrases aloud. For instance, the line giving instructions on how to perform the prekante, "Para segula si azi la marana indo basho sabana," at first made no sense at all. A literal translation would have been, "For a cure, the *marana* is done *indo* bed sheets." Isaac had heard of *merana,* incorrect for *meana,* Turkish for pub; and he was aware of the term *marrano* (converted Jew), and of *marana* (Judeo-Spanish for "a great disturbance"). However, these words were also used incorrectly in the published prekante. He finally realized that *marana* should have been *marona* (early morning), and that the two words, *indo* and *basho,* should have been one, *indibasho* (under). Thus, the correct translation would be, "The cure should be performed in the morning, under the sheets, before [the patient] gets up." In fairness to Elazar and others, we should remark on the particular challenges of working with Judeo-Spanish. The Sephardim, wherever they settled, adopted words from the local language—French, Turkish, Greek, Serbo-Croatian, Italian, Arabic, and Hebrew. Quite often the Sephardim themselves reinterpreted the meaning of these words and changed their pronunciation. Thus, even when one is a native speaker of Judeo-Spanish, there are challenges in working with the language and in translating the texts, which are akin to a gigantic linguistic puzzle.

Yet another complexity involves the interpretation of symbols. For instance, the first line of the following *prekante por espanto* (prekante for fright), which Isaac had collected from his Aunt Rachel in 1968, initially made no sense:

Roka baroka,	*Roka baroka,*
Fiero en la boka,	Iron in the mouth,
Kadenado en los piezes.	Padlock on the feet.
Disho el romero,	Said the rosemary,
"Yo nasi primero."	"I was born first."
Disho la ruda,	Said the rue,
"Ke el Dio de Avram este en su ayuda."	"May the Lord of Abraham come to his aid."

Since symbols, as Victor Turner elucidates, are multivocal—a single symbol may stand for many things (1967, 50)—then *roka* and *baroka* could have several interpretations. The fourth line, "Disho el romero [said the rosemary]" and the sixth one, "Disho la ruda [said the rue]," refer to the plants rosemary and rue, respectively. Possibly *roka* was a reference to the plant by that name in Judeo-Spanish, known as roquette, and as arugula in English. Since plants with strong odors, such as rue and garlic, were used to ward off the evil spirits, especially those attracted to babies, pregnant women, and nursing mothers, then *roka,* with its pungent aroma and spicy taste, might have the same protective powers. Additionally, as Eliyah Arnon notes, *roka* in Hebrew is a plant used by a *roke'a*[*h*] (Hebrew for pharmacist),[37] an individual who heals through the use of the essence of herbs; it also is a Hebrew term for one who makes perfume. Rabbi Yossi Y. Groner agrees with Arnon: "*Roke'a*[*h*], by extension, also refers to a substance, an herb, used by pharmacists for curative purposes."[38] John Reeves remarks that since Isaac's great-great uncle was a biblical scholar from Izmir, Turkey, he must have been aware that *roka* (Hebrew also for ingredient) was a generic term for a special mixture of spices used as "a holy anointing oil, a superior ointment [Hebrew, *mirkahat*] compounded after the art of the perfumer,"[39] as God charged Moses to have prepared as a holy anointing oil (Exodus 30:22, 25).

While the Hebrew for *roka* and *roke'a*[*h*] offers these additional meanings of ointment and healing, there was no definition to be found for *baroka.* None of the Sephardic women with whom we spoke could explain it, except that it was "una koza presioza [a precious thing]." We thought that *baroka* might be a magical word with supernatural powers, and perhaps it may have derived from *beraha,* Hebrew for blessing. Eliyah Arnon explained that *ba,* a Hebrew preposition, together with a word, emphasizes the value of the term. Thus, the seemingly nonsensical first line, comprised of the two words, *roka* and *baroka,* takes on its power by the repetition of the word. As with many verbal art forms, and specifically with many prekantes, the repetition of words and phrases builds the power and convinces the hearer of its importance. In this case, the preposition *ba* along with *roka* strengthens the value of the term. Thus, an accurate translation of the first line would be, "Roquette, a valued [blessed] plant," "Spices, blessed spices," or "Healing, a real cure."

The last two lines of this prekante are similar to the popular "Komplas de las flores" (The couplets of the flowers), which we collected in Ashdod in 1990. The recitation of these verses was customary during the celebration of Tu BiShevat (Jewish Arbor Day), which takes place on the fifteenth day of the Jewish month of Shevat. On that day, people celebrate by eating fruit and planting trees.[40] Among the Sephardim, rue was considered to be "la reina de las yervas [the queen of all herbs]," due to its curative powers and magical potency. In the following couplet, after listening to the other flowers laud their own merits, rue jumps in and brags about her own powers, especially in guarding an individual against the evil eye:

> Great is my fame,
> I am the rose of newly delivered mothers.
> They place me on their beds,
> And all the evil eye
> I consume with my plants.
> I guard the soul
> Of the one who wears me.

The rue, as well as the other flowers, realizes that the true praise must go to the *kreador,* the Creator. Thus, the following refrain is repeated at the end of each couplet: "Sovre todo es de alavar / Al hay tsur olamim. [Above all it is to praise / The Living God, the Eternal Rock]."

Sarota Musafir, Isaac's grandmother, often told him, "El prekante era koza presioza i ayudava muncho [the prekante was a precious thing and it helped a lot]." Yet when even the most complex prekante did not bring the desired relief, the Sephardim made recourse to *saradura,* the complex ritual of enclosure, which we take up in the next chapter.

9 Saradura: *The Ritual of Enclosure*

The most complex cure, that of ritual enclosure, was reserved for those who did not respond to simpler remedies. The cause of illness was the same as for the simpler ones, as indicated by the terminology: *espanto mucho* (great *espanto*), *puro espanto* (pure *espanto*), *espanto negro* (dreadful *espanto*). The curative procedure was intricate, performed several days prior to Rosh Hodesh, the new month, which for the Jewish lunar calendar was also the new moon. It involved enclosing the afflicted in a house with the *maestra* and her helpers for at least three days and nights, and sometimes more. Special precautions had to be observed: no fire was allowed in the house, and the afflicted was kept in bed, ritually bathed, and fed a specific bland diet. This included bread, but there could be no oil, no onion, no garlic, no meat, and no fish, the latter forbidden for the entire month. As we were told, "Nothing with an odor is eaten." The procedure caused so much fear that the neighbors on both sides had to move out for the duration of the cure. In her 1891 work *The Women of Turkey and Their Folk-Lore,* Lucy Garnett described such a ritual: "Another method of exorcising demons is . . . called *indulgéncia,* or coaxing, and is employed in the case of a violent shock, or any mental excitement, as this is believed to be caused by some demon having gained mastery over the sufferer. The patient is washed, dressed in white linen, and laid on a white bed. . . . The sufferer . . . must remain as much alone as possible, eating nothing but bread, butter, and milk, and taking as medicine occasional small doses of pulverized mummy, dissolved in sugar water" (2:67–68).

This ritual cure of enclosure was denoted by two terms, *endulko* and *saradura,* both of which were pronounced differently according to the place of origin of the informant. In Edirne and in Celebria, near Istanbul, *endulko* was rendered *aldurko;* in Bulgaria, as *indulko,* and also as *indulto.* It was known as *asaradura, saradura, seradura,* as related by people from Rhodes and Boudroun, Turkey. It was also known as *saladura, asaladura,* or *salvadura* in Rhodes. The following exchange between Rosemary, Isaac, and his mother, Caden Lévy Israel, shows two modifications of the term:

Rosemary: Mother, what happens if a woman wants to have a baby and she can't have a baby, does she do anything special?
Caden: They used to do things, *la izian por ispantu* [they performed espanto for her], *asaladura* that's it.
Isaac: Is it the regular asaladura that they would shut someone up for three days?
Caden: *Saladura,* as they did. In order to know what the [woman] had . . . , they believed in that.

In similar fashion, Isaac's grandmother, Sarota Musafir, originally from Milas, Turkey, also corrected him when he asked, "What do they do for asaradura?" She responded, "Saladura," and then continued, "they take three different types of sugar." The following exchange between Isaac; his step-father, Baruch Israel; and Bohora Biton shows further variation of terms:

Isaac: My grandmother only gave half of it. She did not remember the whole thing, of seradura. Of a woman or a man being enclosed.
Baruch: Saladura, not seradura.
Bohora: Not man, a woman. . . . Asaradura.

At times in our fieldwork, the very pronunciation of the term made the difference between a lack of comprehension and a willing response. When we interviewed Mary Algrante in Izmir, Turkey, Isaac asked her, "Do you remember something for *endulcho,* that they enclosed someone for three days, for the evil eye?" The interview continued:

Mary: Three days, what? I don't know.
Isaac: That's what I want to know, I don't remember it.
Mary: What is it?
Isaac: They called it endulcho.
Mary: Ahh! Endulko! Endulko, endulko.

A man sitting in the lounge nearby immediately interrupted Isaac and Mrs. Algranate: "Endulko, it happened to me." One way to avoid such confusion in our fieldwork was simply to provide a listing of the various terms, as Isaac did in the following question, which he posed to a woman who was originally from Istanbul: "Have you heard of asaradura, *indulcho?* Some call it seradura, others call it indulcho. When they would enclose a person for three days."

The etymology of the two terms, *endulko* and *saradura*, provides a key to an understanding of this ritual cure. *Endulko, endulcho, indulgo,* and *indulto* derive from the Latin verb, *indulgere,* to be benevolent. In Latin, *indulgĕo* means to be indulgent or lenient, to have regard for some consideration, to look favorably, to show kindness to a person; to grant a favor, concede, bestow. The Spanish *indulto*—which derives from the Latin, *indultus,* and is the past participle of *indulgere*—also refers to the total or partial pardon granted by a higher power for a transgression. In 1891, Garnett used the term *indulgéncia* to refer to "a particular curing ritual of the Turkish Sephardim" (2:67). While not found in Spanish or Portuguese dictionaries, *indulco* in Latin means to make sweet, or to sweeten. We point, then, to the connection between the intent of the ritual in which one asks pardon of the spirits, and the etymology of *endulko,* and the related words, to grant a favor or a pardon by a higher power. Therefore we suggest that *endulko,* and its variations, refer to the sweetening of the spirits, and to the plea of the Sephardic women that the spirits be *induljentes,* indulgent. While the etymology of *endulko* goes back to the Spanish and Latin roots, the source for the meaning of *saradura* derives from the Hebrew noun *tsar* (צער), which means "distress, fright, danger, anguish" (Nehama 1977, 497). Additionally, in Judeo-Spanish, *seradura* means "lock"; and in modern Spanish, *cerradura,* means "lock, closure, act of shutting or locking" (Cuyas 1953, 113). The Judeo-Spanish verb *serar* and the Spanish verb *cerrar* have the additional meaning "to inclose" (Cuyas, 113). Finally, *salvadura* derives from the Judeo-Spanish verb *salvar,* to save (Nehama 1977, 494), and refers to the state of being saved or delivered. Thus, the etymological meaning of *endulko, endulcho,* and *indulto* emphasized the goal of the ritual, to seek pardon from a superior; *salvadura* also emphasized the goal, being delivered from the danger of the spirits; *saradura* stressed the emotional state of the person, "to be in fright or distress"; and *seradura,* the chief characteristic of the ritual, "to inclose."

In our survey of the scholarship on this ritual, we find that authors have attached their own definitions to these terms and have provided little or no evidence that the people were in accord. In his otherwise engaging study on "Sephardic Folk-Curing in Seattle" (1962), Melvin Firestone delineates a broad definition for what he terms *endurcos,* which, for him, encompassed all of folk curing: "The Sephardim brought with them from the Near East procedures which were used in curing the sick. This body of practice, known as *endurcos,* lies outside the normative religion and is performed for the most part by women" (301). In "The Sephardic Community of Los Angeles" (1980), Stephen Stern draws from Firestone in the reference to "*endurcos.*" Unfortunately, Stern also uses this term with the same imprecision as does Firestone, to designate cures that do not involve ritual enclosure. In "*Indulco* and *Mumia,*" Raphael Patai (1964) aligns himself with his "good friend, Michael Molho" of Salonika, in regarding "the usual form of the name of the magic cure [as] *indulco*" (3), rather than the term used by Firestone, *endurcos* (Firestone 1962, 303). In this alliance, Patai is ignoring the variation of pronunciation according to the geographical origin of the speaker. From our extensive interviews with Sephardic informants from numerous geographical locations throughout the former Ottoman Empire, we can say without hesitation that there is nothing that would make Molho's and Patai's term, *indulco,* more correct than Firestone's *endurcos.* In still another interpretation, Albert Adatto uses the term *aldurko,* in reference to "incantation sessions" held by Jews from Rhodes. As Adatto writes, "Oftentimes these sessions last for many hours. *Aldurkos* are group gatherings for the purpose of joint prayer or incantation for the relief of the enchanted or afflicted person" (1939, 303). For us, Adatto's term *aldurko* makes sense, but his designation of what it entails is misleading. We assume he is referring to ritual enclosure, though his discussion of "group gatherings" for prayer is not an accurate portrayal of what takes place.[1]

In his work on ritual enclosure, Raphael Patai draws extensively from a Jerusalem scholar of the nineteenth century, Manasseh Matlub Sithon, who designated two types of *indulcos,* "a 'great' one and a 'small' one," which he called *matoq,* from the Hebrew, sweet (or, possibly, *mittuq,* from the Hebrew, sweetening) (Patai 1964, 3).[2] According to Sithon, "the Jews in all Muslim lands" performed *indulcos* as a cure for illness, for female infertility, for miscarriage, death of infants, eye disease, and mental illness (4). As Patai notes, "The wide prevalence of the *indulco* is attested by the fact that the . . . 'unmasking' [by Sithon] of its superstitious practices was approved of by the rabbis of all the Sephardi and Ashkenazi communities in Palestine (Jerusalem, Safed, Hebron, Tiberias, Jaffa, Haifa), as well as the Sephardi rabbis of Smyrna, Damascus, and Beirut, and the chief rabbi of Egypt" (5). Thus, Patai and Sithon were not addressing the procedure as practiced in the Balkans or Turkey. For the "great one," Sithon described a procedure that resembled the ritual we have studied in the following ways: the enclosure of the women curers and the stricken one for a certain period of time (three, seven, or nine nights); the moving out of the neighbors; the ritual cleansing of the house; the use of honey, sugar, and mumia as cures; and the repeated use of blessings.

However, there was a significant difference between the "great" ritual described by Sithon and those we studied. Whereas for the people with whom we spoke, the ritual enclosure and all other cures were always done in the name of God, the patriarchs, and the matriarchs, Sithon found the deliberate exclusion of all things sacred. He wrote: "All the Holy Books are taken out from the house, and some go so far as to remove even the *Mezuzoth* . . . from the doors, so that there be no hindrance there to prevent the demons from entering the house. . . . And the patient is warned and doubly warned to say neither the *shema* nor any other prayer, to recite neither a long nor a short benediction, not even the after-meal grace . . . , nor to utter the name of God, nor any other holy thing, from neither the written nor the oral Torah, neither aloud nor in a whisper, so that the demons should enter the house and join him and appear to him in his dream" (Patai 1964, 4; quoting Sithon). The woman curer prostrated herself before the demons and implored them to take pity on the stricken one. She then broke eggs and offered them to the demons as "a sacrifice to you, a soul for a soul . . . so that you may return to us the soul of this patient." With this, the woman curer poured the eggs on the ground, prostrated herself again, and kissed the floor several times. "All this is done three times, and then repeated for three nights, for each patient. Some, however, insist that it has to be done as often as seven or even nine times, as well as at noontime on Friday. . . . Also, on certain other nights of the week, which are the fixed time for this procedure, because in them many Liliths and demons are abroad, and go up and down" (Patai 1964, 4; quoting Sithon). For those who could not afford such a lengthy procedure, and for all who sought a ready appeal to the spirits, there was, according to Sithon, "the Small Sweet," which Patai classifies as the small *indulco.* This involved going to the pits and the tanners where the evil spirits dwelled and "pouring water and salt for the demons. And this being easy to perform, is found so frequently, every day, that there is no day in which this would not be performed several times. And some throw sugar and mumia and spices. And this libation is the slightest of all the works of Satan, and it is called in several places 'The Small Sweet'" (Patai 1964, 5; quoting Sithon).

Patai also refers to the work of Abraham Moshe Luncz (1882), which followed Sithon's by eight years. A member of the small Ashkenazi community of Jerusalem, Luncz based his study of the ritual on Sithon's but added, as Patai notes, "several details which show that he had personally observed the ritual which does not seem to have been given up by the people in spite of the stern rabbinical warnings against it" (Patai 1964, 5). Luncz referred to these ritual procedures as *indulco* and, with the adjective, *indulcado.* In what appears to us an erroneous if fanciful explanation, Patai suggested that "these names . . . were originally applied to abandoned and desolate houses, and then transferred to the ritual for whose duration the patient's house must be abandoned by all the other residents" (Patai 1964, 5). According to Luncz, *indulco* was used to treat "only impermanent diseases such as lunacy, blindness, sudden fright, barrenness of women, difficulty in childbirth, loss of children, epilepsy, and the like" (Patai 1964, 5; quoting Luncz).

Both Sithon and Luncz agreed that the *indulco* "was performed either in a vacated house, or in a place of impurity" (Patai 1964, 6; quoting Sithon and Luncz). Additionally, they reported that sometimes it was performed in "holy places, such as in a synagogue, or in the Cave of the Prophet Elijah on Mt. Carmel, or in the House of Study which is over the Tomb of Ezra the Scribe in Baghdad" (6). Luncz continued, "'The patient is left lying alone in that place. And when the purpose of the ritual is to give children to childless couples, the man and woman will stay alone overnight in the sacred place, while the woman who performs the ceremony for them leaves the place upon its conclusion and locks them in'" (Patai 1964, 6; quoting Luncz).

Taking exception to Sithon and Luncz, both of whom regarded this ritual held in sacred space as a variant of the *indulco,* Patai stresses that "whatever the formal similarity of the performance itself—the two are based on two completely different, in fact, contrasting, motivations." Patai regards the "great one" as reported by Sithon as a variety of the "true *indulco*"; its aim was to propitiate the demons, to avoid all things holy, and not to bring "the patient into close contact with the holiness of a sacred site in order thereby to rid him of the baneful influence of the demons" (Patai 1964, 6). Noting that the *indulco* practiced in Salonika also called on holy names and involved guarding the patient against the evil spirits, Patai writes: "However, the second variety, too, was and remained known under the name *indulco.* Michael Molho describes this second type of the *indulco* which was practiced in Salonica. Although in this ritual, too, everybody must leave the house, three or four women remain with the patient 'to guard him against the evil spirits who might attack him.' Moreover, and more importantly, in the Salonica *indulco,* . . . the old woman who administers the *indulco* invokes Abraham, Isaac, Jacob, and other saints to intercede with God" (7). In this circuitous and engaging route, Patai arrives at the ritual of enclosure as described by Michael Molho in *Usos y costumbres de los Sefardíes de Salónica* (1950).

While Patai regards the "great sweet" as described by Sithon as the "true *indulco,*" we are not so disposed to judge the merits of the ceremonies described to us by our informants. Rather than seeking the "true" ritual of enclosure, we have attempted to arrive at an understanding of the nuances in this ritual practice by paying close heed to what the people have related about variation in performance.

Bienvenida Gabay told us that *aldurko pezgado* (heavy aldurko), also known as *aldurko de miel* (aldurko of honey), was only done "if the patient is truly very sick." Stressing the serious nature of the cure, Zimbul Maya Suzi referred to *aldurko puro* (pure aldurko) as "*muy fuerte* [very strong]." In her various explanations, Caden Lévy Israel emphasized both the severity of the cure and the importance of enclosure: "You perform asaradura for *puro espanto* [pure espanto] when someone is very ill"; "You enclose him in a house"; and "Lu insiro pur ispantu [She locked him up for the performance of espanto]." In relating specific cases, our mother again stressed the importance of enclosure, though the length of time for it might vary: "[The stricken one] was three days home, *inserada* [enclosed]"; "The curer enclosed him for the [cure of] espanto for four days in a house only the two together, with the young man who was sick. And she performed what is called asaradura."

Enclosure and isolation of the stricken one were the crucial components of the ritual. Everyone who lived in the house had to pack up and leave for the three- or four-day duration of the cure, as did the neighbors in the houses on either side. Melvin Firestone stipulates that "neighbors who lived in dwellings whose walls touched the walls of the house in which the *cerradura* was being performed" would move out (1962, 307). If the neighbors lived on "the other side of an archway," as Rebecca Amato Levy notes, they did not have to move out but they probably would (1987, 72). Diana Cadranel, originally of Rhodes, explained, "I know in the *seradura* one puts the sick one in a closed place." Her husband, Marco Cadranel, interjected, "Isolated," and she continued, "Isolated, yes. This person . . . is enclosed for seven days. . . . Everyone leaves. Even those around the house leave theirs. All the neighbors must leave."

Sol Azuz, originally of Istanbul, told of the cure performed for her during her second pregnancy to protect her unborn child from an illness that had struck her first offspring. While the neighbors did not move out, still the emphasis was on enclosure and isolation: "My mother said, 'You give birth, you get pregnant. . . . I am going to do something so that the child who is going to be born will not be sick any more.' . . . What did she do? . . . When I was already seven months pregnant, . . . she enclosed the complete house [for an] endulko, . . . the complete house, the windows, everything. The house was enclosed. No neighbors should come. No one! Only my husband. Only my husband. They closed all the draperies. And the neighbors from upstairs, no one could enter. No one. . . . We told [the neighbors] not to enter because we were doing a strong endulko. And in this way, eight complete days no one saw me. I was stuck inside the house with the windows closed. With everything closed."

Sol Konfino told of her childhood memories from Bitola, Yugoslavia: "They did other things for fright, but I was a young child. I don't remember what they did. My mother was frightened. . . . They removed us from the house. . . . We all had to leave." Rosa Avzaradel also recollected from her childhood in Rhodes: "We used to hear that they were going to enclose someone, and we left the house." This had a side benefit for the children who had to leave home: "We went to the house of some relatives. I recall taking our . . . mattresses to . . . Aunt Rahel, who lived on the Kay Ancha. I wanted saraduras to take place because there were six girls there and I was the seventh one. And it was a party." Mrs. Avzaradel concluded, "That I recall. We left the house. But what the ladies did [was serious]."

Throughout the duration of the ritual cure, the stricken one was expected to rest quietly in bed. As Bohora Biton said, "She did not even walk, not even to the toilet. She lay there in bed." Sol Konfino remarked about the cure for her mother, "Everything had to be very quiet . . . , a lot of silence. A lot of rest for her." Zimbul Maya Suzi commented on the care for the stricken one: "When she sleeps, they must keep her completely quiet. The house must be quiet."

Often two women were in charge of the cure, though sometimes there was a third. They were, as Bohora Biton said, *bravas*, strong, courageous, capable of performing the saradura and of speaking with the *sheddim*, the spirits. Rosa Avzaradel remembered that in Rhodes, "There were two women. They always went together with the sick one. . . . These two women enclosed themselves [with the sick one] and every day they would make some medicine." Caden Lévy Israel recalled, "They closed everything. And the women who performed it and the sick person were the only ones there." Bienvenida Gabay, originally of Edirne, Turkey, told us of the strict procedure for the cure done with honey, which she called *aldurko de miel*. The period of enclosure was lengthy and the isolation was rigidly enforced: "The patient must be home nine days and nine nights locked up in the house with the maestra. The draperies must be drawn, the doors must be closed. No cooking can be done in the room, because of the odor. Neither of the two can leave the room. Only the person who takes care of them can come and go, because she has to bring something to eat."

Since the stricken one should also be protected from menstruating women, the women curers should be past menopause. Melvin Firestone remarked on this, "Only women who are past menopause may practice *cerradura*. . . . The patient must have contact with only the specialist and women past menopause" (1962, 302, 307). As Mary Algrante cautioned, "And you will not let, pardon me, *alguna dama suzia* [any (unclean, dirty) menstruating woman] see the patient." Another person told us that "no pregnant woman or young women who had contact with their husbands could see" the sick one. In a similar vein, though with delicacy, Lucy Garnett recorded that "on some occasions the presence of women is considered harmful." Additionally Garnett noted, "All kinds of animals . . . especially poultry, must be kept away from the house" (1891, 2:67–68). Firestone observed that the patient "should not see other people because they would not be keeping the food taboos and may have been smoking. . . . And he must see no other man because he might have seen someone in mourning in the synagogue" (1962, 307).

The cure was performed, as Bohora Biton recalled, "about four, five days before the end of the month"; and then she stipulated, "The Jewish [lunar] month, not the *franko* [French/Christian]." As if spontaneously emphasizing the importance of the moon in determining the time for the cure, Rosa Avzaradel said, "They did it at the end of the moon, on the twenty-fourth of the moon, of the moon. With the moon. When she is getting smaller." Caden Lévy Israel gave this explanation for the timing of the cure: "It was in the *minguanti* [waning moon], after the fifteenth of the month . . . before Rosh Hodesh [the new month]. Zimbul Maya Suzi stipulated that the cure should be performed only when "the moon gets smaller, not when the moon increases," and she added, "Not on Rosh Hodesh [the beginning of the Jewish month]. God forbid! From Rosh Hodesh until the fifteenth of the month, it is not done!" For one young girl, the cure was performed each month until she was cured, as we were told, "Each month they did it, at the end of the moon."

In preparation for the saradura, the house was thoroughly cleaned. The women were particularly careful to remove all foods that would be forbidden during the duration of the cure. As Rosa Avzaradel said, "They did not leave any onion, garlic, not any form of fish, such as *saladu* [salted fish], or such things." During the days of the cure, the patient was forbidden strong food, or food with an odor, and was fed only mild foods. Zimbul Maya Suzi said, "The meal should not include eggs, nothing burnt [because of the odor], no garlic, no onion, not even fish." In exaggeration, but with definite emphasis, Diana Cadranel said, "This person does not eat anything for the seven days that he is *enseradu* [enclosed]. He does not eat but uncooked foods, such as [strong] cheese, yogurt. During the seradura, they do not build a fire in the house." Rosa Avzaradel placed the same emphasis on the absence of food: "These eight days, no one ate anything. No meat, no onion, nothing."

Caden Lévy Israel also stressed the limited diet. In response to Isaac's question "What did they give him to eat?" she responded, "What did they give him to eat? Nothing. Cheese with bread. Nothing, nothing, almost nothing to eat. He couldn't eat fish, no saladu, nothing of this kind for a whole month." In answer to Isaac's question "What food do they serve?" his grandmother, Sarota Musafir, said, "They give spaghetti and cheese. No oil." Isaac continued, "How about meat and fish?" and his grandmother quickly responded, "No, no, no, no. Fish he cannot eat all month long. Meat only after he is washed [when the cure is over]. They give him a bath. He is clean, and then he can eat meat. . . . The person [who] is sick, without strength, . . . for nine days, he doesn't eat. But no fish all month long." In recalling the cure performed for her mother when she was a young girl, Mrs. Avzaradel said, "They brought her home. They told her to go to sleep and not to eat onions, garlic, and fish, for one month. . . . Well, they put her to bed, they told her to sleep. My mother used to tell us that she was dreaming that someone went [to their home] with a dish of fish. She is dreaming [that the man was saying], 'Eat.' 'No, no,' said my mother because the ladies told me to be careful. He would bring onions, 'No, no, no.'" While tempted in her dreams, the young girl avoided these forbidden foods until, at the end of the month, the women said, "'Now you can eat whatever you want." Bienvenida Gabay explained that for the ritual enclosure performed with honey (aldurko de miel), "Both the patient and the maestra must keep the same diet, because we are under the same breath."

During the period of ritual enclosure, the women performed specific cures on the first, second, and third nights. The cures were first administered in the early evening, which was in keeping with the Jewish ritual calendar where the new day began when the moon appeared. They were often given in three portions, at nightfall, at midnight, and at dawn. While each woman with whom we spoke gave a different combination of cures, still there was a standard set of components from which to choose. These usually involved a sequence of three of the following: sugar water, rose water, marjoram, rue, powdered coffee, honey, and *mumia tapada.* When giving the cures, the maestra would bless the stricken one, with the following:

Kon el nombre del Dio,
De muestros padres i madres
Yo te do la melezina
I el Dio ke te de la komplida.

In the name of God,
Of our patriarchs and matriarchs
I give you the medicine
And my God give you the total cure.

As Bohora Biton told us, "One night for each ingredient." For instance, in one account, the women gave three sugar packets to the stricken one at the established intervals throughout the night; on the second night, they gave mashed marjoram as a drink and then rubbed the person's entire body with it; and on the third night, they gave three packets of powdered coffee. In another account, the women administered the mashed marjoram on the first night; the powdered coffee on the second; and poured rose water into the sea on the third. These cures were in essence a compounding of the simpler ones performed for espanto and the evil eye, such as sugar and coffee blessed at the mezuzah and administered in packets at three intervals during the night, sugar and rose water poured with a blessing at the spot where the victim had taken fright, marjoram and sugar water placed in the night air and taken with a blessing in the morning, and mumia tapada given secretly to cure espanto. There was, however, a distinction. For example, with the simpler cures, the rue was used in sprigs, here it was mashed; no additional preparation had been given the coffee, here the powdered coffee was mashed to an even finer consistency. The marjoram, as well, was treated differently according to the severity of the illness. As Caden Lévy Israel explained, "When it is for puro espanto [pure espanto] when someone is very ill, and you perform the asaradura, the marjoram is mashed, and the whole body is covered with it. When it is for *espanto mas liviano* [lighter espanto], you boil the water, you remove the water from the stove, you put the marjoram inside and cover it. Let it cool, and give it to drink."

In Bohora Biton's account, marjoram was administered on the first night. As she recounted, "I had this done to me. They took marjoram and they rubbed the body with marjoram. The marjoram was not boiled. They mashed it under the mezuzah. At the door of the mezuzah, they mashed it and said [a blessing]. And they rubbed marjoram all over the body." On the next night, they took powdered coffee "from Egypt, which is more efficacious. They took a little, they toasted it, they mashed it, they formed three packets. And they gave these three packets to me to drink." Mrs.

Biton stressed that the coffee was "powder, powder, powder." The packets were placed under the pillow at the head of the bed, and they were given in the evening, at midnight, and at dawn. On the third night, rose water was used as the cure. While the stricken one remained quietly in bed, the women "poured it into the sea or wherever he was frightened." Following this, the women washed the patient with "water boiled with *ruda.*" Mrs. Biton continued, "The next morning, early to the bath house to remove the *solombra* [shadow]." Thus, the end of the ritual cure was a final purification to wash away the shadow that remained as a trace of the unhealthy contact with the spirits.

Bienvenida Gabay explained the very serious ritual enclosure with honey (aldurko de miel). At midnight, the maestra washed her hands to purify herself for the cure she was undertaking. Then she took some honey and inserted three burning coals in it until they were extinguished. The maestra dipped her finger in the honey and had the stricken one lick it. She repeated this three times, while intoning the following blessing: "Esto lo ago en el nombre del Dio. Kero la melezina, kero la salud i la salvasion de esta persona [This I am doing in the name of God. I want the healing, I want the health, and the salvation of this person]." She put honey on her finger and rubbed it on the palm, the heart, and both knees of the stricken one, and she repeated this three times with an accompanying blessing. Mrs. Gabay remarked that during the course of the cure, the patient screamed a lot because the women "pressed [massaged, rubbed]" the patient in order to remove the espanto.

Sol Konfino recalled her mother performing this ritual cure with honey. After putting the burning coals in the honey, her mother rubbed her body and recited blessings. "She rubbed me, and she used to rub me on top. And she would give me little tastes of honey. The top she would rub, the stomach, she would rub. All of that she did to me for eight days." Of this cure, Zimbul Maya Suzi remarked, "When someone is very ill, one takes honey and rubs it all over the body, all the way to the feet. Then the patient is covered with a sheet."

For Mrs. Gabay, the enclosure ended on the tenth day, but the sense of isolation was maintained: the maestra and the patient went to the Turkish bath near the house, but no one should see them. Mrs. Gabay instructed, "You must be the first ones in the bath, before anyone sees you there, even the help"; and she cautioned that the two could not be seen until the whole ritual bath was completed. The maestra would go to the first basin and let some water run into a container, to which she added sugar; she poured this on the patient and said, 'I give you [the spirits] the sweetness, you give me the release.'" This was repeated at each basin in the bath. "If this is a Jewish bath," Mrs. Gabay added, "and there is a *tevila* [mikvah, ritual bath], the last one is done in the *tevila.* That's it. After the Turkish bath is completed, people can come in." If there was no Turkish bath available, she said, "it's not the best, but you can do it at home."

Caden Lévy Israel recalled a ritual enclosure that was performed for a man who had journeyed from Adalia [Antalya], Turkey, to Rhodes by boat, and thus had been exposed to the danger of the spirits at sea during a storm: "There was a man who was quite sick. He was coming from Adalia. While he was on the boat, there was a big storm. . . . The man reached home after many hours. But he started to suffer. He was releasing blood through the mouth. All the doctors checked him up and there was no remedy. A lady came and enclosed him for the cure for espanto for four days in a house, only the two together. . . . And she performed what is called asaradura. . . . First she asked the young man, 'Were you frightened in a specific place?' And he said, 'When we were coming in the sea, we had a terrible storm and naturally I got frightened.'" The woman mixed water with sugar; went to the seashore, where she cast a portion of the sugar water in the sea; and said, "Here I pour this sugar, let it be the cure for his fright." When she came home, she took the remaining sugar water and, as our mother said, "gave him three times to drink. She covered him well and put him to sleep." On the next day, the woman mixed mumia with sugar and divided it into three packets, gave them to the stricken one, and then she "let him sleep." At the end of the cure, as our mother said, "The young man felt very good, and he left the house, and he was cured of espanto."

In another account, Caden Lévy Israel told of a women who had offended the spirits, or as she said, "los de abajo [those from below], by throwing dirty water into the street." Isaac asked, "Mama, tell me about that woman in Milas, was she Jewish or Turkish? Tell me about the stones."

Caden: She was Jewish. A young woman. She was home. Suddenly she perceived that they were throwing stones at her. She was inside the house. Suddenly the stones . . . fell on her. No one knew the cause of it.

Isaac: And people were near her?

Caden: Yes, there were a lot of people. But it didn't touch anyone else. Only her. And after a good while, they would remove her from one house and take her to another house, and they would change from another one to another one. Still the stones kept falling.

At first, people thought that stones might have been falling because of something wrong with the houses, but then they realized that they were falling only on this one woman. It was decided that the spirits were the cause:

> Isaac: Who did they say was throwing the stones?
> Caden: *Lus buenus de mozotros* [the good among us]. They said that it was from *lus di abashu* [those from below]. . . .
> Isaac: Mama, give me the reason why the stones were falling.
> Caden: She was indisposed [menstruating]. She washed . . . the rags that she was changing. The water, she threw it away into the street. And they say that this water harmed those who should not do any harm to us [the spirits]. And for that reason they threw stones at her.

Isaac asked his mother for further clarification, "You were explaining the difference between now and then." His mother responded, "Is this nice to include it there?" meaning in what we were writing, and then reluctantly continued, "Before they did not have what women use now for cleanliness. They used rags. When they washed them, they poured the water away. It was dirty and this *azia danyu a lus buenus di mozotrus* [insulted the good among us (the spirits)]." When it was discovered that the spirits were angry with her, "They poured water with sugar in a spot where they said she got espanto. She was three days home, ... they enclosed her and she was cured."

The women with whom we spoke had varying interpretations about the curative power of the ritual enclosure. Sol Konfino reflected on this cure, which had been performed for her mother in Bitola, Yugoslavia: "It helped a little. Is it because of what they did? Is it from—I don't know, maybe just the rest she needed?" After telling us of the isolation of the patient and the strict diet, another woman affirmed the curative power of enclosure by quoting her son, who was a medical doctor: "I told this to Sammy; he told me that 'it is probably something that is good. This person is calm . . . , no one bothers him, they let him rest. It is very good.'" For Bohora Biton, there was no question that the cure was in the "words," or blessings, of the women: "These women spoke with the *sheddimis* [the spirits], 'You are good people, you have pity and you are merciful. Give health to this one, daughter of so-and-so. She did not cause, nor will she cause you any harm.' . . . All of this they spoke orally. With this they got cured." To emphasize her point, Mrs. Biton raised her voice and repeated, "With this, the sick got well!"

For saradura, the crucial aspects of enclosure and isolation were marked by the initial divestment of everyday clothing and by a ritual cleansing. Zimbul Maya Suzi recalled the endulko performed for her, "I was in a room with one woman. She removed everything that I was wearing and put the clothes on the roof. For nine days you cannot leave that room." As Lucy Garnett had observed, "The patient is washed, dressed in white linen, and laid on a white bed" (1891, 67–68). In a symbolic sense, the body of the patient was treated like a corpse. This cleansing, separation, and isolation were combined with the repetitive use of specific cures on each day and the compounding of cures built up over the course of the days of the ritual. In their preparation, the cures were pounded to an essence: the coffee was ground not just fine but to a "powder, powder, powder," as Mrs. Biton emphasized; the marjoram and the rue were mashed to a fine paste. The cures were administered both internally and externally: the stricken one drank the sugar water or the mashed marjoram water, and her whole body was rubbed with these; she ate the honey, and she was covered with it.

With this enclosure and isolation, the compounding of the cures, and the rendering to their powdered and mashed essence, there was also the quietness, the stillness, the absence of quotidian life. The stricken one and the women curers were set apart from others, both literally and symbolically. They were removed from the life of the community for a prescribed number of days. Indeed, as noted for most saraduras, the family members and the neighbors temporarily moved away. In the stillness of the enclosure, with no sounds from the house or from the outside, and with little light coming through the window coverings, the stricken one was required to stay in bed, to sleep, and to rest when she was not sleeping. The timing of the ritual enclosure was such that even the light from the moon was minimal, since it was waning—and in symbolic fashion, as the moon grows smaller, so should the illness diminish.[3] The person's diet was characterized more by what she could not eat—no garlic, no onion, no fish, no meat, nothing with odor—than by what she could. In a sense, the stricken one and the curers with her—since they were under the same breath—were in suspended animation.

Following the analysis of the folklorist Arnold van Gennep and the anthropologist Victor Turner, we might say that the stricken one, and to an extent the curers as well, was in the liminal state, the period of ritual that is "betwixt and between," a time of great danger precisely because it is apart from the ordinary and associated with the sacred. During this time, the ritual participants were placed in closer contact with the dangerous realm of the spirit world. They were, as we were frequently told, "*asolombradas,*" shadowed, or in the presence of the spirits. In answer to Isaac's question about why the neighbors and family members moved out, his mother said, "Because they said that it was *asolombrado* [shadowed, presence of the spirits]." Both Melvin Firestone and Rebecca Amato Levy note that in Rhodes, even those who were not strictly required to move out did so "because it was felt that the place was invaded by demons" (Firestone 1962, 307; R. Levy 1987, 72, 228) and that "the spirits visited the streets of those who were ill." Even the taboo against eating onion reflected the connection with the spirits, for it was said that "the skin of the onion was their clothing."

Bienvenida Gabay told of a man who had been paralyzed on his wedding night because the bridal chamber was asolombrada. She said she had visited the house of her relatives:

> And everybody was crying, everybody was sad. I said, "What's wrong?" They told me that the man couldn't walk, that he had great pain in the small of his back. Since the day he got married, he couldn't walk. After the wedding, he entered the bridal chamber, and he was never able to walk again. I said, "Don't cry. Leave me alone with the patient, and I, God willing, am going to cure him." I performed the *kura de miel* [cure of honey, saradura with honey]. On the tenth day, he was fine. . . . In the house there had been a young girl, who had been sick and had died there. They performed an aldurko on that young girl in that room but they didn't do it properly, the room was still asolombrada, and the couple moved in. To the bride they didn't touch, all to the groom. He went to sleep that night, and the way he went to sleep, that's the way he remained, without walking, with a lot of pains, and always screaming, "My back! My back!"

The ritual bath at the end of the enclosure was intended to remove the shadow, for as Mrs. Biton had said, "The next morning, early to the bath house to remove the *solombra.*" Firestone also remarks on this: "According to one specialist the patient bathed after the *cerradura* 'in order to get rid of the *salombra'* [*sic*] (literally, shadow or shade)" (1959, 25). Just prior to the ritual bath, the woman curer might boil *ruda* and rub it on the body of the patient, then "some of the water is sprinkled on the floor so that the *salombra* will leave" (26). While Firestone suggests that *solombra* "may refer to the demon," we would refine this by translating *solombra* as the shadow cast by the evil spirits. The plural in this instance is important, for it was not "the demon" in the singular that had caused the harm, but rather the plethora of evil spirits that had descended on the unfortunate one to bring about the disastrous state.

In essence, the ritual of enclosure was a way of removing the evil done by the spirits by appealing to them and by purifying the body and the soul. As Raphael Patai remarks: "The intention of the ritual is thus clear: to propitiate, appease, the demons who are believed to have caused the disability, to appeal to their goodwill, sympathy, pity" (1964, 3). The success of the ritual, Patai says, "is based on giving something 'sweet' to the demons who cause these diseases and misfortunes, and thereby propitiating them" (3–4). In the course of the cures, the maestra spoke directly to the spirits. As Mrs. Biton said, "These women spoke with the *sheddimis* [the spirits]"; and they spoke gentle words of pleading, "I give you the sweetness, you give me the release," and of praise, "You are good people, you have pity and you are merciful."

Conclusion

When Isaac was a young child, his grandmother, Sarota Amato Musafir, used to bless him with the following: "Ki kreskas i munchigues komo la algranada [May you grow and multiply like the pomegranate]." The pomegranate with which we began the introduction brings us to a close. Whether boiled as a cure for a stomachache by *muestras madres* (our mothers) or used as a blessing by our grandmother, the pomegranate and the other ritual medical cures of the house were the rich treasures of the Sephardim. In opening this glistening pomegranate, we have looked at the makings and the meanings of these treasures. In the course of examining them, we have also met the people for whom these beliefs comprised a way of life. We found that during our interviews, the past lived again, if only for a moment, in that space created for it between those who tell their lives and those who are there to listen and to record. But those who spoke with us were not without a consciousness of the present, and of its near-total break with the past. Bienvenida Gabay sadly remarked on this break when telling us about the *prekantes:* "Esto es de mil anyos, ma aora ya paso. Todo se murio [This is a thousand years old, but now it is all gone. Everything is dead]." She concluded, "There was much to teach, but with the new life, this generation laughs at the old ways." Zimbul Maya Suzi said it more succinctly, "The old women died and everything left also."

In this same vein, our friend and colleague Krinka Vidaković Petrov observed, "My generation of Sephardic people do not speak Judeo-Spanish, they don't even understand Judeo-Spanish. They understand a few words which they learned when they were small, from their parents. But

I don't think there will be anything left. This is probably the last moment to save what can be saved." However, Vidaković Petrov was not sounding a simplistic death knell for past ways. Speaking in 1990 of the Jews of Yugoslavia, she said, "They are simply more interested in the future than in the past." By way of illustration, she referred to a Sephardi friend who knew no Judeo-Spanish but who was very interested in the Sephardic community. She concluded, "He is more interested in Israel as Israel, and has an emotional and spiritual response to Jewish identity in general, not specifically to Sephardic identity."[1]

Even for those who retained their Sephardic identity, the creation of the state of Israel changed their lives. One man told us that there were no evil spirits in Israel because people were reciting prayers "twenty-four hours a day": "I am going to tell you something that you should pay attention to. Here in Israel, there is no fear. We read the *Sefer Tehilim* and this is a guard. Before beginning the reading of the *Tehilim*, there is a complete chapter. . . . All that there is outside of Israel, it does not exist here because of the benedictions that we read in the *Tehilim*. Here there is a guard and it does not strike at all." Others perhaps did not share his faith that there were no evil spirits in Israel, for as Isaac pointed out to him, "I hear that in Bat Yam [Israel], there are women who still perform for *ayin arah* [evil eye]. How can this be?" When his wife concurred, "There are a lot of women who do!" the man explained, "These are people who came from Turkey, from such places. They still keep what they learned from their mothers, from their grandmothers." Then he concluded, "Here it does not exist, in Israel. We have belief in God." Like a contrary echo, the wife interjected, "There are many who say that they believe in it," and Isaac turned to her to ask, "Do you believe that the spirits exist in Israel?" She responded, "Of course, they exist here." To bridge this divide between husband and wife, Isaac observed, "I have heard here both sides of the story. A woman at a Bet Avot told me that in Israel the spirits do not exist because Salomon, the king, cast them out."

For us and for the people with whom we spoke, the interviews were an investment in the soul and the past of the Sephardim, a shared venture in their rediscovery. This look into the past, this rediscovery, was done through the lens of the present. It was, in Lillian Hellman's terms, a *pentimento.* As Hellman explained on the first page of her book of the same name (1973), "Old paint on canvas, as it ages, sometimes becomes transparent. When that happens it is possible, in some pictures, to see the original lines: a tree will show through a woman's dress, a child makes way for a dog, a large boat is no longer on an open sea. That is called pentimento because the painter 'repented,' changed his mind. Perhaps it would be as well to say that the old conception, replaced by a later choice, is a way of seeing and then seeing again. That is all I mean about the people in this book. The paint has aged now and I wanted to see what was there for me once, what is there for me now." In this metaphor of *pentimento,* Hellman describes older images on a canvas seeping through the newer layer. The strength of line, the original creation, repented of by the artist, is visible in the new. This "old conception, replaced by a later choice" allows one to see and then see again. In just such a way did our work with the Sephardim allow us to see and then see again. The images of a life earlier lived, never to be revisited, emerged in the process of what can only be termed a recreation of time past.

The domesticated religion of the Sephardim ranged from the belief in the profoundly important power of speech to the disruptive influence of the evil eye; from the unsettling upset of *espanto* to the malevolent workings of *echizo* (witchcraft). Equipped with the medicines of the house and with the ritual medical cures of the lyrical *prekante* or the awesome *saradura,* the Sephardic woman worked to maintain a balance in life—between family members, with neighbors, and with the ever-envious denizens of the spirit world. Her words were sweetened with blessings, her cures with sugar and honey.

In the spirit of the Sephardic women of whom we have written, we close with a blessing and a prayer that they would say for those who departed on a journey:

Senyor del Mundo,	Lord of the Universe,
Ke vaiga i venga,	May I go and return,
Mal ke no tenga.	May nothing bad happen to me.
Kaminos de leche i miel,	Paths of milk and honey,
Kaminos buenos,	Good paths,
Ke me guarde el Dio de todo mal.	May the Lord guard me from all evil.

Appendix: Interviewees

Alajef, Julie (née Cohen): born in Rusçuk, Bulgaria, c. 1910. Interviewed at Bet Avot Bulgaria in Rishon LeZion, Israel, April 1990.

Algrante, Mary: born in Izmir, Turkey, in 1906; father, Yakov Algrante, a businessman well versed in biblical studies; sister, Esther Morguez Algrante, the well-known Sephardic poet. Interviewed at the Bet Avot in Izmir, March 1990.

Alkalay, Violette: born in Sofia, Bulgaria. Interviewed at Bet Avot Bulgaria in Rishon LeZion, April 1990.

Alkanli, Ester: born in Istanbul in 1946. Interviewed in Istanbul, March 1990.

Alvas, Kalina (née Zalma): born in Bulgaria, c. 1920. Emigrated to Israel in 1949. Interviewed at Bet Avot Bulgaria in Rishon LeZion, April 1990.

Amram, Lea (née Lucy Misrahi): born in Kuskunjuk, Turkey, in 1902 or 1903. Married Moshe Amram, who was a Hazan and an owner of a small store with his father. Emigrated to Israel in 1968, after her husband's death. Interviewed at Bet Avot Kryat Segal in Ramat Efal, Israel, May 1990.

Arogeti, Regina: born in Rhodes c. 1900. Emigrated to Atlanta, Georgia, in the 1920s. Interviewed 1991, 1992, and 1997.

Avraami, Lili: born in Bulgaria, c. 1930. Secretary of the Union of Bulgarian Jews in Israel. Interviewed in Jaffa, June 1990.

Avzaradel, Izachar: born in Rhodes. Emigrated to Israel in the 1960s. Interviewed in Ashdod, July 1990.

Avzaradel, Rosa: born in Rhodes in 1912. Interviewed in Ashdod, July 1990.

Azuz, Sol (née Zalma): born in Istanbul. Emigrated to Israel when she was twenty-four years old. Interviewed in her home in Herzelia, Israel, May 1990, in company with Korin Madem.

Bardavid, Beki: born in Istanbul. Interviewed 1982, 1990, and 1997.

Benatar, Mary: born in Rhodes c. 1910s. Emigrated to Atlanta in the 1920s. Interviewed 1991.

Benmayor, Leon and Jilda: born in Salonika, Greece. Leon was the president of the Salonika Community. Interviewed 1982, 1984, and 1990.

Biton, Bohora: born in Rhodes c. 1890. Emigrated to Atlanta in the 1920s. Interviewed 1965 and 1968.

Biton, Marie: born in Rhodes c. 1905. Emigrated to Atlanta c. 1920. Interviewed in 1957, 1962, and 1965.

Bohor, Buka (now called Buka Berta Luis Alkuser): born in Kustendil, Bulgaria, in 1909. Emigrated to Israel in 1948. Interviewed at Bet Avot Leon Recanati, April 1990.

Brudo, Rafael Itzhak: born in Salonika in 1903. He was the grandchild of Harbi Manuel Brudo, the chief rabbi of Salonika and judge of the Bet Din. He, his wife, mother-in-law, and son were hidden by a Christian family in Athens during World War II. Interviewed at the Bet Avot in Salonika, March 1990.

Cadranel, Marco and Diana: born in Rhodes c. 1905. Emigrated to Tangiers, Morocco, in 1939 and to Israel in 1950s. Interviewed in Ashdod, 1985.

Danon, Clara: born in Zeniça, Bosnia, in 1907. Interviewed in New Belgrade, February 1990.

Danon, Dina: born in Izmir in 1912. Emigrated to Israel in 1930. Interviewed at Bet Avot Leon Recanati in Kryat Matalon, April 1990.

Dasa, Lisa: born in Jerusalem. Interviewed 1968.

Di Bero, Rosa: born in Rhodes in 1884. Emigrated to the United States in 1919. Interviewed in Seattle, Washington, 1974.

Djrasi, David: born in Israel in 1939 of Salonikan parents. Interviewed May 1990.

Elazar, Paolina: born in Sofia in 1926. Emigrated to Israel in 1948. Interviewed at Bet Avot Bulgaria in Rishon LeZion, Israel, April 1990, in company with Ida Varsano.

Eskenazi, Victoria: born near Edirne, Turkey, in 1910. Interviewed March 1990.

Farji Clara: born in Edirne, Turkey, in 1925. Emigrated to Tel Aviv. Interviewed in 1990.

Franco, Reina: born in Rhodes c. 1880. Emigrated to Atlanta in 1920s or 1930s. Interviewed in Atlanta 1957, 1959, and 1962.

Franko, Lena: born in Istanbul in 1929. Interviewed in 1990.

Gabay, Bienvenida: born in Edirne, Turkey, in 1897. She married Benjamin Gabay in Istanbul and emigrated to Israel in 1946. Interviewed May 1990.

Gross-Gefen, Ella: born in Yugoslavia. Emigrated to Israel. Interviewed in Bat Yam, Israel, May 1990.

Hen, Simha (née Grasiani): born in Trachia, Greece, in 1906, during the reign of the sultan. She lived in Bulgaria for approximately seven or eight years (around 1923). Her father was a Rav. This is why, she said, they remained alive. Emigrated to Israel around 1928, where she was a pioneer.

Israel, Baruch: born in Rhodes c. 1890s. Emigrated to Brooklyn, early 1910s; moved to Atlanta in 1960s. Interviewed periodically between 1965 and 1975.

Israel, Caden Lévy (née Musafir): born in 1905 in Milas, Turkey, lived in Rhodes and Tangiers, Morocco. Emigrated to Atlanta in 1945. Interviewed periodically between 1957 and 1995.

Kabiljo, Isaac: born in 1912, in Sarajevo. Interviewed at the Sarajevo synagogue, February 1990.

Kerido, Senyora: born in 1913, Burgas, Bulgaria, near the Black Sea. Her father was from Orta Köy, Turkey. Interviewed in 1990.

Konfino, Sol: born in Bitola (Monastir), Yugoslavia, in 1921. Emigrated to Israel in 1936, and lived in Jaffa. Interviewed 1990.

Levi, Isaac: born in Yugoslavia. President of the Jewish Community of Sarajevo. Interviewed at Sarajevo synagogue, February 1990.

Levi, Kalo (née Baron): born in Gallipoli c. 1905. Interviewed at the Bet Avot in Istanbul, March 1990.

Levi, Luna: born in Edirne, Turkey. Emigrated to Israel. Interviewed at Bet Avot Leon Recanati, August 1985.

Levy, Rebecca Amato: born in Rhodes. Emigrated to Tangiers, Morocco, in 1939, and to Los Angeles in 1946. Interviewed in 1974, 1987, and 1990.

Lusi, Josifov: born in Bulgaria. Emigrated to Israel. Interviewed in 1990.

Madem, Korin: originally from Istanbul. Interviewed in Herzelia, May 1990, in company with Sol Azuz.

Matia, Avram: born in Salonika in 1904. He was a shoemaker. Emigrated to Israel in 1934. Interviewed at Bet Avot Leon Recanati, April 1990.

Meloh, Inez (née Filos): born in Edirne, Turkey, in 1910; went to Istanbul as a young child. Married in Istanbul and lived there until she was forty years old. Second husband was Shaul Meloh. Interviewed March 1990.

Meshula, Bela: born in Turkey c. 1915. Emigrated to Israel. Interviewed in Herzelia, June 1990.

Mipusi, Rita: born in Turkey c. 1910. Emigrated to Israel. Interviewed in Herzelia, June 1990.

Missistrano, Estrella: born in Ortay Köy, Istanbul. Emigrated to Israel. Interviewed in Bat Yam, May–June 1990.

Missistrano, Isaac: born in Istanbul in 1920s. Emigrated to Israel. Interviewed in Bat Yam, May–June 1990.

Mizan, Vera: born in Turkey. Interviewed at Bet Avot Leon Recanati, August 1985.

Mizrahi, Yakov and Fortuna: born in Istanbul, Turkey. Yakov was born in 1924. Emigrated to Israel with his family in 1980. Interviewed May–June 1990.

Musafir, Dolsa: born in Milas, Turkey, in 1890s. Interviewed in Izmir, March 1990.

Musafir, Nissim: born in Izmir. Interviewed in Izmir, March 1990.

Musafir, Rachel: born in Izmir. Interviewed several times from 1968 to 1990.

Musafir, Sarota (née Amato): born in Milas, Turkey, in 1888; lived in Rhodes. Moved to Tangiers, Morocco, in 1939 and emigrated to Atlanta, Georgia, in February 1945. Interviewed from 1956 until 1970.

Musafir, Yeoshua: born in Milas, Turkey. Moved to Izmir, Turkey. Interviewed several times from 1968 to 1990.

Nahmias, Benny: born in Israel. Interviewed in Bene Brah, Israel, July 1990.

Nair, Sara: born in Edirne in 1926. Moved to Istanbul where she became a renowned spirit medium. Interviewed 1990 and 1997.

Nar, Duka: born in Salonika in 1907. Emigrated to Israel in 1932. Interviewed at Bet Avot Leon Recanati, April 1990.

Reuven, Shelomo: born in Salonika. Emigrated to Israel. Interviewed in Tel Aviv, 1982, 1984, 1985.

Roberts, Fannie: born c. 1925. Interviewed in Seattle, April 1975.

Sarfati, Deborah (née Noah): born in Salonika c. 1905. Emigrated to Israel the same year. Interviewed at Bet Avot Leon Recanati, April 1990.

Sarfati, Rivka (née Lahan): born in Salonika in 1912. She was a survivor of the Holocaust. Emigrated to Tel Aviv in 1990. Her husband, Alberto Sarfati, also a Holocaust survivor, painted tableaux of the tragedy.

Sephiha, Solomon: born in Salonika, Greece. Interviewed at the Bet Avot, March 1990.

Shaul, Moshe: born in Istanbul, Turkey. Emigrated to Israel. He was the commentator of the Judeo-Spanish section of Kol Israel Radio. Presently he is the editor of the journal *Aki Yerushalayim.*

Shemaria, Dora: born in Rhodes, moved to Israel. Interviewed in Ashdod, 1990.

Suzi, Zimbul (née Maya): born in Celebria, Turkey, near Istanbul in 1905. She went to Cuba two months after her marriage, when she was sixteen or seventeen. She emigrated to Israel from Cuba in 1971. Interviewed in Tel Aviv, 1990.

Tuvi, Bohor Albert: born in Turkey. Emigrated to Israel in 1956. Interviewed in Netanya, May 1990.

Tuvi, Luna (née Haleo): born in Chanakali, Turkey in 1925. Her father was a peddler who traveled to villages. Emigrated to Israel in 1956. Interviewed in Netanya, May 1990.

Tuvi, Margalite: born in Israel c. 1970. A student of Sephardic studies. Interviewed in Herzelia, 1990.

Varsano, Ida: born in Yambul, a small town outside of Sofia, Bulgaria, in 1925. She moved to Sofia in 1932. After her marriage and the birth of two children, she emigrated to Israel. Interviewed at Bet Avot Bulgaria in Rishon LeZion, Israel, April 1990, in company with Paolina Elazar.

Notes

Introduction

1. Anonymous, Bet Avot Leon Recanati, Kryat Matalon, Israel, 1985.

2. The Judeo-Spanish orthography differs from that of contemporary Spanish. Since our goal has been to represent the way in which the people enunciated Judeo-Spanish, we have adhered strictly to the spoken word in our transcription of interviews. There is variation in the language itself according to the geographical area and the educational background from which one comes. Additionally, an individual might use different phrases and pronunciation within a single conversational exchange. Thus, there are variations in the spelling of the same word or phrases throughout this work. Note also that when the words "Torah" and "mezuzah" are rendered in Judeo-Spanish, they will be spelled following the orthography to represent their pronunciation, "Tora" and "mezuza." All translations of foreign-language materials are by the authors, unless otherwise indicated.

3. Isaac conducted one of the earliest interviews in 1957, when he spoke with his grandmother, Sarota Amato Musafir, originally of Milas, Turkey, and the island of Rhodes, then living in Atlanta, about the use of *prekantes*. In 1965 and again in 1968, he spoke with Bohora Biton, originally from Rhodes, and living in Atlanta, about the same topic. On a trip to Israel in 1968, he interviewed Lisa Dasa, a Sephardic woman of Jerusalem. In 1985, Isaac and Rosemary carried out research in Jerusalem, and in Kryat Matalon, Israel, at Bet Avot Leon Recanati.

4. Nineteenth- and early twentieth-century anthropological and folklore theories were replete with supposed means for arriving at the origin of customs. For a review of these theories and of their limitations, see Zumwalt (1988, 103–12).

5. For a discussion of the combination of insider and outsider perspectives in conducting fieldwork, see Dundes and Falassi (1975, xvi).

6. Personal communication, 1997. In his earlier work, Isaac Jack Lévy referred to this complex of belief as "A Domesticated Supernatural: Home Magic of the Sephardim" (1985).

Chapter 1: Keeping the Spirits Happy, Keeping the Family Healthy

1. Ben-Yehuda's *English-Hebrew, Hebrew-English Dictionary* defines *shed* and *sheddim* (שׁדים, plural masculine) as "devil" (1964, 289).

2. "Euphemism" comes from the Greek, *euphēmismos,* for "the use of an auspicious word for an inauspicious one," which derives from *euphēmo,* "of good sound or omen," from "*eu,* good, and *phēmē,* voice from *phanai,* to speak." For a comparison to Judeo-Spanish euphemisms, see Charles E. Kany's collection of Spanish euphemisms in the Americas (1960).

3. Personal communication, Rav Rafael Hillel, Director of Or Hachayim Institutions, Benei Berah, Israel, 1990.

4. Don Yoder (1974, 5) makes this determination. See the entire article for a discussion of the sources for the study of folk religion, which Yoder traces to two sources, German *Religiöse Volkskunde* and anthropology.

5. For a poignant example of this name-changing ritual, see *In Her Own Time,* a videotape by Vikram Jayanti and Barbara Myerhoff concerning Myerhoff's fieldwork in an Orthodox Jewish community in Fairfax, California, during the course of which she discovers she has cancer. The video ends with the ritual of the name change in front of the open ark and Myerhoff's toss of a bouquet of flowers into the air; a concluding caption indicates her birth and death dates.

6. Hayim Palache was a prolific writer who published under several additional spellings of his name. For his last name, these were Palacci, Palachi, Palagi, and Pallagi; for his first name, Haïm, Hayim, and Hayyim. We thank Avner Perez, a biblical scholar and a Judeo-Spanish poet from Jerusalem, for the translation from Hebrew to English.

7. See Molho (1950, 163) for another version of "Kuatro Kantonadas." According to Benbassa-Dudonney, the Sephardic women utter the prayer "Kuatro kantonadas ay en esta kaza" after reciting the "Kriat Shema" (1982, 26–29). It should be pointed out, however, that in many cases, "Kuatro kantonadas" in Judeo-Spanish was the only prayer used by women before going to sleep since they could not read Hebrew, the language of "Kriat Shema." This prayer was popular not only in the Sephardic centers of the Balkans, Turkey, and the Dodecanese Islands, but also in Christian Spain and other localities, such as France and Portugal. In the *Kriat Shema al Hamitah,* the Shema for the Night Prayer, found in the *Daily Prayer Book,* the four angels referred to in "Kuatro kantonadas" are specifically named: "In the name of the Lord God of Israel, may Michael be at my right hand, and Gabriel at my left; before me Uriel; behind me Raphael; and above my head the divine presence" (Birnbaum 1949, 784). The Israeli-Sephardic singer Yoram Gaon performed for the welcoming of the new week, "Eli-Eliyahu," in Hebrew, save for the following four lines, which are in Judeo-Spanish: "A la derecha Mihael, / I a la siedra Gabriel, / Sovre la kavesa Shehina de El, / Kada dia i kada noche [To the right Michael, / And to the left Gabriel, / Above the head the Presence of Him, / Each day and each night]" (Gaon, n.d.). José Manuel Pedrosa writes about the night prayer in Christian Spain (2000, 30–42). According to Pedrosa, "Certain determined common traits . . . allow us to affirm that the formulas concerning *Las cuatro esquinas* [The four corners] must be multi-cultural protective expressions of a magical rite against the spirits that in many countries are believed to

surround an individual and his environment . . . in moments of carelessness, such as sleep" (1995, 187–220).

8. Jamila Ventura, Brusa, Turkey; Israeli National Sound Archives, tape Y 5479 [6].

9. Anonymous, Israeli National Sound Archives, tape Y 3980 [24].

10. Jamila Ventura, Brusa, Turkey; Israeli National Sound Archives, tape Y 5479 [6].

11. Ibid.

12. Israeli National Sound Archives, tape Y 3980 (24).

13. Israeli National Sound Archives, No. 7 (a).

Chapter 2: The Sephardim of the Ottoman Empire

1. Barnai quotes Capsali (1976, 218–19). See also Shaw (1991, 32–33).

2. Biblical accounts in Genesis (10:2–5) and 1 Chronicles (1:5–7) refer to Javan, the son of Japheth, who, after the flood, settled with his family on the Hellenic mainland and in the Ionian region. The sons of Javan resided in Cyprus (biblical Kittim) and Rhodes (biblical Rodanim) (Lévy 1989b, 17–18). Benyamin Arditi suggests that many Israelites, particularly of the tribes of Asher and Zebulun, came as sailors to the Balkan Peninsula to trade with the Phoenicians and "subsequently settled permanently both north and south of the Danube, in Dacia and Moesia" (Tamir 1979, 3). Molho (1962, 376–83) places the arrival of the Jews in Greece at the end of the second millennium and beginning of the first B.C.E. Baruch Schiby (1970, 92) dates their arrival to the eighth and seventh centuries B.C.E. with the exodus during the time of Jeremiah (92). For Macedonia, Alexandar Matkovski (1982, 10) writes, "There are those who claim that the Jews came after Darius' campaign against the Scythians (approximately 513 B.C.); others date their presence to after the campaign of Alexander the Great in Asia Minor (approximately 330 B.C.); yet a third opinion is that they arrived after the conquest of the Balkan Peninsula by the Romans, particularly after the capture of Jerusalem (circa 130 B.C.)."

3. For an excellent study of the literature and for photographs of the costumes worn by the Jews in the Ottoman Empire, see Juhasz (1990, 121–72).

4. Whether the Jews moved from one urban center of the empire to another willingly or by force is a contested topic. The repopulation was not restricted only to Romaniot Jews since the Ottomans also transferred Armenians, Turks, Greeks, Slavs, and Jewish immigrants from Italy, Sicily, France, Hungary, and Spain. In the case of Jews, the move was not only to rebuild the urban commercial centers, but also because the Sultans viewed the Jews as more reliable than the local Christian Greeks and Slavs. See A. Levy (1992, 21–23) and Hacker 1978.

5. Raphaela Lewis states that one of the first acts of Mehmed II after the conquest of Constantinople "was to re-people the city. Many who had fled were promised protection of property and religion, but thousands were deported to Adrianople, Gallipoli and Anatolia. On the other hand thousands were brought to Constantinople from Serbia, Albania, and Greece, and many more arrived from all parts as slaves, immigrants, prisoners of war and refugees. The largest settlements were those of Anatolian Turks who were brought into the city to stabilize it" (1971, 16).

6. In the fifteenth century, due to the concern for the *limpieza de sangre* (purity of blood) and the influence of the Inquisition, the situation in the peninsula changed drastically. Castro writes that "the ferocious persecution of the Jews modified the traditional relations between the nobles, the clergymen, the peasants and the Jews" (1948, 538). Christian families were now linked by marriage not to Jews, but rather to converts and to their children and grandchildren, who were born as Christians.

7. See the discussion in Baer (1966, 252).

8. For a discussion and clarification of the dilemma in defining "coexistence" and "living together," see Romano (1995, 359–81). Scholars have neglected the topics of the composition of the Hispano-Jewish family and the interaction of the Jewish working class with people from Christian and Muslim society. Perhaps this is due in great part to the lack of documentation, with manuscripts still buried in monasteries and municipal libraries. Only a scant number of these were published in the *Boletín de la Academía de Historia* in the 1800s. Additionally, not enough attention has been paid to the *responsa* literature of medieval rabbis and to the Jewish communal accounts. The few records that have been studied have made available remarkable information on the Jews and *conversos* in the Iberian Peninsula and their rapport with the non-Jewish communities. For more information on the life of the Jews and *conversos* in Spain, see Adreth (1539), Epstein (1925), Fernández (1964), and Gerondi (1984). For the position of Jewish or Cypto-Jewish women in Spain see Assis (1988), Melammed (1991, 1992, and 1999) and in nineteenth-century Turkey, Bortnick (1993) and Zumwalt (1993). On the Jewish family see Goitein (1978).

9. In 1281, a formal ban was issued in the community of Toledo against sexual immorality. Yet, some rabbis, such as Nahmanides, preferred men to have one concubine and to acknowledge her publicly "rather than resorting to indiscriminate relations with a number of women" (Assis 1988, 39, 40). The problem with sexual morality was also a major preoccupation of the northern European Jewish communities and their rabbis. The *Takana* (communal ordinance) of Forli (1418) charged the officials of cities and provinces to convince those who sinned to mend their ways and to turn aside from forbidden women, prostitutes, and married Jewish women. It warned that affairs with Christian women were unlawful. "The rigor of the proposed sanctions demonstrate how these abuses were spread" (Schwarzfuchs 1986, 137–38).

10. On the background of the persecution of 1391, see Kayserling (1898, 257).

11. David Gitlitz made these observations in a letter dated April 10, 2000.

12. See Padilla (1981, 1982b, 1983). Padilla's study is based on the archives dealing with the trials before the *Santo Oficio* located in the Audience and Council Seminary of the City of Zaragoza and in those of the *Protocolos Notariales* of Zaragoza and Calatayud. The articles are valuable not only because they confirm the normal contact between the converts and the Jews, but also for the rich information on the traditions of each, such as the use of magic and home remedies, and the belief in the evil eye.

13. For a derivation of the term *aljama*, see Cargas (1946, 91–93). Lacave writes, "The *aljama* was a legal institution which grouped together all the Jews from a specific locality and directed their lives, determined its own statutes and by-laws, which once approved publicly in the synagogues and obtained royal sanction,

served as the civil and penal codices for the internal life of Jewry. These ordinances, naturally, were based on rabbinic laws" (1991, 38).

14. Fernández is citing Document R.G.S. 1477-VII, fol. 317, p. 16. For more information on the attitude of the Catholic monarchs toward the Jews see Gerber (1992, 129); and Norman Roth (1995, 306–7).

15. Birnbaum (1991, 48) states that in addition to "swine," the Spanish term for *marranos* "is derived from the Aramaic phrase *maran atha* (our Lord has come), which the unfortunate were compelled to repeat on frequent occasions. *Anusim,* the Hebrew equivalent of *marranos,* signifies *those who were compelled.*"

16. Cecil Roth, quoting Llorente, the former Secretary of the Holy Office, writes, "These figures are so enormous as to seem highly suspicious. It must be recalled, however, that at the outset, the activity and the violence of the Holy Office was [so] boundless . . . this high estimate does not appear to be out of the question" (1964, 123). Amador de los Ríos, as quoted by Cecil Roth, estimates that between the years 1484 and 1525, "the number of [those] burned in person came to 28,540, those in effigy to 16,520, and those penanced to 303,847" (123). See also Burke (1900).

17. With no definite records, it is difficult to determine the exact number of Jews living in the Iberian Peninsula at the time of the expulsion. One can arrive at an estimate of Jewish households by using religious and fiscal documents, and one can multiply that number by the average number of people per household. The latter, however, is not a simple matter of mathematics, since scholars dispute the average number of people in a household, whether it be three, five, or seven. We feel it likely that these numbers are too small, for scholars fail to allow for married children who often lived with their parents. Additionally, for tax purposes, the whole family was regarded as one. Thus, in order to avoid paying the fully assessed poll tax, those in the household found it to their advantage not to report the exact number of families living under one roof.

18. It should be mentioned that the figures given by Cecil Roth and Baron refer to the Jews from Castile and Aragon and do not refer to those living in the other regions of the peninsula, including Andalusia, the Balearic Islands, Galicia, Leon, Extremadura, Cataluña, and Valencia. Moreover, these figures do not include the number of *conversos* who also left the peninsula in the sixteenth century. Following are the opinions given by other scholars: Yitzhak Baer proposes a maximum of 170,000 from Castile and Aragon (1966, 438). Stanford Shaw estimates, unfortunately without giving any sources, that "as many as 250,000 Jews came from the Iberian Peninsula to the Ottoman Empire in the late fifteenth century," and he adds that "the exact numbers will probably never be known" (1991, 34–35). According to Graetz, "At least three hundred thousand Jews left the country they had loved so ardently, and wandered in part to the north, to the contiguous kingdom of Navarre, in part to the south, in order to reach Africa, Italy or Turkey" (1941, 222). Haim Beinart acknowledges that the number is problematic. Yet, he offers some rough estimate: "Castilian Jews (not conversos) thought to have numbered between 120,000 and 150,000 persons; Aragonese Jewry is estimated to have been about 50,000. Thus the total Spanish Jewish population was about 200,000" (1997, 93). He, too, disregards the other Jewish communities in Spain.

19. For the type of community in Spain, see Epstein (1925, 33–70). For those in medieval Europe, see the chapter on "Les institutions de la communauté" (Schwarzfuchs 1986).

20. For the names of congregations founded in the Ottoman Empire, see Shaw (1991, 66–68). Shaw divides them according to "Place of origin," "Method of arrival in the Ottoman Empire," "Name of Ottoman locale," "Profession of founders," "Names of founders or donors," "Distinguishing characteristics," and "Aim or purpose of foundation."

21. This custom was quite often duplicated in the twentieth century by their descendants who emigrated to Africa, the Americas, and elsewhere. They, too, named their synagogues after their former homes—Istanbul, Monastir, Rhodes. See Zimmels (1976, 44).

22. Moreover, the officials were responsible for the protection of married women. See "Resolution of the Romaniots of Vidin," dated October 19, 1377 (Tamir 1979, 288–89), which addresses the rights of married women. The charitable organizations looked after the welfare of the poor, widows, orphans, the elderly, and the infirm, as well as of those stranded on journeys or captured by pirates and highwaymen. For a discussion of Jewish communal organizations, see Lévy (1989b, 28).

23. As in the case of the Romaniot period and of Spain, the Sephardic officials in the Ottoman Empire were preoccupied with the contact between their coreligionists and the non-Jewish population, their personal comportment, and bodily decorations. This was true mainly among those who arrived from Castile, where the Valladolid Conference of 1432, which took place in the "Large Synagogue" under Don Abraham Benveniste, the doctor of King John II, warned against wearing lavish garments and excessive luxury. See Schwarzfuchs (1986, 129–31) and Loeb (1886, 194); also see Lacave (1991, 41).

24. See Shaw (1991, 70–71). Isaac recalls that as late as 1938 in his native island of Rhodes, the functions of the *samas* were similar to the ones described here (Lévy 1989b, 39).

25. There were two types of excommunications: the *niddui* (minor excommunication) and the *herem* or *shamta* (major excommunication). For the power of the anathema, see Epstein (1968, 71–78). For a description of the *herem*, and the responsibility of the *Bet Din*, see Schwarzfuchs (1986, 84–108).

26. For a study dealing with *converso* ethnicity in the *conversos'* new homes, see Glick (1997).

27. Eschewing the explanation based on numerical advantage, Gerber credits the assimilation to "the higher social, cultural, and economic position of the Sephardic congregations [which] attracted members of other groups" (1992, 60).

28. See also Shaw (1991, 51–58), and Benbassa and Rodrigue (1995, 11–16).

29. On the taxes paid by the community see, Danon (1895, 52–60).

30. Along with the elite and the educated came the poor. In his trip to Istanbul in 1555, Hans Dernschwam, a German, remarked that most of the Jewish population worked in ordinary and modest menial trades. He encountered skilled artisans, apothecaries, weavers of cloth, lapidaries, masons, woodworkers, physical laborers, boatmen, broom vendors, dock workers, and woodcutters.

31. On the Hamon family, see H. Gross (1908, 1–26).

32. Avigdor Levy writes, "The growing impoverishment of the Ottoman Jewish communities at the end of the eighteenth century, and their increased isolation from European culture and the new Jewish centers of Europe, resulted in a general decline in scholarship and intellectual creativity" (1992, 92). The increase in the use of Judeo-Spanish was also due to the desire to reach the common people. With westernization of the Ottoman Empire in the nineteenth century and

the advent of foreign schools, there were translations of novels and dramas from the French, Italian, English, and Russian. The use of Latin characters was adopted. For a list of newspapers and periodicals in Judeo-Spanish, see Benbassa and Rodrigue (1995, 268–69).

33. For the attitude of the Janissaries toward the Jews and Jewish life in Turkey in the nineteenth century, see Franco (1893, 110–30). According to Franco, the Janissaries caused a great deal of harm to the Jews with the least pretext. For more than three centuries, "they set fire to the Jewish quarters of Istanbul without any scruples, even though often Jew and [Janissary] fraternized" (111). Their actions were not restricted to Turkey. In 1688, they plundered and burned the Jewish areas of Austria.

34. Lewis is quoting Ebüzziya, *Kütübhane-i Ebüzziya*, no. 66 (Istanbul, 1305/1888).

35. For an excellent study on the Alliance Israélite Universelle, see Rodrigue (1990).

36. As a youth, Isaac left his native island of Rhodes, traveled to Italy, and then took refuge with his mother and grandmother in Tangier, Morocco (September 1939 to December 1944), where he attended the Alliance school for boys. The director, Mr. Israel, originally from Milas, Turkey, understanding that his students would not be able to continue with their academic program after graduation due to World War II, enrolled approximately twelve students, Isaac among them, at the Remington International Business School. Twice a week, they took classes in shorthand, accounting, and typing. By so doing, this administrator was ensuring that upon graduation, the pupils would be able to secure jobs for themselves.

37. Daniel Elazar estimates that at the beginning of the twentieth century there were over 300,000 Sephardim living in the countries of Yugoslavia, Bulgaria, Greece, and Turkey (1984, 1–11). While it is impossible to establish the exact number of Jews in the Ottoman Empire, scholars have proposed a figure of a third of a million before World War II, with approximately 37,000 to 50,000 still living in this area. It is impossible to determine how many were carried to their final destination in the frightening cattle cars. "Of the six million Jews who perished, at least 160,000 were Sephardim" (Lévy 1989a, 9).

38. This is a translation from the Judeo-Spanish text that Isaac obtained in Israel in 1968: "Desde el dia ke fuimos los eskojidos, fue muestro destino de ser odiados, de ser ronjados de lugar en lugar. Dezmudos mos fuimos, ma no sin muestras tradisiones, muestras kreyensas, i el lavoro de muestras manos. Este fue muestro legado."

Chapter 3: Memories of Time Past

1. For an exquisite and provocative discussion of the role of the senses in fieldwork, of smell, sound, and taste, see Stoller (1990).

2. For a superb example of the interpretive approach as applied to the study of narrative, see Narayan (1989). For a critique of aspects of Myerhoff's reflexive approach, see Whaley (1993) and the response from Atkinson (1993). See Prell (1989) for a positive critique of Myerhoff's life history approach and the reflexive nature of her work. For a poignant study of Myerhoff's works, see Kaminsky (1992).

In *Folklore, Culture, and Aging,* David Shuldiner writes of interviewing the elderly as "an individual embodiment of a remembered past" and "the product of a collective memory" (1997, xiv). Elaborating on the collective nature of memory, Mary Hufford refers to the "generational 'cohort'" as an age group who participated "in history from the same position in the life cycle." Thus, Hufford argues, "elderly contemporaries share understandings to which younger generations are not privy, and these shared understandings and memories are a resource that the . . . elders produce with and for each other" (1996, 13). For additional discussion of the "cohort," see Hufford, Hunt, and Zeitlin (1987, 28). While we find Hufford's discussion of the "generational 'cohort'" persuasive, we should note that in our own fieldwork there was much less evidence of the elders' "engaging each other, shaping and affirming their generation's reality," and much more of their vying individually for our attention. Certainly this could have been an artifact of the collecting situation in which the two of us were the primary hearers at that particular moment, to listen to, to record, and thus, to validate the memories of the elderly. Shuldiner remarks on this aspect of fieldwork: "Perhaps one of the most vital roles played by the folklorist is that of stimulating the very process of reflection among interview subjects" (1994, 217). For a superb annotated bibliography on folklore and aging, see Shuldiner (1997). For an annotated bibliography of *Anthropology of Aging*, see Schweitzer (1991). Patrick Mullen (1992, 10–21) and Barbara Kirshenblatt-Gimblett (1989a, 136, 138–39) provide good synopses of theories on aging. Specifically, Kirshenblatt-Gimblett points to the stunning work of Hufford, Hunt, and Zeitlin (1987): "Most recently, folklorists have been exploring indigenous forms, processes, and occasions of life review. *The Grand Generation: Memory, Mastery, Legacy*, an exhibition and book, breaks new ground by revealing the wide variety of ways that elderly individuals recover earlier experiences" (1989a, 139). For cross-cultural studies on aging, see Fry (1980) and Myerhoff and Simic (1978). For a clinical perspective on the functions of reminiscence in the lives of the elderly, see Sherman (1991). The classic, consummate works on narratives and the elderly are those by Myerhoff (1978, 1986), and Myerhoff and Ruby (1992).

3. The concept of "young" is relative. At the time of the fieldwork in 1990, Isaac was sixty-two and Rosemary was forty-six.

4. The woman was describing the practice of going to the synagogue, pouring oil in a small container, either of brass or glass, and lighting a wick that floats in the oil. *Echar azeite* is an idiom meaning to thank God for saving someone from a grave sickness or danger.

5. In 1990, when we were conducting the interviews, Bitola and Monastir (Mostar) were part of Yugoslavia. They are now, respectively, in Macedonia and Bosnia Herzogovina.

Chapter 4: The Power of Speech

1. The Temple was first destroyed by the Babylonians in 586 B.C.E., and then by the Romans in 70 C.E.

2. For a discussion of the tetragrammaton and the names for God, see Birnbaum (1991, 35, 608–9).

Chapter 5: "Let It Go to the Garlic!"

1. Account given by a man in the audience at the Judeo-Spanish hour, a program hosted by Moshe Shaul, in Jerusalem, on June 8, 1982. Isaac had been invited to speak about his research on Sephardic magic and home remedies.

2. *Ojo kui: ojo,* Spanish, eye; *khouï,* Turkish, evil character; thus, eye of evil character.

3. Scholarship on the evil eye is extensive, including Gifford (1958), Maloney (1976), and Dundes (1981), as well as other works related to the evil eye, such as Donaldson (1938), Molho (1950), Galanté (1935), Firestone (1959), Dahbany-Miraglia (1975), and Rebhun (1995).

4. National Sound Archives, Jerusalem, Y 5479 (6).

5. According to our informant, a Greek Orthodox priest, the expression "*Skata sta moutra sou* [Greek, feces in your expression/feces in your face]" is used in the villages, while the more educated class in the city would say, "*Apo tisou nou satana* [Greek, In the back, Satan!]."

6. National Sound Archives, Jerusalem, Y 3980 (24).

7. In *Island of Roses: The Jews of Rhodes in Los Angeles,* a video by Rebecca Amato Levy's grandson, Gregori Viens (1995), Rebecca Levy is shown preparing rue with gold leaf for a baby's *brit milah.*

8. Our good friends and colleagues Moshe Shaul, Shmuel Refael, and Avner Perez provided the following commentary on this informant's explanation: It was a general custom among Jews, including the Sephardim, to leave a piece of the eastern wall in a room, often close to the ceiling, unpainted in memory of the destruction of the Temple. In this place one would hang a *Mizrah* (east), a picture with the Hebrew passage, "If I forget, thee Jerusalem, I will lose my right hand" (*Talmud Bavli, Baba Batra,* p. 60, col. 2; *Midrash Tehilim,* Ch. 137, paragraph 6).

9. National Sound Archives, Jerusalem, Y 3980 (24). *Namusias* translates most correctly as "mosquito netting," though this literal rendering should not overshadow the aesthetic beauty of the netting that fell in graceful folds around the bed.

10. A *minyan* is a group of not less than ten men required for reciting certain prayers.

11. National Sound Archives, Jerusalem, Y 3980 (24).

12. Muslims were called *vedres,* meaning "green." The Ottoman ruling issued in 1622 forbade Jewish women from wearing green *chintiyan* (wide, baggy pants) or green belts (Matkovski 1982, 49).

13. National Sound Archives, Jerusalem, Y 3980 (24).

14. The following version was recorded in Sarajevo by Jakov Maestro in 1933:

Te lambo, te lambo
Komo lambe el bezero a su biserik'o;
No te lampo [*sic*] por lamber
Otro ke por kitar el ožo malo i ajin raa,
I mandar a las profondinas de la mar.

I lick you, I lick you
As the calf (cow) licks her young calf;

I do not lick you just to lick (wash/clean)
Rather to remove *ojo malo* (Spanish, evil eye) and *ayin arah* (Hebrew, evil eye)
And send it to the bottom of the sea. (1933, 113)

The ancient Greeks warded off the evil eye and restored sexual potency by applying saliva to the forehead, though this was done by licking the middle finger and then touching the forehead (Onians 1954, 233 n. 5). The Sephardim would lick the extended index finger and touch the Adam's apple three times as a protection against *espanto* (fright).

15. In a talk on Sephardic folk beliefs and magic given at the Sephardic synagogue in San Francisco, Isaac reported on this incident. The next day, Isaac spoke long distance to the person who was arranging for his lecture in Los Angeles. The individual told Isaac that the rabbi in San Francisco had called him to tell him about Isaac's talk. The rabbi said that when he had returned home after the talk, he had found his infant son "crying, crying, crying." He did what Isaac's grandmother had done, licked the baby's forehead three times, and it worked. The baby went to sleep. Thus our initial fears were allayed about the rabbi's reception of Isaac's talk on magical beliefs, delivered as it was with Isaac directly in front of the Holy Arc of the Covenant and immediately beneath the Eternal Light.

16. National Sound Archives, Jerusalem, Y c 930 (12).

17. Rabbi Joseph Telushkin explains the mezuzah as follows: "The Hebrew word for doorpost is *mezuzah,* and for thousands of years Jews have posted small boxes, also known as *mezuzot,* on their doorposts. Inside each box is a small scroll, which must be written by a scribe" (1991, 633). The verses, from Deuteronomy 6:4–9, comprise a portion of the *Shema,* one of the most important prayers in Judaism. This begins, "Hear O Israel: the Lord is our God, the Lord is One," and ends with the commandment, "And thou shalt write them upon the door-posts of thy house, and upon thy gates." The remainder of the *Shema* is from Deuteronomy 11:13–20.

18. Firestone records the following story told by a woman from Rhodes: "A demon in the guise of a woman attempted to snatch a newborn child from her arms." The woman tried to cry out but could not "for the demon had its hand on her heart, rendering her speechless." She tried to awaken her sleeping children by nudging them with her foot "because demons flee when other people are present and awake" (1962, 305).

19. As noted in *The Western Medical Tradition, 800 B.C. to A.D. 1800,* "The historical Hippocrates was a contemporary of Socrates. The Hippocratic Corpus was largely written during the period 420–350 B.C.; what, if anything, Hippocrates himself wrote of it is hotly disputed" (Conrad et al. 1995, 7 n. 1).

Chapter 6: Narrating Health, Marking the Social

1. This is a pseudonym.

2. *Kendiziko* is the English word, candy, with the diminutive *-iko,* meaning little.

Chapter 7: The Treasured Medicine and the Blessed Cure

1. See Nehama (1977); Molho (1960, 391). We disagree with the definition offered by Passy (1994, 216), who defines *segula* as "a magic cure for one who is possessed." Since in all cases save *echizo* (witchcraft), we eschew the use of the term "magic," we would be loath to apply it here to the cures that were regarded by the people as operating always in God's name. Additionally, a *segula* was not always performed for one who was possessed, though occasionally this was the case.

2. See Dundes (1968) for the significance of the number three in magic.

3. Patai refers to Moshe Reischer, *Sepher Sha'are Yerushalayim* (Jerusalem, 1870), no pagination; Patai translated it from Hebrew. He also refers to the chapter "Mummy as a Drug," in Warren R. Dawson, *The Bridle of Pegasus* (London, 1930).

4. This same form of divination was practiced by Muslim Turks. The following was taken from the Folklore Archives of the University of California, Berkeley. Molten lead is poured into cold water and forms shapes that are then interpreted. "A common practice in the villages among the older generations. Not seen much in the cities." Collected from Denise Tukennez in 1988, by Kim Pruett.

5. For the use of sugar and honey as medicine, see also Mintz (1996, 60–63, 88).

6. *Yauch* or *jauch* refers to the Turkish term *yaur.* Nehama defines it as "A non-Moslem, an infidel. It is a term of contempt used by the Turkish people, the believers, when referring to the Christians" (1977, 600). Rebecca Amato Levy informs us that it refers to the Greek Orthodox.

Chapter 8: Prekante

1. We are indebted to Professor Charles Faulhaber, a specialist in medieval Spanish literature at the University of California at Berkeley, for consulting the Archivo Digital de MSS y Textos Espannoles (ADMYTE). With a data base of 150 medieval and early modern Spanish texts, ADMYTE contained no references to the term *prekante* or the verb *prekantar.*

2. José Manuel Pedrosa (1998, 156 n. 8) writes, "La etimología de todas estas designaciones populares [*percante, precante, precantar* o *aprecantar*] de los ensalmos que los sefardíes suelen emplear en los tratamientos de diversas enfermedades nunca se ha explicado de manera convincente. Aunque resulta obvio el parentesco con la familia de la voz *encanto* (y con *en-cantar*), la anteposición del prefijo *per-* o *pre-* en el ámbito sefardí no tiene paralelos en el resto de las lenguas y dialectos ibéricos. [The etymology of all these popular designations of the *ensalmos* that the Sephardim tend to use in the treatment of various infirmities was never explained in a convincing manner. Even though the relationship with the term *encanto* (and *con en-cantar*) is obvious, the placing of the prefix *per-* or *pre-* in the Sephardic usage has no parallel in the rest of the Iberian languages and dialects]."

3. Translations from the Spanish are by Isaac Jack Lévy: "se explican por las fórmulas cantadas o recitadas que usaban los hechiceros" (Corominas and Pas-

cual 1980–91, 812). Samuel Elazar suggests that the term *prekantar* comes from the infinitive *cantar,* to sing (1966, 161).

4. All translations from the Spanish are by Isaac Jack Lévy.

5. Samuel Elazar (1966), Michael Molho (1950), Joseph Nehama (1977), Albert Passy (1994), and Albert Adatto (1939) wrongly associate the *prekante,* as well as the *endulko* (ritual enclosure), with the performance of a shaman, an enchantress, or a witch.

6. Personal communication from David Bunis, March 2000. The article, entitled "Melamed" (Teacher), was originally published in *El dia de Plovdiv* and later was reprinted in *El Meseret de Izmir* 2, no. 23 (1989): 180.

7. This is our translation of the Spanish, "acostumbraba pasar la mano por la cara abajo y escupia" (Padilla 1983, 259).

8. Collected from a Sephardic professor in Istanbul at *Nochada espanyola,* a Judeo-Spanish group sponsored by *Shalom* newspaper.

9. National Sound Archives, Jerusalem, Y 5479 (6); recorded in Tel Aviv, 1985; told by Gamila Ventura, born in Brusa, Turkey.

10. As Trachtenberg notes, this practice was also followed by the Greeks and Arabs, and in post-Talmudic Aramaic and medieval incantations (1939, 115).

11. None of the nine *prekantes* collected in the 1930s by Samuel Elazar (1966) mentions the name of the stricken one. The rituals were annotated by his sister, Sara Elazar (S. Elazar 1987), from the oral tradition in Sarajevo. Unfortunately, the author included the *prekantes* under the title of "Sortilejos" ("Sorceries").

12. The woman, originally from Izmir, Turkey, was a participant at the Judeo-Spanish gathering in Jerusalem, sponsored by Moshe Shaul, the editor of *Aki Yerushalayim,* in June 1982.

13. Isaac interviewed his step-father, Baruch Israel, and Bohora Biton in 1965 and 1966, in Atlanta, Georgia.

14. Born in Cairo, Egypt, Albert Hemsi was Isaac's uncle. An ethnomusicologist, he was known for his collection of Judeo-Spanish ballads and songs and for writing the accompanying music. For a collection of his works, see Hemsi (1995); for a study of his *coplas,* see Menascé (1993).

15. Interview with Mary Algrante, Izmir, 1990.

16. This information was conveyed to us by Arthur Benveniste who, at our request, interviewed Rebecca Amato Levy at her home in Los Angeles on February 22, 1998. In the remarkable video *Island of Roses: The Jews of Rhodes in Los Angeles,* Rebecca Levy is shown performing a *prekante* (Viens 1995).

17. Personal communications from Rebecca Levy, August 1999; Michael K. Toumazou, Professor of Classics, Davidson College, September 1999; and Beki Bardavid, Istanbul, Turkey.

18. The following is the Spanish entry under *pelo:* "Significa también una enfermedád, que dá à mugéres en los pechos, causada de congelarse la leche, con que se malicia y daña. . . . Hácense en las tetas de la mugéres inflamaciones, y apostémas, y zaratanes, y otras enfermedades que consisten en la disposición de la leche, ò en su generación, assi como falta, abundancia, ò congelamiento, à quien llaman pelo" (*Diccionario de Autoridades* 1979, 196). Juan Fragóso's original version, *Cirugía Universal,* appeared in Madrid in 1570 under the title *Erotemas chirurgicos.* It underwent several revisions. See also *Diccionario de la lengua española,* where *pelo* is defined as follows, "A sickness that women suffer in the

breasts, when they are nursing, from the obstruction of the milk ducts" (1956, 1000).

19. This phrase can also be translated as, "I pray and implore you."

20. Elazar added parenthetically the word for snake at the end of "Protiv groznice-zmijuljice (colebrica)."

21. Personal communication from Professor Kuzmanovich, Davidson College, September 1999. We are grateful to him for translating Elazar's article from Serbo-Croatian.

22. The following is the Spanish version from a 1977 facsimile edition of the original 1611 work: "Cierta enfermedad intercutánea a manera de empeine, que suele nacer comúnmente en la barba." Covarrubias also lists the same skin condition in different categories:

a. *Lichen* (*enis*) Lat. Tetter [a skin disease, eczema], ringworm. For Pliny (23–79 A.D.), it refers to a lichen-like eruptive skin disease.

b. *Impetigo* (*inis*) Lat. A kind of eruption on the skin, a sort of scab, tetter, ringworm.

c. *Mentagra* Lat. A foul tetter or scab, which begins on the chin and spreads over the face.

d. *Impeine* (*empeine*) Span. Tetter, ringworm.

23. Depending on the historical period and region, the disease was referred to by any of the following terms: *decipela* (*dessipela, decipola, disípula, isípula*), as well as *erisipela, empeine* (*enpeyne*), impedigo, and *usagre* (Lis Quibén 1980, 48).

24. While the *prekante* gives seventy as the number of Sanhedrim, the members of the highest court of the ancient Jewish nation, the actual number was seventy-one. The word *demiza,* requires exegesis. Our informants suggested one possible interpretation: *d'mezuza,* meant the entrance to heaven, also known as *Yeshiva shel mala* (the sitting, assembly above), where it was believed that the court met. The second interpretation could be *d'mizrah,* from the east, referring to the Eastern Wall of Jerusalem, or to the most important section of a synagogue, and by extension, of heaven. Thus the line "ke estan sentados en la demiza de ganeder" could mean either those "who are seated at the entrance of heaven," where the souls are judged, or those "who are seated on the most prominent section of heaven."

25. Personal communication, Rabbi Yossi Y. Groner, Lubavitch Synagogue, Charlotte, North Carolina, October 1999.

26. In an unpublished paper entitled "Kreyensas populares djudeo-espanyolas," presented to the members of the Sirkolo de Aki Yerushalayim in 1986, Koen-Sarano gave a longer version of "El prekante kontra el áyin ará."

27. In his article about Gad Nassi's work, Moshe Shaul notes that Nassi copied the *prekante* from Moise Franco's *Sciences Mystiques chez les Juifs de l'Orient* (Paris, 1900).

28. Personal communication from the Reverend Doctor Alan Corré, October 17, 1997.

29. Translated from the French by Isaac Jack Lévy.

30. Pedrosa conducted fieldwork in collaboration with José María Sanz and José Luis González in La Nava de Francia (Salamanca) on July 31, 1989. He conducted additional fieldwork in Asturias, Badajoz, Cáceres Deón, and Léon. In addition, Pedrosa carried out archival and bibliographic research. In sum, he found *ensalmos*

from Portugal and from the following provinces in Spain: Asturias, Cáceres Deón, and Salamanca (Pedrosa 2000).

31. Translated from the Hebrew by Rabbi Howard Kosovske.

32. For a study of the fourth key, which some consider to be the same as the key of rain, see *The Talmud, Tractate Ta'anit* (1989), 13–14.

33. For the theme of the transference of harm to the sea, and of the transference to a place where "no rooster crows or dog barks," see Pedrosa (2000, 63–111). Pedrosa located allusions to both themes as far back as the eighth century in Asturias, Spain, and even to Sicily and to Serbo-Croatia.

34. Personal communication, Rabbi Samuel Benaroya, Sephardic Bikur Holin Congregation, Seattle, Washington, April 23, 1975.

35. Schrire notes that the mere mention of Joseph in late oriental Jewish amulets was expected to be efficacious based on the interpretation that Joseph's descendants have immunity from the evil eye (1966, 114). Use of the full verse, "'Joseph is a fruitful bough, a fruitful bough by a spring; whose branches run over the wall,' . . . or portions of the verse, or the first letters of the individual words of the verse . . . , are important in the writing of amulets and *prekantes*" (Schiffman and Swartz 1992, 121).

36. The last four lines of this *prekante* are from Genesis 49:18 and are included as well in the Night Prayer (Birnbaum 1949, 784).

37. Personal communication, Eliyah Arnon, Center for Jewish Studies, Graduate Theological Union, Berkeley, California, April 1996.

38. Personal communication, Rabbi Groner, Lubavitch Synagogue, Charlotte, North Carolina, October 1998.

39. Personal communication, John Reeves, Professor of Judaic Studies, University of North Carolina, Charlotte, April 1998.

40. For a study of this day and of the verses, see Molho (1950, 237–42). Also see Armistead and Silverman (1968, 395–98). For the complete song, see Uziel (1956, 66–78). Molho (1950, 238) attributes this song to the eighteenth-century Salonikan poet Judah Kali, while Armistead and Silverman (1968, 396–97) point to its similarities with Greek verses.

Chapter 9: Saradura

1. The profusion of terms does not cease here, for in a variation of what we render as *saladura* and *saradura,* Abraham Galanté (1935) refers to as *saladoura* and *saradoura;* Rebecca Amato Levy, as *ensaradura* (1987, 72); and Rabbi Marc Angel, as *enseredura* (1978b, 132).

2. Patai was quoting Sithon, *K'nesiyah l'Shem Shamayim* (Gathering for the sake of heaven) (Jerusalem, 1874).

3. See also Firestone 1962, 306, for a discussion of the influence of the moon on the cure: "as the moon wanes at the end of the month the sickness will also wane."

Conclusion

1. Personal communication, Krinka Vidaković Petrov, Belgrade, Yugoslavia, 1990.

Bibliography

Adatto, Albert. 1939. "Sephardim and the Seattle Sephardic Community." M.A. thesis, University of Washington.

Adreth, Solomon ben. 1539. *Sheelot u-Teshuvot.* Vol. 1. Bologna: n.p.

Alfasi, R. Isaac ben Jacob. 1781. *Sefer Sheelot u-Teshuvot. Livorno: Bi-defus ha-shutafim.*

Alkalay, Arye. 1984. Imrot Ve-Pitgamim shel yeudei Sefarad (*Dichos i refranes sefaradíes*), edited by David Benveniste. Jerusalem: Ed. Moreshet.

Altabe, David Fintz. 1993. *Spanish and Portuguese Jewry: Before and after 1492.* Brooklyn, N.Y.: Sepher-Hermon Press.

Altamira, Rafael. 1949. *A History of Spain.* Translated by Muna Lee. New York: D. Van Nostrand.

Angel, Marc D. 1978a. *The Jews of Rhodes: The History of a Sephardic Community.* New York: Shepher-Hermon Press and the Union of Sephardic Congregations.

———. 1978b. "Segulot in a Manuscript from the Island of Rhodes." *Estudios sefardíes* 1:84–89.

———, trans. 1991. *The Essential Pele Yoetz: An Encyclopedia of Ethical Jewish Living.* New York: Sepher-Hermon Press.

Ankori, Zvi. 1977. "Greek Orthodox-Jewish Relations in Historic Perspective: The Jewish View." *Greek Orthodox Theological Review* 22 (1): 533–73.

Anonymous. 1989. "Melamed." *El Meseret of Izmir* 2 (23): 180.

Arditti, Lily. 1988. Letter to the Editor. *Sephardic Home News* 41 (3): 2.

Armistead, Samuel. 1992. "Judeo-Spanish Traditional Poetry in the United States." *American Jewish Archives* 44:357–77.

Armistead, Samuel, and Joseph H. Silverman. 1968. "Las 'Complas de las flores' y la poesía popular de los Balcanes." *Sefarad* 28:395–98.

———. 1981. "La orasion de una mujer sefaradi." *Aki Yerushalayim* Year 3, 11:16–17.

Assis, Yom Tov. 1986. "Crime and Violence among the Jews of Spain (Thirteenth–Fourteenth Centuries)" (in Hebrew). *Zion Jubilee Volume* 50:221–40.

———. 1987. "Social Unrest and Class Struggle in Hispano-Jewish Society before the Expulsion" (in Hebrew). In *Tarbut ve-historyah (Culture and History)*, edited by J. Dan, 121–45. Jerusalem: Misgav Yerushalayim.

———. 1988. "Sexual Behaviour in Mediaeval Hispano-Jewish Society." In *Jewish History: Essays in Honour of Chimen Abramsky*, edited by Ada Rapoport-Albert and Steven J. Zipperstein, 25–59. London: Peter Halban.

Atkinson, Paul. 1993. "Ethnography or Fiction: A False Dichotomy. Response to Whaley." *Linguistics and Education* 5:53–60.

Avigad, Nahman. 1989. "The Inscribed Pomegranate from the 'House of the Lord.'" *Israel Museum Journal* 8:7–16.

Avraham Yitshak Kastilo ve Eliezer Sa'dum. 1968. Reprint. Jerusalem: n.p.

Babcock, Barbara. 1977. "The Story in the Story: Metanarration in Folk Narrative." In *Verbal Art as Performance*, edited by Richard Bauman, 61–79. Prospect Heights, Ill.: Waveland Press.

Baer, Yitzhak. 1966. *A History of the Jews in Christian Spain*. Vol. 2. Philadelphia: Jewish Publication Society of America.

Barnai, Jacob. 1990. "On the History of the Jews in the Ottoman Empire." In *Sephardi Jews in the Ottoman Empire*, edited by Esther Juhasz, 19–35. Jerusalem: The Israel Museum.

Barocas, David N. 1976. *A Study on the Meaning of Ladino, Judezmo and the Spanish Jewish Dialect*. New York: Foundation for the Advancement of Sephardic Studies and Culture.

Baron, Salo Wittmayer. 1967. *A Social and Religious History of the Jews: Late Middle Ages and Era of European Expansion*. Vol. 12. New York: Columbia University Press.

Basgöz, Ilhan. 1986. "Digression in Oral Narrative: A Case Study of Individual Remarks by Turkish Romance Tellers." *Journal of American Folklore* 99:5–23.

Battaglia, Salvatore. 1984. *Grande Dizionario della Lingua Italiana*. Vol. 12. Torino: Unione Tipografico.

Bayley, Harold. 1992. *The Lost Language of Symbolism: An Inquiry into the Origin of Certain Letters, Words, Names, Fairy-Tales, Folklore, and Mythologies*. Vol 2. London: Williams and Norgate.

Behar, Nissim. 5746 (1993). *Guide for the Practice of Judaism: Based on the "Shulhan Aruch" and Its Commentaries*. Translated by H. Dunner. Bnei Berak, Israel: Or-Hahaim Educational Center.

———. n.d. *The Solemn Days of Rosh Hashanah and Kipur: Testimony of Sages, Laws, Concerning Rosh Hashanah and Kipur, Tales about Miracles*. Bnei Berak, Israel: Or-Hahaim Educational Center.

Beinart, Haim. 1997. "Order of the Expulsion from Spain: Antecedents, Causes, and Textual Analysis." In *Crisis and Creativity in the Sephardic World, 1391–1648*, edited by Benjamin R. Gampel, 79–94. New York: Columbia University Press.

Benardete, Mair José. 1952. *Hispanic Culture and Character of the Sephardic Jews*. New York: Hispanic Institute in the United States.

Benbassa, Esther, and Aron Rodrigue. 1995. *The Jews of the Balkans: The Judeo-Spanish Community, Fifteenth to Twentieth Centuries*. Cambridge, Mass.: Blackwell.

Benbassa-Dudonney, Esther. 1982. "El ojo malo." *Aki Yerushalayim* Year 3, 12:26–29.

Ben-Yehuda, Ehud. 1964. *English-Hebrew, Hebrew-English Dictionary.* New York: Pocket Books.

Birnbaum, Philip. 1949. *Daily Prayer Book, Ha-Siddur Ha-Shalem.* New York: Hebrew Publishing Company.

———. 1991. *Encyclopedia of Jewish Concepts.* New York: Hebrew Publishing Company.

Bivach, A. 1992. "El judaismo español antes del destierro." In *Los judíos de España,* edited by Henry Méchoulan, 31–47. Valladolid: Editorial Trotta.

Bortnick, Rachel Amado. 1993. "The Jewish Women of Turkey." *Jewish Folklore and Ethnology Review* 15 (2): 96–103.

Budge, Ernest A. 1930. *Amulets and Superstitions.* London: Humphrey Press.

Bunis, David M. 1981. "The Hebrew and Aramaic Component of Judezmo: A Phonological and Morphological Analysis." Ph.D. diss., Columbia University.

———. 1993. *A Lexicon of the Hebrew and Aramaic Elements in Modern Judezmo.* Jerusalem: Magnes Press, the Hebrew University, Misgav Yerushalayim, and the Institute for Research on the Sephardi and Oriental Jewish Heritage.

Burke, Ulick Ralph. 1900. *A History of Spain: From the Earliest Times to the Death of Ferdinand the Catholic.* New York: Longmans, Green.

Capsali, Eliyahu. 1976. *Seder Eliyahu Zuta.* Jerusalem: Ben Zvi Institute.

Cargas, Isidro de las. 1946. "Tres cartas públicas de Comanda." *Sefarad* 6:73–93.

Castro, Américo. 1948. *España en su historia: Cristianos, moros y judíos.* Buenos Aires: Editorial Losada.

Conrad, Lawrence. 1995. "The Arab-Islamic Medical Tradition." In *The Western Medical Tradition, 800 B.C. to A.D. 1800,* edited by Lawrence I. Conrad, Michael Neve, Vivian Nutton, Roy Porter, and Andrew Wear, 93–138. Cambridge: Cambridge University Press.

Conrad, Lawrence I., Michael Neve, Vivian Nutton, Roy Porter, and Andrew Wear. 1995. *The Western Medical Tradition, 800 B.C. to A.D. 1800.* Cambridge: Cambridge University Press.

Corominas, Joan. 1954. *Diccionario crítico etimológico de la lengua castellana.* 4 vols. Madrid: Editorial Gredos.

Corominas, Joan, and José Pascual. 1980–91. *Diccionario crítico etimológico castellano e hispánico.* 6 vols. Madrid: Editorial Gredos.

Covarrubias Horozco, Sebastían de. 1977. *Tesoro de la lengua castellana o española.* Madrid: Ediciones Turner. Facsimile edition of the original work published in 1611 in Madrid.

Crawley, Ernest. 1934. *Oath, Curse, Blessing.* London: Watts.

Crombie, J. E. 1892. "The Saliva Superstition." In *The International Folk-Lore Congress, 1891,* edited by Joseph Jacobs and Alfred Nutt, 249–58. London: David Nutt.

Cuyas, Arturo. 1953. *Diccionario revisado: Inglés-Español y Español-Inglés.* New York: Appleton-Century-Croft.

Dahbany-Miraglia, Dina. 1975. "Verbal Protective Behavior among Yemenite Jews." In vol. 13, *Working Papers in Yiddish and East European Jewish Studies.* New York: Max Weinreich Center for Advanced Jewish Studies of the YIVO Institute for Jewish Research.

Danon, Abraham. 1895. "Etude historique sur les impôts directs et indirects des communautés israélites en Turquie." *Revue des études juives* 31:52–61.

———. 1896. "Recueil de romances judéo-espagnoles chantées en Turquie." *Revue des études juives* 32:102–23, 32:263–75, 33:122–139, 33:255–68.

———. 1897. "Les Superstitions des Juifs Ottomans." *Actes du Onzième Congrès International des Orientalistes*, Section 7, Paris. Reprinted in *Section Ethnographie et Folk-lore d'Orient*, 259–70. Nendeln/Liechtenstein: Kraus Reprint, 1968.

———. 1899–1900. "La comunauté juive de Salonique au XVIe siècle." *Revue des études juives* 40:206–30, 41:98–117, 250–65.

———. 1925. *Sa vie et ses oeuvres.* Paris: Imprimerie H. Elias.

Dawson, Warren R. 1930. *The Bridge of Pegasus; Studies in Magic, Mythology and Folklore.* London: Methuen.

Diccionario de Autoridades. 1979. Dir. Dámaso Alonso. Edición Facsímil. Madrid: Editorial Gredos.

Diccionario de la lengua castellana. 1914. Por La Real Academia Española, 14th ed. Madrid: Imprenta de los Sucesores de Hernando.

Diccionario de la lengua española. 1956. Real Academia Española. Madrid: Editorial Espasa-Calpe.

Dobrinsky, Herbert C. 1986. *A Treasury of Sephardic Laws and Customs.* Hoboken, N.J.: KTAV Publishing House.

Domínguez Ortiz, Antonio. 1984. "La mujer en el tránsito de la Edad Media a la Moderna." In *Las mujeres en las ciudades medievales, Actas de las Jornadas de Investigación Interdisciplinaria,* edited by Cristina Segura Graiño, 171–78. Madrid: Seminario de Estudios de la Mujer, Universidad Autónoma de Madrid.

Donaldson, Bess Allen. 1938. *The Wild Rue: A Study of Muhammadan Magic and Folklore in Iran.* London: Luzac.

Donin, Hayim Halevy. 1972. *To Be a Jew.* New York: Basic Books.

Douglas, Mary. 1966. *Purity and Danger: An Analysis of Concepts of Pollution and Taboo.* London: Routledge and Kegan Paul.

———. 1973. *Natural Symbols: Explorations in Cosmology.* New York: Random House.

Dundes, Alan. 1966. "Metafolklore and Oral Literary Criticism." *The Monist* 50:505–16.

———. 1968. "The Number Three in American Culture." In *Every Man His Way: Readings in Cultural Anthropology,* edited by Alan Dundes, 401–24. Englewood Cliffs, N.J.: Prentice-Hall.

———. 1981. "Wet and Dry, the Evil Eye: An Essay in Indo-European and Semitic Worldview." In *The Evil Eye: A Folklore Casebook,* edited by Alan Dundes, 257–312. New York: Garland.

———, ed. 1981. *The Evil Eye: A Folklore Casebook.* New York: Garland.

Dundes, Alan, and Alessandro Falassi. 1975. *La Terra in Piazza: An Interpretation of the Palio of Siena.* Berkeley: University of California Press.

Elazar, Daniel. 1984. "The Sunset of Balkan Jewry." In *The Balkan Jewish Communities: Yugoslavia, Bulgaria, Greece and Turkey,* edited by Daniel Elazar et al., 1–11. Lanham, Md.: University Press of America.

Elazar, Daniel, Harriet Pass Friedenreich, Baruch Hazzan, and Adina Weiss Liberles. 1984. *The Balkan Jewish Communities: Yugoslavia, Bulgaria, Greece and Turkey.* Lanham, Md.: University Press of America.

Elazar, Samuel. 1966. "Narodna medicina sefardskih jevreja u Bosni." In *Spomenica 400 Godina od dolaska jevreja u Bosni i Hercegonivu, 1566–1966,* edited by Samuel Kamhi, 155–66. Sarajevo: Oslobodjenje.

———. 1987. *El Romancero judeo-español: Romances y otras poesías.* Sarajevo: "Svjetlost," Oour Izdavačka Djelatnost.

Eliade, Mircea, ed. 1987. "Domestic Observances." In *The Encyclopedia of Religion,* 400–417. New York: Macmillan.

Elnecavé, David. 1963. "Folklore de los sefardíes de Turquía." *Sefarad* 23, fasc. 1: 121–33 and 325–34.

———. 1964. "Folklore de los sefardíes de Turquía." *Sefarad* 24:12–136.

Elworthy, Frederic Thomas. 1958. *The Evil Eye: The Origins and Practices of Superstition.* New York: Julian Press.

Encyclopaedia Judaica. 1971. 16 vols. Jerusalem: Keter Publishing House.

Entralgo, Pedro Laín. 1970. *The Therapy of the Word in Classical Antiquity.* Edited and translated by L. J. Rather and John M. Sharp. New Haven: Yale University Press.

Epstein, Isidore. 1925. *The Responsa of Rabbi Solomon ben Adreth of Barcelona: 1235–1310.* London: Kegan Paul, Trench, Trubner.

———. 1968. *Studies in the Communal Life of the Jews of Spain: The "Responsa" of Rabbi Solomon ben Adreth of Barcelona (1235–1310) as a Source of the History of Spain.* New York: Hermon Press.

———, ed. 1980. *Talmud Hullin* (Hebrew-English Edition of the Babylonian Talmud). London: Soncino Press

Estrugo, José. 1958. *Los sefardíes.* Havana: Editorial Lex.

Fernández, Luis Suarez. 1964. *Documentos acerca de la expulsion de los judíos.* Burgos: Ediciones Aldecoa.

Firestone, Melvin M. 1959. "Magical Curing in the Seattle Sephardic Community." M.A. thesis, University of Washington.

———. 1962. "Sephardic Folk-Curing in Seattle." *Journal of American Folklore* 75:301–10.

Foster, George M. 1953. "Relationships between Spanish and Spanish-American Folk Medicine." *Journal of American Folklore* 66:201–17.

———. 1965. "Peasant Society and the Image of Limited Good." *American Anthropologist* 67:293–315

———. 1966. "Euphemisms and Cultural Sensitivity in Tzintzuntzan." *Anthropological Quarterly* 39 (2): 53–59.

———. 1994. *Hippocrates' Latin-American Legacy: Humoral Medicine in the New World.* Langhorne, Pa.: Gordon and Breach.

Fragóso, Juan. 1570. *Erotemas chirurgicos.* Madrid: n.p.

Franco, Moise. 1893. "Les juifs de l'Empire Ottoman au dix-neuvième siècle." *Revue des études juives* 26:110–30.

———. 1897. *Essai sur l'Histoire des israélites de l'Empire Ottoman depuis les origines jusqu'à nos jours.* Paris: Librairie A. Durlacher.

Frankel, Ellen, and Betsy Platkin Teutsh. 1992. *The Encyclopedia of Jewish Symbols.* Northvale, N.J.: Jason Aronson.

Frazer, James George. 1890–1915. *The Golden Bough: A Study in Magic and Religion.* 12 vols. New York: Macmillan.

———. 1968. "The Roots of Magic." In *Every Man His Way: Readings in Cultural Anthropology,* edited by Alan Dundes, 79–118. Englewood Cliffs, N.J.: Prentice-Hall.

Freud, Sigmund. 1959. "The 'Uncanny.'" In *Collected Papers,* vol. 4, 368–407. New York: Basic Books.

Fry, Christine L. 1980. *Aging in Culture and Society.* Brooklyn, N.Y.: J. F. Bergin.

Galanté, Abraham. 1930. "The Blood Libel in Damascus and Rhodes." *Mizrah Umaarav* 5:47–51.

———. 1931. *Documents officiels turcs concernant les juifs de Turquie.* Istanbul: Haim Rozio.

———. 1935. *Histoire des juifs de Rhodes, Chios, Cos, etc.* Istanbul: Société Anonyme de Papeterie et d'Imprimerie (Fratelli Haim).

———. 1937. *Histoire des Juifs d'Anatolie: Les Juifs d'Izmir.* Istanbul: Imprimerie M. Babok.

———. 1954. *Quatrième recueil de documents concernant les juifs te Turquie, Proverbes judeo-espagnols.* Istanbul: Fakülteler.

Gampel, Benjamin R. 1989. *The Last Jews on Iberian Soil: Navarrese Jewry 1497/1498.* Berkeley: University of California Press.

———, ed. 1997. *Crisis and Creativity in the Sephardic World: 1391–1648.* New York: Columbia University Press.

Gaon, Yoram. n.d. "Eli-Eliyahu." *Shabbath Songs in the Sephardic Tradition,* CBS 40-82760.

García de Diego, Vicente. 1985. *Diccionario etimológico español e hispánico.* Enlarged by Carmen García. Madrid: Espasa Calpe.

Garnett, Lucy M. J. 1891. *The Women of Turkey and Their Folklore: The Jewish and Moslem Women.* Vol. 2. London: David Nutt.

Gaster, Theodor. 1968. "Additional Notes." In *Every Man His Way,* edited by Alan Dundes, 114–19. Englewood Cliffs, N.J.: Prentice-Hall.

———. 1980. *The Holy and the Profane: Evolution of Jewish Folkways.* New York: Morrow.

Gennep, Arnold van. 1960. *The Rites of Passage.* Translated by Monika B. Vizedom and Gabrielle L. Caffe. Chicago: University of Chicago Press.

Gerber, Jane S. 1992. *The Jews of Spain: A History of the Sephardic Experience.* New York: Free Press.

Gerondi, Nissim ben Reuben. 1984. *Sheelot u-Teshuvot.* Edited by Aryeh L. Feldman. Jerusalem: Moznaim Pub.

Gevirtz, Stanley. 1959. "Curse Motifs in the Old Testament and in the Ancient Near East." Ph.D. diss., University of Chicago.

Gifford, Edward S. 1957. *The Evil Eye: Studies in the Folklore of Vision.* New York: Macmillan.

Glick, Thomas F. 1997. "On Converso and Marrano Ethnicity." In *Crisis and Creativity in the Sephardic World,* edited by Benjamin R. Gampel, 59–76. New York: Columbia University Press.

Goitein, Shlomo D. 1978. "The Family." In *A Mediterranean Society: The Jewish Communities of the Arab World as Portrayed in the Documents of the Cairo Geniza.* Berkeley: University of California Press.

Goldstein, Kenneth. 1964. *A Guide for Field Workers in Folklore.* Hatboro, Pa.: Folklore Associates.

Graetz, Henrich. 1891–92. *History of the Jews from the Earliest Times to the Present Day.* Edited and translated by Bella Löwry. 5 vols. London: David Nutt.

———. 1941. *History of the Jews.* Vol. 4. Philadelphia: Jewish Publication Society of America.

Greenberg, Blu. 1983. *How to Run a Traditional Jewish Household.* New York: Simon and Schuster.

Gross, Henri. 1908. "La famille juive des Hamon: Contribution a l'histoire des juifs en Turquie." *Revue des études juives* 56:1–26.

Gross, Morris. 1934. "The Relation of Blessing and Cursing in the Psalms to the Evolution of Hebrew Religion." Ph.D. diss., University of Chicago.

Gunkel, Hermann. 1933. *Einleitung in die Psalmen.* Göttingen: Vandenhoeck and Ruprecht.

Hacker, Joseph. 1978. "The Jewish Community of Salonika from the Fifteen [*sic*] to the Sixteen [*sic*] Century" (in Hebrew). Ph.D. diss., Hebrew University of Jerusalem.

Hand, Wayland. 1960. "Jewish Popular Beliefs and Customs." In *Studies in Biblical and Jewish Folklore,* edited by Raphael Patai, Francis Lee Utley, and Dov Noy, 309–26. Bloomington: Indiana University Press.

———. 1980. *Magical Medicine.* Berkeley: University of California Press.

Haskell, Guy H. 1994. *From Sofia to Jaffa: The Jews of Bulgaria and Israel.* Detroit: Wayne State University.

Hassán, Iacob M. 1970. *Actas del I Simposio de estudios sefardíes.* Madrid: Instituto Arias Montano.

Hemsi, Alberto. 1995. *Cancionero sefardí.* Edited by Edwin Seroussi. Jerusalem: Jewish Music Research Centre, Hebrew University of Jerusalem.

Hertz, J. H., ed. 1990. *The Pentateuch and Haftorahs.* London: Soncino Press.

Hillers, Delbert R. 1964. *Treaty-Curses and the Old Testament Prophets.* Rome: Pontifical Biblical Institute.

Holy Scriptures. 1943. Philadelphia: Jewish Publication Society of America.

Hufford, Mary. 1996. "Aging, Folklore and." In *American Folklore: An Encyclopedia,* edited by Jan Harold Brunvand, 12–14. New York: Garland.

Hufford, Mary, Marjorie Hunt, and Steven Zeitlin, eds. 1987. *The Grand Generation: Memory, Mastery, Legacy.* Seattle: University of Washington Press.

Ibn Khurradadhbih, Ubayd Allah. 1889. *Kitab al Masalik wa'l Mamalik.* Vol. 6. With French translation; edited by Michael Jan de Goeje. Leyden: Bibliotheca Geographorum Arabicorum.

Juhasz, Esther. 1990. *Sephardi Jews in the Ottoman Empire: Aspects of Material Culture.* Jerusalem: The Israel Museum.

Kaganoff, Benzion C. 1978. *A Dictionary of Jewish Names and Their History.* New York: Schocken Books.

Kamhi, Djina. 1980. "Medisina Popular." *Aki Yerushalayim* 7:17–20.

Kaminsky, Marc. 1992. "Introduction." In *Remembered Lives: The Work of Ritual, Storytelling, and Growing Older,* edited by Barbara Myerhoff, 1–97. Ann Arbor: University of Michigan Press.

Kany, Charles, ed. 1960. *American-Spanish Euphemisms.* Berkeley: University of California Press.

Kayserling, M. 1898. "L'Arçhidiacre Ferrand Martinez et les persécutions de 1391." *Revue des études juives* 37:257–73.

Kendall, Laurel. 1985. *Shamans, Housewives, and Other Restless Spirits: Women in Korean Ritual Life.* Honolulu: University of Hawaii Press.

Kirshenblatt-Gimblett, Barbara. 1987. "Introduction." In *The Grand Generation: Memory, Mastery, Legacy,* edited by Mary Hufford, Marjorie Hunt, and Steven Zeitlin, 12–15. Seattle: University of Washington Press.

———. 1989a. "Authoring Lives." *Journal of Folklore Research* 26 (2): 123–49.

———. 1989b. "Objects of Memory: Material Culture as Life Review." In *Folk*

Groups and Folklore Genres: An Introduction, edited by Elliott Oring, 329–38. Logan: Utah State University Press.

Koen-Sarano, Matilda. 1982. "Las maldisiones." *Aki Yerushalayim* Year 4, 13–14:36–37.

———. 1983. "Rekordos i refleksiones sovre el 'ainarah.'" *Aki Yerushalayim* Year 5, 18:23–24.

———. 1989. "El aynara en el reflan djudeo-espanyol." *Aki Yerushalayim* Year 10, 40:42–45.

———. 1992. "Las maldisiones djudeo-espanyolas de Yerushalayim." *Aki Yerushalayim* Year 13, 46:54–55.

Kowalchik, Claire, and William H. Hylton, eds. 1987. *Rodale's Illustrated Encyclopedia of Herbs.* Emmaus, Pa.: Rodale Press.

Lacave, José Luis. 1991. "Judíos en España." In *La vida judía en Sefarad,* edited by Elena Romero, 17–42. Madrid: Ministerio de Cultura.

Laredo, Abraham Isaac, and David Gonzalo Maeso. 1944. "El nombre de 'Sefard.'" *Sefarad* 4:349–63.

Lauterbach, Jacob Z. 1932. "The Naming of Children in Jewish Folklore, Ritual and Practice." *Yearbook of the Central Conference of American Rabbis* 42:316–60.

Leroy, Beatrice. 1986. *L'Aventure Sefarade.* Paris: Albin Michel.

Levack, Brian P., ed. 1992. *Articles on Witchcraft, Magic and Demonology: Possession and Exorcism.* Vol 9. New York: Garland.

Levy, Avigdor. 1992. *The Sephardim in the Ottoman Empire.* Princeton, N.J.: Darwin Press.

Levy, Bernard. 1952. *Notes and Documents from the Turkish Archives: A Contribution to the History of the Jews in the Ottoman Empire.* Jerusalem: Central Press.

Lévy, Isaac Jack. 1969. *Prolegomena to the Study of the Refranero Sefardí.* New York: Las Americas Publishing Company.

———. 1985. "A Domesticated Supernatural: Home Magic of the Sephardim." *Shofar* 3 (3): 12–19.

———. 1989a. *And the World Stood Silent: Sephardic Poetry of the Holocaust.* Urbana: University of Illinois Press.

———. 1989b. *Jewish Rhodes: A Lost Culture.* Berkeley: Judah L. Magnes Museum.

Lévy, Isaac Jack, and Rosemary Lévy Zumwalt. 1987. "The Evil Eye and the Power of Speech among the Sephardim." *International Folklore Review* 5:52–59.

———. 1993. *Sephardic Folklore: Exile and Homecoming.* Special issue, *Jewish Folklore and Ethnology Review* 15 (2).

Levy, Rebecca Amato. 1987. *I Remember Rhodes.* New York: Sepher-Hermon Press.

Lewis, Bernard. 1984. *The Jews of Islam.* Princeton, N.J.: Princeton University Press.

Lewis, Raphaela. 1971. *Everyday Life in Ottoman Turkey.* New York: Dorset Press.

Lis Quibén, Victor. 1980. *La medicina popular en Galicia.* Madrid: Fareso.

Lloyd, G. E. R. 1964. "The Hot and the Cold, the Dry and the Wet in Greek Philosophy." *Journal of Hellenistic Studies* 84:92–106.

Loeb, Isidore. 1886. "Règlement des juifs de Castille." *Revue des études juives* 13:182–216.

———. 1887. "La correspondance des juifs d'Espagne." *Revue des études juives* 40:262–76.

Luncz, Abraham Moshe. 1882. *Yerushalayim: Year-book for the Diffusion of an Accurate Knowledge of Ancient and Modern Palestine.* Jerusalem (Vienna, Austria): Carta.

Maestro, Jakov. 1933. "Praznovjerje kod sefardskih Jevreja." *Yearbook,* 110–16. Sarajevo, Belgrade: Godišnahk Izdahu La Benevolencia i Potpora Štamparija Menahem Papo.

Maloney, Clarence, ed. 1976. *The Evil Eye.* New York: Columbia University Press.

Mandelbaum, David. 1966. "Transcendental and Pragmatic Aspects of Religion." *American Anthropologist* 68:1174–91.

Mann, Vivian B., Thomas F. Glick, and Jerrilynn D. Dodds, eds. *Convivencia: Jews, Muslims, and Christians in Medieval Spain.* New York: George Braziller and the Jewish Museum.

Martínez, Nicolás López. 1954. *Los judaizantes castellanos y la Inquisición en tiempos de Isabel la Católica.* Serie A, vol. 1. Burgos: Seminario Metropolitano de Burgos.

Matisoff, James A. 1979. *Blessings, Curses, Hopes, and Fears: Psycho-Ostensive Expressions in Yiddish.* Philadelphia: Institute for Study of Human Issues.

Matkovski, Alexandar. 1982. *A History of the Jews in Macedonia.* Skopje: Macedonian Review Editions.

Mayer, N. 1913. *The Jews of Turkey. A Lecture Delivered before the Jewish Society at Beth Hamidrash on Saturday, March 29, 1913.* London: n.p.

Méchoulan, Henry, ed. 1992. *Los judíos de España: Historia de una diáspora (1492–1992).* Valladolid: Editorial Trotta.

Melammed, Renée Levine. 1991. "Sephardi Women in Medieval and Early Modern Periods." In *Jewish Women in Historical Perspective,* edited by Judith R. Baskin, 115–34. Detroit: Wayne State University Press.

———. 1992. "Women in Post 1492 Spanish Crypto-Jewish Society." *Judaism* 41 (162): 156–68.

———. 1999. *Heretics or Daughters of Israel? The Crypto-Jewish Women of Castille.* New York: Oxford University Press.

Menascé, Fintz Esther. 1992. *Gli ebrei di Rodi: Storia di un'antica comunità annientata dai nazisti.* Milano: Edizioni Angelo Guerini e Associati.

———. 1993. "Alberto Hemsi and His *Coplas Sefardíes.*" *Jewish Folklore and Ethnology Review* 15 (2): 62–69.

Middleton, DeWight R. 1986. "The Production and Management of Fear in Urban Contexts." In *Sociophobics: The Anthropology of Fear,* edited by David L. Scruton, 122–41. Boulder, Colo.: Westview Press.

Mintz, Sidney W. 1985. *Sweetness and Power: The Place of Sugar in Modern History.* New York: Viking.

———. 1996. *Tasting Food, Tasting Freedom.* Boston: Beacon Press.

Mitchell, Christopher Wright. 1987. *The Meaning of BRK "To Bless" in the Old Testament.* Atlanta, Ga.: Scholars Press.

Miyake, Hitoshi. 1972. "Folk Religion." In *Japanese Religion,* edited by Hori Ichiro, 121–43. Tokyo and Palo Alto: Kodansha International.

Moliner, María, ed. 1970. *Diccionario de uso del español.* 3 vols. Madrid: Editorial Gredos.

Molho, Michael. 1950. *Usos y costumbres de los sefardíes de Salónica.* Madrid-

Barcelona: Consejo Superior de Investigaciones Científicas, Instituto Arias Montano.

———. 1960. *Literatura sefardita de Oriente.* Madrid-Barcelona: Consejo Superior de Investigaciones Científicas, Instituto Arias Montano.

———. 1962. "Dos necropolis sobrepuestas en Salonica." *Sefarad* 22:376–83.

———. 1973. *In Memoriam: Hommage aux victimes juives des nazis en Grèce.* 2d ed. Salonica: Communauté Israélite de Thessalonique.

Moss, Leonard W., and Stephen C. Cappanari. 1976. "The Mediterranean 'Mal'occhio, Ayn hara, Oculus fascinus, Judelblick': The Evil Eye Hovers Above." In *The Evil Eye,* edited by Clarence Maloney, 1–15. New York: Columbia University Press.

Mullen, Patrick B. 1992. *Listening to Old Voices: Folklore, Life Stories, and the Elderly.* Urbana: University of Illinois Press.

Myerhoff, Barbara. 1978. *Number Our Days.* New York: Simon and Schuster.

———. 1983. *Number Our Days.* Direct Cinema Ltd. Videocasette.

———. 1986. "'Life Not Death in Venice': Its Second Life." In *The Anthropology of Experience,* edited by Victor W. Turner and Edward M. Bruner, 261–86. Urbana: University of Illinois Press.

———. 1992 [1988]. "Surviving Stories: Reflections on *Number Our Days.*" In *Remembered Lives: The Work of Ritual, Storytelling, and Growing Older,* edited by Barbara Myerhoff, 277–304. Ann Arbor: University of Michigan Press.

Myerhoff, Barbara, and Jay Ruby. 1992 [1982]. "A Crack in the Mirror: Reflexive Perspectives in Anthropology." In *Remembered Lives: The Work of Ritual, Storytelling, and Growing Older,* edited by Barbara Myerhoff, 307–40. Ann Arbor: University of Michigan Press.

Myerhoff, Barbara, and Andrei Simic, eds. 1978. *Life's Career—Aging: Cultural Variations on Growing Old.* Beverly Hills, Calif.: Sage Publications.

Narayan, Kirin. 1989. *Storytellers, Saints, and Scoundrels: Folk Narrative in Hindu Religious Teaching.* Philadelphia: University of Pennsylvania Press.

Nebrija, Antonio. 1973. *Vocabulario de romance en latín. Transcripción crítica de la edición revisada por el autor (Sevilla, 1516).* Introduction by Gerald J. Macdonald. Philadelphia: Temple University Press.

Nehama, Joseph. 1935–59. *Histoire des israelites de Salonique.* Vols. 1–5, Salonica: Librairie Molho; vols. 6–7, Salonica: Communauté Israélite de Thessalonique.

———. 1977. *Dictionnaire du Judéo-Espagnol.* Madrid: Consejo Superior de Investigaciones Científicas, Instituto Benito Arias Montano.

Netanyahu, B. 1995. *The Origins of the Inquisition in Fifteenth Century Spain.* New York: Random House.

Noy, Dov. 1980. "Is There a Jewish Folk Religion?" In *Studies in Jewish Folklore,* edited by Dov Noy and Frank Talmage, 273–85. Cambridge, Mass.: Association for Jewish Studies.

Nutton, Vivian. 1995. "Medicine in the Greek World, 800–50 B.C." In *The Western Medical Tradition, 800 B.C. to A.D. 1800,* edited by Lawrence I. Conrad, Michael Neve, Vivian Nutton, Roy Porter, and Andrew Wear, 11–38. Cambridge: Cambridge University Press.

Onians, Richard Broxton. 1954. *The Origins of European Thought about the Body, the Mind, the Soul, the World, Time and Fate.* Cambridge: Cambridge University Press.

Ortner, Sherry. 1973. "On Key Symbols." *American Anthropologist* 75:1338–46.

Padilla, Encarnación Marín. 1981. "Relación judeoconversa durante la segunda mitad del siglo XV en Aragón: Nacimientos, hadas, circunsiciones." *Sefarad* 41:273–300.

———. 1982a. "Relación judeoconversa durante la segunda mitad del siglo XV en Aragón: Matrimonio." *Sefarad* 42:243–98.

———. 1982b. "Relación judeoconversa durante la segunda mitad el siglo XV en Aragón: Nacimientos, hadas, circunsiciones." *Sefarad* 42:59–77.

———. 1983. "Relación judeoconversa durante la segunda mitad del siglo XV en Aragón: Enfermedades y muertes." *Sefarad* 43:251–344.

Palache, Hayim [Hayyim Palaggi]. 1874. *Refua ve-Hayim (Melizina i vida).* Izmir: Aaron Yeoshua de Sigura.

Papo, Joseph M. 1987. *Sephardim in Twentieth-Century America.* San Jose, Calif.: Pelé Yoetz Books.

Passy, Albert Morris. 1994. *Sephardic Folk Dictionary, English to Ladino, Ladino to English,* 2d ed. n.p.: AMPCO.

Patai, Raphael. 1960. "Jewish Folklore and Jewish Tradition." In *Studies in Biblical and Jewish Folklore,* edited by Raphael Patai, Francis Lee Utley, and Dov Noy, 11–24. Bloomington: Indiana University Press.

———. 1964. "*Indulco* and *Mumia.*" *Journal of American Folklore* 77:3–11.

Pedrosa, José Manuel. 1993. "Conjuros y ritos májicos sobre la dentición infantil." *Revista de Dealectología y Tradiciones Populares* 48:155–67.

———. 1995. "Correspondencias cristianas y judías de la oración de Las cuatro esquinas." In *Las dos sirenas y otros estudios de literatura tradicional (De la Edad Media al siglo XX),* 187–220. Madrid: Siglo XXI de España Editores.

———. 1998. "Las tres llaves y los huevos sin sal: Versiones hispanocristianas y sefardíes de dos ensalmos mágicos tradicionales." *Sefarad* 58:153–65.

———. 1999. "La candela nocturna: canción de alba sefardí, oración cristiana panhispánica y canción piadosa del Siglo de Oro." *Studia Neophilologica* 7:97–102.

———. 2000. *Entre la magia y la religión: Oraciones, conjuros, ensalmos.* [Oiartzun (Guipuzkoa)]: Sendoa Editorial.

Prell, Riv-Ellen. 1989. "The Double Frame of Life History in the Work of Barbara Myerhoff." In *Interpreting Women's Lives: Feminist Theory and Personal Narratives,* edited by the Personal Narratives Group, 241–58. Bloomington: Indiana University Press.

Rabbinowitz, J., trans. 1983. *Rabbah* [Deuteronomy, Perasha 7:6]. London: Soncino Press.

Rabinow, Paul. 1977. *Reflections on Fieldwork in Morocco.* Berkeley: University of California Press.

Rapoport-Albert, Ada, and Steven J. Zipperstein, eds. 1988. *Jewish History: Essays in Honour of Chimen Abramsky.* London: Peter Halban.

Rebhun, Linda-Anne. 1995. "Contemporary Evil Eye in Northeast Brazil." In *Folklore Interpreted: Essays in Honor of Alan Dundes,* edited by Regina Bendix and Rosemary Lévy Zumwalt, 213–33. New York: Garland.

Redfield, Robert. 1934. "Culture Changes in Yucatan." *American Anthropologist* 36:57–69.

———. 1941. *The Folk Culture of Yucatan.* Chicago: University of Chicago Press.

———. 1947. "The Folk Society." *American Journal of Sociology* 52:293–308.

———. 1956. *Peasant Society and Culture.* Chicago: University of Chicago Press.

Reinach, Solomon. 1900. "L'Inquisition et les juifs." *Revue des études juives* 40:50–64.

Reischer, Moshe. 1870. *Sepher Sha'are Yerushalayim.* Jerusalem: n.p.

Ríos, Amador de los. 1984. *Historia social, política y religiosa de los judíos de España y Portugal.* Vol. 3. Madrid: Ediciones Turner.

Rodrigue, Aron. 1990. *French Jews, Turkish Jews: The Alliance Israélite Universelle and the Politics of Jewish Schooling in Turkey, 1860–1925.* Bloomington: Indiana University Press.

———. 1992. "The Sephardim in the Ottoman Empire." In *Spain and the Jews,* edited by Elie Kedourie, 162–88. London: Thames and Hudson.

Rodrígues Marín, Francisco. 1927. *Ensalmos y conjuros en España y América: Conferencia leída en la Unión Ibero-Americana el día 17 de febrero de 1927.* Madrid: Tip. de la Rev. de Archivos, Bibliotecas y Museos, Olózaga.

Róheim, Gésa. 1952. "The Evil Eye." *American Imago* 9:351–63.

Romano, David. 1995. "Coexistenza/convivenzia tra ebrei e cristiani ispanici." *Sefarad* 55:359–81.

Romero, Elena, ed. 1991. *La vida judía en Sefarad.* Madrid: Ministerio de Cultura.

Roth, Cecil. 1964. *The Spanish Inquisition.* New York: Norton.

Roth, Norman. 1995. *Conversos, Inquisition, and the Expulsion of the Jews from Spain.* Madison: University of Wisconsin Press.

Sachar, Howard M. 1994. *Farewell España: The World of the Sephardim Remembered.* New York: Knopf.

Sacks, Karen Brodkin. 1989. "What's a Life Story Got to Do with It?" In *Interpreting Women's Lives, Feminist Theory and Personal Narratives,* edited by the Personal Narratives Group, 85–95. Bloomington: Indiana University Press.

Saporta y Beja, Enrique. 1979. *Selanik i sus djidyos (Salonique et ses juifs).* Paris: Association Vidas Largas.

———. 1982. *En torno a la Torre Blanca.* Paris: Vidas Largas.

———. n.d. *Salonika and Her Jews.* Translated by Lilian Beraha. n.p.

Schauss, Hayyim. 1950. *The Lifetime of a Jew throughout the Ages of Jewish History.* New York: Union of American Hebrew Congregations.

———. 1978. *The Jewish Festivals: History and Observance.* New York: Schocken Books.

Schiby, Baruch. 1970. "Notes sur les juifs de Thessalonique." In *Actas: I Simposio de estudios sefardíes,* edited by Iacob M. Hassán, 92–94. Madrid: Instituto Arias Montano.

Schiffman, Lawrence H., and Michael D. Swartz. 1992. *Hebrew and Aramaic Incantation Texts from the Cairo Genizah: Selected Texts from Taylor-Schechter Box K1.* Sheffield, Eng.: JSOT Press.

Schrire, T. 1966. *Hebrew Amulets: Their Decipherment and Interpretation.* London: Routledge and Kegan Paul.

Schwarzfuchs, Simon. 1986. *Kahal: La communauté juive de l'Europe médievale.* Paris: Maisonneuve et Larose.

Schweitzer, Marjorie, ed. 1991. *Anthropology of Aging: A Partially Annotated Bibliography.* New York: Greenwood Press.

Sephiha, Haim Vidal. 1977. *L'Agonie des judéo-espagnols.* Paris: Editions Entente.

———. 1981. "Bendisiones i maldisiones arekojidas por el 'Atelier Judeo-Espagnol' de Paris." *Aki Yerushalayim* Year 3, 9:44–47.

———. 1986. *Le ladino (judéo-espagnol calque): Structure et évolution d'une langue liturgique.* 2 vols. Paris: Association Vidas Largas.

Sered, Susan Starr. 1992. *Women as Ritual Experts: The Religious Lives of Elderly Jewish Women in Jerusalem.* Oxford: Oxford University Press.

———. 1994. *Priestess, Mother, Sacred Sister: Religions Dominated by Women.* Oxford: Oxford University Press.

Shaul, Moshe. 1979. "Saludos i bendisiones para okaziones determinadas." *Aki Yerushalayim* 3:36–37.

———. 1980. "Perkante para ojo malo sigun el livro 'Refua behaim' de Harbi Haim Palachi." *Aki Yerushalayim* 5:47.

———. 1981. "Saludos i bendisiones." *Aki Yerushalayim* Year 3, 11:31–32.

———. 1982. "Maldisiones en djudeo-espanyol." *Aki Yerushalayim* Year 4, 13–14:33–35.

———. 1986. "El sefer refuot (Livro de milizinas) (Izmir, 1878)." *Aki Yerushalayim* Year 8, 44:47.

———. 1993. "Prekante." *Aki Yerushalayim* Year 14, 47:49.

Shaw, Stanford J. 1991. *The Jews of the Ottoman Empire and the Turkish Republic.* London: Macmillan.

Sherman, Edmund. 1991. *Reminiscence and the Self in Old Age.* New York: Springer.

Shuldiner, David P. 1994. "Promoting Self-Worth among the Aging." In *Putting Folklore to Use,* edited by Michael Owen Jones, 214–25. Lexington: University of Kentucky Press.

———. 1997. *Folklore, Culture, and Aging: A Research Guide.* Westport, Conn.: Greenwood Press.

Simpson, D. P. 1959. *Cassell's New Latin Dictionary, Latin-English, English-Latin.* New York: Funk and Wagnalls.

Siskin, Edgar E. 1987. "Transcendental and Folk Aspects of Judaism." *Judaism* 36 (3): 283–95.

Sithon, Manasseh Matlub. 1874. *K'nesiyah l'Shem Shamayim.* Jerusalem: n.p.

Sitton, David. 1985. *Sephardi Communities Today.* Jerusalem: Council of Sephardi and Oriental Communities.

Sola Pool, David de, ed. 1936. *Book of Prayer According to the Custom of the Spanish and Portuguese Jews.* New York: Union of Sephardic Congregations.

Sorić, Ante. 1989. *Jews in Yugoslavia.* Zagreb: Muzejski prostor.

Stern, Stephen. 1980. *The Sephardic Community of Los Angeles: A Study in Folklore and Ethnic Identity.* New York: Arno Press.

Stillman, Norman. 1979. "Aspects of Jewish Life in Islamic Spain." In *Aspects of Jewish Culture in the Middle Ages,* edited by Paul E. Szarmach, 51–84. Albany: State University of New York Press.

Stoller, Paul. 1990. *The Taste of Ethnographic Things: The Sense in Anthropology.* Philadelphia: University of Pennsylvania Press.

Sumner, William Graham. 1906. *Folkways.* Reprint, New York: Dover, 1959.

Talmud, Tractate Ta'anit. 1989. Part 1, vol. 13. The Steinsaltz Edition. New York: Random House.

Tamir, Vicki. 1979. *Bulgaria and Her Jews: The History of a Dubious Symbiosis.* New York: Sepher-Hermon Press.

Tcherikover, Victor. 1961. *Hellenistic Civilization and the Jews.* Translated by S. Applebaum. 2 vols. Philadelphia: Jewish Publication Society of America.

Telushkin, Joseph. 1991. *Jewish Literacy.* New York: Morrow.
Thompson, R. Campbell. 1971. *Semitic Magic: Its Origin and Development.* New York: KTAV Publishing House.
Tousignant, Michael. 1979. "*Espanto:* A Dialogue with the Gods." *Culture, Medicine and Psychiatry* 3:347–61.
Trachtenberg, Joshua. 1939. *Jewish Magic and Superstition: A Study of Folk Religion.* New York: Behrman's Jewish Book House. Reprint, New York: Atheneum, 1970.
Turner, Victor. 1967. *The Forest of Symbols: Aspects of Ndembu Ritual.* Ithaca, N.Y.: Cornell University Press.
Ulmer, Rivka. 1994. *The Evil Eye in the Bible and in Rabbinic Literature.* Hoboken, N.J.: KTAV Publishing House.
Uziel, Baruh. 1956. "Ha-komplas ba-širāh ha-'āmāmit ha-sĕfāraddit." *Yeda-'Am* 4:66–78.
Vidaković-Petrov, Krinka. 1986. *Kultura* Španskih Jevreja na Jugoslovenskom Tlu. Sarajevo: Svjetlost.
———. 1994. "Spanish Folklore and the Balkan Cultural Environment." In *History and Creativity in The Sephardi and Oriental Jewish Communities,* edited by Tamar Alexander, Abraham Haim, Galit Hasan-Rokem, and Ephraim Hazan, 285–300. Jerusalem: Misgav Yerushalayim.
Viens, Gregori. 1995. *Island of Roses: The Jews of Rhodes in Los Angeles.* Paradox Productions. Videocassette.
Vocabulario de Romance en Latin. 1973. Edited by Gerald J. Macdonald. Philadelphia: Temple University Press.
von Grunebaum, Gustave E. 1955. "The Problem: Unity in Diversity." In *Unity and Variety in Muslim Civilization,* edited by Gustave von Grunebaum, 17–37. Chicago: University of Chicago Press.
Waddington, Raymond B., and Arthur H. Williamson. *The Expulsion of the Jews.* New York: Garland.
Westermann, Claus. 1978. *Blessing in the Bible and the Life of the Church.* Translated by Keith Crim. Philadelphia: Fortress Press.
Westermarck, Edward A. 1907. "L'Ār, or the Transference of Conditional Curses in Morocco." In *Anthropological Essays Presented to Edward Burnett Tylor in Honour of His Seventy-fifth Birthday, Oct. 2, 1907,* 361–74. Oxford: Clarendon Press. Reprint, New York: AMS Press, 1978.
———. 1968. *Ritual and Belief in Morocco.* 2 vols. Reprint, New Hyde Park, N.Y.: University Books. Originally published London: Macmillan, 1926.
Whaley, Terrence R. 1993. "Ethnography or Fiction: An Essay on Confounding Reader Response in Barbara Myerhoff's *Number Our Days.*" *Linguistics and Education* 5:39–51.
Wirth, Louis. 1964. "Urbanism as a Way of Life." In *On Cities and Social Life,* ed. Albert J. Reiss Jr., 60–83. Chicago: University of Chicago Press.
Yoder, Don. 1965–66. "Official Religion Versus Folk Religion." *Pennsylvania Folklife* 15 (2): 36–52.
———. 1974. "Toward a Definition of Folk Religion." *Western Folklore* 33:2–13.
Zimmels, Hirsch Jacob. 1952. *Magicians, Theologians and Doctors: Studies in Folk Medicine and Folklore as Reflected in the Rabbinical Responsa (Twelfth–Nineteenth Centuries).* London: E. Goldston.

———. 1976. *Ashkenazim and Sephardim: Their Relations, Differences, and Problems as Reflected in the Rabbinical Responsa.* London: Marla Publications.

Zumwalt, Rosemary Lévy. 1988. *American Folklore Scholarship: A Dialogue of Dissent.* Bloomington: Indiana University Press.

———. 1993. "*Las buenas mujeres:* The Keepers of Sephardic Health and Home." *Jewish Folklore and Ethnology Review* 15 (2): 107–12.

———. 1997. "'Let It Go to the Garlic!' Evil Eye and the Fertility of Women among the Sephardim." *Western Folklore* 55:233–44.

Index

ISAAC JACK LÉVY is Distinguished Professor Emeritus of Spanish Literature at the University of South Carolina. He is the author of *And the World Stood Silent: Sephardic Poetry of the Holocaust, Jewish Rhodes: A Lost Culture,* and other works and is the founder of the American Society of Sephardic Studies.

ROSEMARY LÉVY ZUMWALT is Vice-President of Academic Affairs and Dean of the College at Agnes Scott College. She previously was the Paul B. Freeland Professor of Anthropology at Davidson College. Her books include *American Folklore Scholarship: A Dialogue of Dissent* and *Wealth and Rebellion: Elsie Clews Parsons, Anthropologist and Folklorist.* She is president of the Fellows of the American Folklore Society.

University of Illinois Press
1325 South Oak Street
Champaign, IL 61820-6903
www.press.uillinois.edu